Interaction within the
Brain-Pituitary-Adrenocortical System

Based on Papers given at a satellite symposium of the Vth International Conference on Hormonal Steroids held at Varanasi, India, in November 1978.

Interaction within the Brain-Pituitary-Adrenocortical System

Edited by

MORTYN T. JONES
Sherrington School of Physiology,
St. Thomas's Hospital Medical
School, London,
U.K.

BRIAN GILLHAM
Department of Biochemistry,
St. Thomas's Hospital Medical
School, London,
U.K.

MARY F. DALLMAN
Department of Physiology,
U.C. Medical Center,
San Francisco, California,
U.S.A.

SUKUMAR CHATTOPADHYAY
Department of Physiology,
Institute of Medical Sciences,
Banaras Hindu University,
Varanasi, India.

1979

ACADEMIC PRESS London New York San Francisco

A Subsidiary of Harcourt Brace Jovanovich, Publishers

ACADEMIC PRESS INC. (LONDON) LTD.
24–28 OVAL ROAD
LONDON NW1

U.S. Edition published by
ACADEMIC PRESS INC.
111 FIFTH AVENUE
NEW YORK, NEW YORK 10003

British Library Cataloguing in Publication Data

Interaction within the brain–pituitary-adrenocortical
    system.
    1. Adrenal cortex – Congresses
    2. Brain – Congresses
    3. Pituitary body – Congresses
    I. Jones, Mortyn T II. International Conference
    on Hormonal Steroids, *5th, Varanasi, 1978*
    612'.82   QP188.A28   79-40759

    ISBN 0–12–389150–7

Typeset by Reproduction Drawings Ltd., Sutton, Surrey
Printed by Photolithography in Great Britain by
Whitstable Litho Ltd, Whitstable, Kent

PREFACE

Advances in medicine depend equally on observations made by basic scientists and by clinicians. Nowhere is this fact better illustrated than in the studies directed towards an understanding of the complex interactions that occur within the brain–pituitary–adrenocortical system. It is appropriate therefore that the contributors to this book include anatomists, biochemists, pathologists, pharmacologists and physiologists.

In preparing their chapters, authors were asked to provide a review of their particular field of interest that placed their own experimental results in a wider context. The result is a broad view of the functions of the axis in health and disease. The book reflects the way in which the once somewhat circumscribed view of the axis, consisting simply of the hypothalamus, anterior pituitary and zonae reticularis/fasciculata of the adrenal cortex, is currently being widened. Thus due place is given to the whole brain, not just the hypothalamus, and to the intermediate and posterior lobes of the pituitary.

The book opens with a review of the variety of peptides synthesized and secreted by the cells of the pituitary, and this view of a gland producing several related peptides of possibly complementary or overlapping functions has an echo in the chapters dealing with the unresolved nature of the hypothalamic peptides involved in the regulation of corticotropin (ACTH) secretion. The behavioural effects of pituitary peptides and adrenal steroids are reported, as are current views on neural pathways and neurotransmitters regulating ACTH and melanotropin (MSH) secretion. The role of corticosteroid negative feedback control of ACTH release in man and in experimental animals is assessed. Developmental aspects of the axis are discussed by several contributors. The potentially important, but as yet unresolved, role of 18-hydroxydeoxycorticosterone is aired, as is the possible role that corticotropin-like-intermediate-lobe peptide (CLIP) may play in insulin secretion. The recent advances in the treatment of Cushing's disease are outlined as is the way the axis is influenced by mental disease and the practice of yoga.

An opportunity for scientists and clinicians to exchange information and ideas is provided by Symposia and the series of chapters is the result of a Satellite Symposium of the Vth International Congress in Hormonal Steroids. The hosts of the Symposium were the local organising committee of the Institute of Medical Sciences, Banaras Hindu University (BHU), Varanasi, India. The Editors would like to thank the contributors for submitting their manuscripts within the time limits.

It is a pleasure to thank the various companies and organizations which provided financial support to the Symposium and to Academic Press for their useful suggestions. Last, but not least, we would like to thank Mrs Fiona Chandler who re-typed the edited scripts.

May 1979   *The Editors*

FINANCIAL SUPPORT WAS RECEIVED FROM:

U.S.A. – Schering Corporation–Upjohn Corporation

U.K.   – Merck Sharp & Dohme–Imperial Chemical Industries–The British Council

      Beecham Research Laboratories–Wellcome Medical Division–Sandoz Pharmaceutical Division–Lilly Research Centre–Winthrop Laboratories

      Allen & Hanburys Ltd.–Berk Pharmaceuticals–Orth Pharmaceuticals–Schering Chemicals–E.R. Squibb

INDIA – University Grants Commission–Indian National Science Academy–Indian Council of Medical Research

vii

This book is dedicated to the memory
of two of its contributors

Madame Cecile Mialhe
and
Claude J. P. Giroud

CONTENTS

Chapter 1.   Lipotropin- and Corticotropin-Related Peptides of the
Mammalian Pituitary.
P. J. LOWRY, R. SILMAN, S. JACKSON AND F. ESTIVARIZ.   1

Chapter 2.   Behavioural Effects of Neuropeptides (Endorphins, Enkephalins
ACTH Fragments) and Corticosteroids.
B. BOHUS AND E. R. de KLOET.   7

Chapter 3.   Regulation of Corticotropin-Related Peptides in the Intermediate Lobe and their Possible Relation to Obesity.
J. A. EDWARDSON AND AMANDA DONALDSON   17

Chapter 4.   Differential Control of Anterior Lobe and Intermediate
Lobe Corticotropin (ACTH) Secretion in the Rat.
P. G. SMELIK AND F. J. H. TILDERS.   29

Chapter 5.   Perspectives on Corticotropin-Releasing Hormone (CRH)
B. GILLHAM, R. L. INSALL AND M. T. JONES   41

Chapter 6.   The Relationship between Vasopressin and Corticotropin-
Releasing Factor.
G. GILLIES AND P. J. LOWRY   51

Chapter 7.   Corticotropin-Releasing Factor (CRF) and Vasopressin in the
Regulation of Corticotropin (ACTH) Secretion
†C. MIALHE, B. LUTZ-BUCHER, B. BRIAUD,
R. SCHLEIFFER AND B. KOCH.   63

Chapter 8.   Neural Pathways Controlling Release of Corticotropin (ACTH).
D. S. GANN, D. G. WARD AND D. E. CARLSON.   75

Chapter 9.   Changes in Brain Amines During Stress.
M. PALKOVITS.   87

Chapter 10.   The Site of Origin of Corticoliberin (CRF).
               G. B. MAKARA.   97

Chapter 11.   The Secretion of Corticotropin-Releasing Hormone *in vitro*:
               Effects of Neurotransmitter Substances, Drugs and
               Corticosteroids.
               JULIA C. BUCKINGHAM AND J. R. HODGES.   115

Chapter 12.   The Role of γ-Aminobutyric Acid (GABA) in Controlling
               Corticoliberin (CRF) Secretion.
               G. B. MAKARA.   121

Chapter 13.   Modification of the Sensitivity of Receptors Involved in
               the Regulation of the Hypothalamo–Pituitary–Adrenal Axis.
               U. SCAPAGNINI, L. ANGELUCCI, I. GERENDAI,
               P. VALERI, P. L. CANONICO, M. PALMERY,
               F. PATACCHIOLI AND B. TITA.   127

Chapter 14.   Glucocorticosteroid and Mineralocorticosteroid Hormone
               Target Sites in the Brain: Autoradiographic Studies with
               Corticosterone, Aldosterone and Dexamethasone.
               W. E. STUMPF AND M. SAR.   137

Chapter 15.   Adrenal Feedback on Stress-Induced Corticoliberin
               (CRF) and Corticotropin (ACTH) Secretion.
               MARY F. DALLMAN.   149

Chapter 16.   The Characteristics and Mechanism of Action of Cortico-
               steroid Negative Feedback at the Hypothalamus and
               Anterior Pituitary
               M. T. JONES, B. GILLHAM, S. MAHMOUD AND
               M. C. HOLMES   163

Chapter 17.   Observations on Feedback Regulation of Corticotropin
               (ACTH) Secretion in Man.
               J. R. DALY, S. C. J. READER, J. ALAGHBAND-ZADEH
               AND P. HAISMAN.   181

Chapter 18.   The Effects of Intermediates in Cortisol Synthesis on its
               Feedback Control in Man.
               R. V. BROOKS, G. JEREMIAH, CLARA LOWY,
               P. H. SONKSEN AND M. WHEELER   189

Chapter 19.   Secretory Patterns of 18-OH-DOC and Related Steroids and
               their Possible Role in Hypertension.
               M. K. BIRMINGHAM, J. T. OLIVER, A. BARTOVA,
               P. FREI AND S. LEVY.   197

Chapter 20.   Endogenous Levels of 18-OH-DOC and Related Steroids
               in the Brain.
               A. BARTOVA.   213

Chapter 21. The Diurnal Rhythmicity of Brain, Pituitary and
Adrenocortical Hormones.
JANET SADOW. 221

Chapter 22. Possible Roles for Adrenal Lysosomes in Controlling the
Response to ACTH.
VINEETA PRASAD AND SUKUMAR CHATTOPADHYAY. 229

Chapter 23. Studies on the Human Fetal Pituitary–Adrenal Axis in
Tissue Culture.
†C. J. P. GIROUD, C. GOODYER, G. HALL AND
C. BRANCHAUD. 235

Chapter 24. A Role for Cortisone in Human Fetal Development.
BEVERLEY E. PEARSON MURPHY. 247

Chapter 25. Pituitary-Dependent Cushing's Disease.
LESLEY H. REES. 257

Chapter 26. Adrenocortical Functions in Psychiatric Disorders.
SARADA SUBRAHMANYAM, R. CHANDRAMOULI,
S. SIVAKUMAR AND V. S. AMANULLAH BAIG. 265

Chapter 27. Yoga in Relation to the Brain–Pituitary–Adrenocortical
Axis.
K. N. UDUPA AND R. H. SINGH. 273

Chapter 28. An Overall View of the Hypothalamo-Pituitary–Adrenocortical Axis.
L. MARTINI and M. T. JONES 279

Index 287

1

THE LIPOTROPIN- AND CORTICOTROPIN-RELATED PEPTIDES OF THE MAMMALIAN PITUITARY

P. J. Lowry, R. Silman*, S. Jackson and F. Estivariz

Pituitary Hormone Laboratory, Department of Chemical Pathology and Department of Reproductive Physiology*, St. Bartholomew's Hospital, London EC1A 7BE, U.K.

INTRODUCTION

The paper will describe recent work carried out in our laboratory on the nature of the corticotropin (ACTH)- and lipotropin (LPH)-related peptides. Our earlier work has been previously reviewed in detail[1,2]. A family of peptides is found

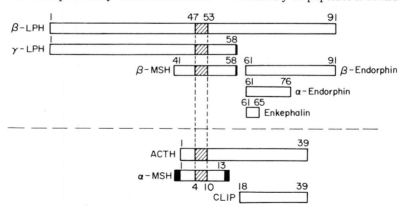

Fig. 1. Peptides in the top half have structural homology with their numbered alignments in the parent peptide β-LPH.
Similarly peptides in the lower half are identical with the appropriate regions of ACTH, except that α-MSH has a N-terminal acetyl group and a C-terminal amide group.
The common heptapeptide core sequence Met-Glu-His-Phe-Arg-Trp-Gly occurs at 47–53 in the LPH series and 4–10 in the ACTH series.

1

in the vertebrate pituitary which consists of two related groups, ACTH and LPH being the parent peptide of each group (Fig. 1). Melanotropin (α-MSH) and corticotropin-like intermediate-lobe peptide (CLIP) eminate from ACTH and β-MSH, γ-LPH, α-, β- and γ-endorphin and *N*-fragment all being post-translational fragments of β-LPH. We suggested that it was the anatomical localization of a common cell, which manufactured both the ACTH- and LPH-related peptides, that dictated the type of peptide the cell secreted. If the cell was located in the pars distalis then only ACTH and LPH were found. If, however, the cell was found in the pars intermedia then all the small peptides could be expected to occur.

HUMAN

Work carried out on the human foetus reinforced this hypothesis[3]. The adult human pituitary is unusual in not possessing a functional pars intermedia and thus some of the peptides normally associated with the pars intermedia e.g. β-MSH, α-MSH and CLIP could not be found. β-Endorphin also cannot be detected in significant quantities in the adult human pituitary (unpublished results). Examination of the human foetus (where a pars intermedia can be found) revealed the presence of the smaller pars intermedia peptides. This led to the suggestion that it was the switch in the types of peptide that caused the qualitative change in steroid production in the adrenal gland. Indeed recently, it has been shown that short-term administration of α-MSH *in vivo* directly or indirectly stimulates the foetal adrenal gland of the rabbit at a time when synthetic 1–24 ACTH is relatively ineffective. In contrast 1–24 ACTH is a potent corticosteroidogenic agent on the newborn adrenal whereas α-MSH is virtually inactive[4].

SHEEP

Recently, ACTH/LPH-related peptides from whole sheep pituitary were compared[5]. Surprisingly, there was no evidence for the presence of CLIP in either the adult or foetal pituitary. There was, however, occasional evidence for the presence of minute amounts of α-MSH. These findings were considered insignificant when compared with the relatively large quantities of α-MSH in the adult rat and the human and monkey foetal pituitary. It is noteworthy that the sheep pituitary has always been thought to contain significant amounts of α-MSH. β-MSH was clearly demonstrated in both the foetal and adult pituitary.

The most dominant form of ACTH in the sheep foetal pituitary was a 'big ACTH', whereas the ratio was reversed in the adult where 1–39 ACTH became the major component.

The occurrence of a common precursor for ACTH and LPH was first suggested after investigation of these peptides in human pituitary glands[1]. The AT20 mouse tumour line has proved an ideal model for studying this precursor and has led to its partial chemical characterization[6]. Two large common precursors were found in the sheep study[5], one appeared to be similar to the 31K peptide found in the mouse tumour and another was rather larger. Other peptides, which were identified tentatively on the basis of chromatographic and immunological characteristics, were β-LPH, γ-LPH, β-endorphin and 1-76 LPH.

MONKEY

The monkey adrenal, in common with the human adrenal, has a foetal zone which involutes at birth. Like the adult human there were insignificant amounts of α-MSH and CLIP in either the infant or adult monkey pituitary. Although β-LPH, γ-LPH and β-endorphin were present in both simian and human pituitary extracts only β-MSH was found in the monkey.

Foetal pituitaries contained increased amounts of β-MSH in relation to β- and γ-LPH. β-Endorphin was also increased relative to β-LPH. Significant peaks of α-MSH and CLIP were also found. The pituitary of a 12h neonate showed substantial amounts of α-MSH and CLIP with a dominant amount of β-endorphin. This last observation may prove of great physiological importance. Although pituitary levels of hormones cannot be transposed to blood and/or brain levels it is interesting to speculate that it might protect the baby from the trauma of birth[7].

RAT

As the two lobes, the pars distalis (PD) and the pars intermedia (PI), were easily separated in the rat, we decided to make a careful survey of the ACTH- and LPH-related peptides in both lobes by using a combination of gel filtration on Bio-Gel P6 and Sephadex G-50 and several radioimmunoassays (RIAs)[8].

A peptide resembling β-endorphin was found both in the PD and the PI. In the chromatogram of the PI there was an additional peak, which was eluted slightly ahead of β-endorphin. This peak also cross-reacted partially in our human β-MSH assay. There is no full cross-reaction in crude extracts of rat pituitaries in our human β-MSH RIA. A peptide with elution and immunological characteristics similar to those of β-endorphin was found in the PI. Conversely, this peptide was absent from the PD. A peptide with the elution characteristics of β-LPH was detected with the β-endorphin assay only in extracts from the PD. It showed partial cross-reaction in the human β-MSH RIA. CLIP was present in much greater quantities in the PI than in the PD whereas the converse was true for 1–39 ACTH. In the chromatogram of the PI extract, there was, however, a large peak of *C*-terminal ACTH immunoreactivity which was co-eluted with the small peak of 1–39 ACTH. This 1–39 peak in the PD (after Sephadex G-50 chromatography) contained more *C*- than *N*-terminal immunoreactivity. Rechromatography of this fraction on Bio-Gel P6 resulted in the separation of a solely *C*-terminal immunoreactive peak, which was eluted ahead of 1–39 ACTH. We have termed this peptide 'big CLIP'. α-MSH, although found mainly in the PI, was present in small but significant amounts in the PD. Three peaks of high-molecular-weight ACTH were detected in the PD and these corresponded to 31K, 23K and 13K. A peak of β-endorphin/LPH activity was eluted in the same position as the 31K ACTH peak. Similarly, a peak containing both ACTH and β-endorphin immunoreactivity was found after chromatography of extracts of PI. Thus it appears that LPH–ACTH prohormone is present in both lobes.

The picture of the pattern of ACTH/LPH peptides in the rat pituitary is therefore more complicated than was originally thought. The common precursor is present in both lobes. In the PD, the larger peptides β-LPH and ACTH predominate, although there are small quantities of some of the smaller peptides i.e. β-endorphin, CLIP and α-MSH.

In the PI, the smaller peptides CLIP, α-MSH, β-endorphin predominate along with exclusive peptides 'big endorphin' and α-endorphin. Big CLIP is present in both lobes in approximately the same amounts.

A peptide resembling γ-LPH was not detected in the rat pituitary.

We have also attempted to characterize these peptides in rat plasma by chromatography of acidified plasma under dissociating conditions. As the elution buffer (1% formic acid) is volatile, resultant fractions can be evaporated to dryness, so permitting the assay of each fraction with increased sensitivity. This method enabled us to identify β-LPH, ACTH and the two forms of β-endorphin in the plasma of ether-stressed rats. A 20-fold concentration of plasma by ODS silica treatment, followed by chromatography on Bio-Gel P6 allowed the detection of α-MSH, CLIP, big CLIP and α-endorphin in addition to the above peptides. These results suggest that the plasma of ether-stressed rats contains significant quantities of all the ACTH/LPH-related peptides identified in extracts of both the PD and PI of their pituitaries.

CONTROL OF THE SECRETION OF ACTH AND LPH

We have proposed previously that the release of ACTH and LPH from the corticotroph of the PD is under the same hypothalamic control[1,2]. This suggestion resulted from several observations:

1. The corticotroph of the PD immunostained for both ACTH and LPH.
2. The immunostaining material was found in the same secretory granules[9].
3. Both peptides can be detected immunologically in the same precursor.
4. Physiologically or pathologically elevated levels of immunoreactive plasma ACTH are always accompanied by similar levels of immunoreactive β-LPH[10].

We decided to investigate the secretion of ACTH and LPH from the corticotroph of the rat using the perfused isolated anterior pituitary cell column[11,12,13].

Rat ACTH, β-LPH, β-endorphin and α-MSH in the cell secretions were measured by RIA. The assay system used for β-LPH could not distinguish between this peptide and β-endorphin.

The stimuli used to release the hormones were stalk median-eminence extracts (SME), arginine vasopressin (AVP) and 45mM potassium. ACTH and LPH/endorphin were released by all three secretagogues. The dose–response curve for LPH paralleled that for ACTH whichever stimulus was used. The less-steep dose-response curve for AVP-stimulated ACTH release also applied to LPH. Preincu-

bation of SME or AVP with an AVP antiserum significantly quenched the activity
with regard to release of both ACTH and LPH/endorphin from the PD cells in an
identical manner. Neither normal rabbit serum nor a non-specific immune serum
impaired the releasing activity of SME or AVP with respect to ACTH or LPH.
Luteinizing hormone-releasing hormone (luliberin) bioactivity of SME was not
affected by preincubation with any of the above antisera.

Immediate acidification of material secreted from the pituitary cell column
after stimulation allowed chromatography (in 1% formic acid) on Sephadex
G-50. The elution pattern of peptides reacting in the LPH/endorphin RIA was
identical whether SME, AVP or 45mM potassium was used as the stimulus. The
major peak of activity coincided with the position of β-LPH and two smaller
peaks were found, one was eluted near the void volume and the other in the
position expected for β-endorphin. Four peaks of immunoreactive ACTH were
detected, the main one being eluted in the position of 1–39 ACTH. The smaller
peaks were eluted near the void volume, and at positions where CLIP and
intermediate ACTH would be expected. When the fractions were monitored with
a specific α-MSH RIA, a small but significant peak was located in the elution
position of α-MSH. Further experiments revealed that SME caused an increase in
α-MSH immunoreactivity from the anterior pituitary cell column and not a
decrease as would be expected if the anterior pituitary cells were contaminated
with PI cells.

These observations confirm that ACTH and β-LPH are secreted concomitantly
from the corticotrophs of the PD and are under the same physiological control.
In addition, the involvement of AVP in the corticoliberin (CRF) release of
ACTH (as inferred from the antisera quenching experiments) has also been
shown to be true for β-LPH. Thus we can say that CRF as we know it releases
ACTH and β-LPH from the corticotroph in an identical manner.

Because of the stimulatory effect of SME on the secretion of α-MSH, we can
preclude contamination with PI cells, thus it appears that α-MSH, β-endorphin
and CLIP are released from the PD by extracts of the stalk median eminence in a
manner parallel to that of ACTH and β-LPH release[13].

CONCLUSION

Our studies with a variety of mammals have shown that the pattern of ACTH
and LPH related peptides is by no means consistent, but some general facts
have emerged.

Studies with primates indicate that the smaller PI peptides are apparent in the
foetal pituitary and decrease or disappear altogether after partuition.

The larger precursor molecules are barely detectable in primate and mouse
pituitaries, whereas large amounts are present in sheep pituitaries and these
change in their amounts relative to the smaller peptides during foetal development. As the above studies were carried out with whole pituitaries it is difficult
to say whether these changes are due to anatomical or biosynthetic changes
within the pituitary.

The rat pituitary is not typical with regard to its ACTH/LPH-related peptides.
Neither γ-LPH nor β-MSH can be found although two peptides, big CLIP and

big endorphin, appear to be exclusive to this species. It is an ideal laboratory animal, however, and we have shown that isolated PD cells do secrete ACTH and β-LPH concomitantly. The physiological significance of this has yet to be elucidated. The small amounts of α-MSH, CLIP and β-endorphin are difficult to explain, but as the concentrations of these are much lower in the PD than in the PI, they are due to either a small amount of PD cells that have the biosynthetic machinery of PI cells, or low level biosynthesis of PI peptides in corticotrophs.

The reason for the many peptides in the PI is not yet clear. No physiological peripheral action has been unequivocally found for any of these peptides. Indeed, preliminary evidence would suggest that their release is controlled by a common mechanism. Thus the simultaneous release of several potentially biologically active peptides is difficult to interpret in simple physiological terms. Most of these peptides, however, have been found to have effects when present in the central nervous system. One could simply postulate that the PI acts as a permanent supply of several centrally active peptides which can be taken up by neural tissue when required and released by specific stimuli to give the effects on behaviour and learning observed with these peptides (see Bohus and de Kloet, this volume). It is noteworthy that in primates, where there is considerable development of the cortex, the PI undergoes partial or complete involution at birth. This would suggest that synthesis of these peptides in the PI plays a minor role in learning and behaviour in animals with a highly evolved intelligence.

REFERENCES

1. Lowry, P. J. *et al.* (1976). *Proc. Vth Int. Congr. Endocrinol.* Hamburg, Excerpta Medica, Amsterdam.
2. Lowry, P. J. *et al.* (1977). *Ann. N.Y. Acad. Sci.* **297**, 49.
3. Silman, R. E. *et al.* (1976). *Nature* **260**, 716.
4. Challis, J. R. G. and Torosis, J. D. (1977). *Nature* **269**, 818.
5. Silman, R. E. *et al.* (1979). *J. Endocrinol. (in press).*
6. Mains, R. E. *et al.* (1977). *Proc. Natl. Acad. Sci. USA* **74**, 3014.
7. Silman, R. E. *et al.* (1978). *Nature* **276**, 526.
8. Jackson, S. and Lowry, P. J. (1979). *J. Endocrinol. (in press).*
9. Phifer, R. F. *et al.* (1974). *J. Clin. Endocrinol. Metab.* **39**, 684.
10. Gilkes, J. J. H. *et al.* (1975). *J. Clin. Endocrinol. Metab.* **40**, 450.
11. Gillies, G. and Lowry, P. J. (1978). *Endocrinology* **103**, 521.
12. Gillies, G. *et al.* (1978). *Endocrinology* **103**, 528.
13. Estivariz, F. E. *et al.* (1979). *J. Endocrinol. (in press).*

2

BEHAVIORAL EFFECTS OF NEUROPEPTIDES (ENDORPHINS, ENKEPHALINS, ACTH FRAGMENTS) AND CORTICOSTEROIDS

B. Bohus and E. R. de Kloet

*Rudolf Magnus Institute for Pharmacology, University of Utrecht,
Utrecht, The Netherlands*

INTRODUCTION

The concept that the brain serves as a target organ for pituitary and hypothalamic peptide hormones stems from observations that showed that pituitary–adrenal system hormones influence adaptive behavioral processes[1,2]. In the last decade it has become evident that the brain is a major endocrine organ both as a source of neuropeptides and as a target for peptides of pituitary origin. These neuropeptides affect learning, memory, motivational, attentional, perceptional, sexual and sleep processes by serving as modulators or transmitters in more-or-less specific brain processes[3,4]. The discovery that some fragments of β-lipotropin (β-LPH) are naturally occuring peptides with opiate-like activity (endorphins) has initiated major efforts to determine the physiological role of these neuropeptides. Some of the behavioral effects of intracranially administered endorphins, like catatonia, led Bloom *et al.*[5] to suggest that subtle derangements in physiological mechanisms regulating β-endorphin homeostasis could result in pathological changes in psychic functions. Jacquet and Marks[6] proposed that β-endorphin may serve as an endogenous neuroleptic.

Recently de Wied[7], proposed that discrete changes in the generation of fragments of β-endorphin, which depend on the site of enzymic cleavage, may assure a well-balanced modulation of behavioral adaptation to environmental events. An imbalance in the biogenesis of these fragments, on the other hand, may lead to disturbances in adaptive processes which may form an etiological basis of mental disorders. Although endorphins have been primarily related to schizophrenia, it has also been hypothesized that deficiency of the neuropeptide vasopressin in the brain may also cause cognitive dysfunctions and thereby may be involved in affective illnesses[8].

The search for an endocrine origin of mental dysfunctioning, which began almost three decades ago, is now reaching the final stages. In contrast to early attempts, which were mainly based on accidental clinical observations, the recent hypotheses stem from extensive basic research. Our present knowledge allows the construction of a picture, although sometimes a fragmentary one, of the physiological significance of hormones in modulating brain functions. We would like to emphasize here that corticotropin (ACTH) and β-LPH-like peptides, which are synthesized from a common precursor molecule in the same anterior pituitary cells[9] and controlled by the same central nervous mechanisms[10], have multiple interactions with brain mechanism serving adaptation. Additionally, the significance of adrenal hormones in the regulation of behavior is reemphasized. Finally, we would like to stress the importance of interactions between the various neuropeptides and corticosteroids in the regulation of behavioral adaptation to environmental changes.

BEHAVIORAL EFFECTS OF ACTH- AND β-LPH-LIKE PEPTIDES: INVOLVEMENT OF TWO PUTATIVE RECEPTOR SYSTEMS?

The involvement of the pituitary gland in the modulation of behavioral adaptation was indicated by the impairment in the acquisition and maintenance of conditioned behavioral responses that follows the removal of the pituitary gland[11-13]. Behavioral abnormalities of hypophysectomized rats can be corrected by the administration of ACTH[11,13], but also by treatment with melanotropin (α-MSH) and fragments of ACTH, which are practically devoid of classical endocrine target effects[1,14]. The absence of endocrine effects of the active sequences such as $ACTH_{1-10}$ or $ACTH_{4-10}$ [1] and the finding that $ACTH_{1-24}$ is effective in the absence of the adrenal cortex[15] clearly indicated the extra-adrenal nature of the behavioral effect of ACTH and related neuropeptides. Subsequently, it was shown that ACTH-like peptides profoundly modulated adaptive behavior of intact rats whether the response was motivated by fear, hunger or sex[16]. We have proposed that these peptides temporarily increase the motivational value of environmental stimuli thereby increasing the probability of the occurance of stimulus-specific behavioral responses[3,16]. Additionally, effects of ACTH-like peptides on brain processes related to memory have also been observed[16].

Attempts to isolate highly active neuropeptides from hog pituitaries indicated the presence of oligopeptides dissimilar to ACTH but more potent in normalizing the impaired avoidance behavior of hypophysectomized rats[17]. Although the structures were not determined, the amino acid composition of two of these peptides resembled β-LPH_{61-69} and β-LPH_{70-79} [18]. The recognition that the C-terminal fragments of β-LPH and related peptides possess opiate-like and other behavioral activities[19,20] stimulated us to investigate whether the endorphins are involved in the modulation of adaptive behavior.

Peripheral administration of α- and β-endorphin (β-LPH$_{61-76}$ and β-LPH$_{61-91}$ respectively) and Met^5-enkephalin (β-LPH$_{61-65}$) and β-LPH$_{61-69}$ in doses of a few micrograms delayed extinction of a pole-jumping avoidance response; similar effects occurred after treatment with ACTH$_{4-10}$[21]. Administration of the peptides into a lateral cerebral ventricle in doses of a few nanograms mimicked the effect of peripherally injected peptides. This observation indicated a central site of action for near-physiological amounts of both β-LPH and ACTH-like neuropeptides. Further, shortening of the peptide chain of β-endorphin increased its potency on avoidance behavior. This suggested that the β-endorphin molecule contained more than one behavioral bit of information. Observations on the effect of various doses of β-endorphin on the retention of a passive avoidance response provided further support of this idea. A smaller amount of the peptide administered subcutaneously (1.5μg) facilitated passive avoidance behavior. On the contrary, a larger dose (10.0μg) affected behavior in a dual way. Facilitation of passive avoidance behavior was only observed in 50 per cent of the investigated rat population. The other half displayed attenuated passive avoidance. It seemed therefore that although β-endorphin has some intrinsic behavioral activity, availability of the peptide in larger concentrations may have yielded metabolic product(s) that might have opposite effects on behavior.

The presence of opiate-like peptides other than β-endorphin both in the brain and the pituitary has been demonstrated[19,22]. Further, metabolic transformation of β-endorphin may yield γ- and α-endorphin and Met^5-enkephalin[23]. Because α-endorphin and Met^5-enkephalin also facilitate avoidance behavior, γ-endorphin (β-LPH$_{61-77}$) or related peptides seemed to be reasonable candidates to cause opposite effects on avoidance behavior. Indeed, γ-endorphin markedly facilitates extinction of an active avoidance response[24] and attenuates passive avoidance behavior. β-LPH$_{78-91}$ was practically devoid of behavioral activity. Thus it appears that γ-endorphin within the β-endorphin moiety carries the opposite behavioral information. α-Endorphin is only one amino acid (Leu^{77}) shorter than γ-endorphin and α-endorphin is one of the most powerful endorphins that facilitate conditioned behavior. Since this peptide may be formed in the brain from β- or γ-endorphin, it is tempting to suggest that subtle changes in the biotransformation of endorphins may assure a dynamic control of behavioral adaptation to environmental changes.

The profound behavioral effects of peptides related to the C-terminus of β-LPH such as catatonia, antinociception, wet shaking episodes, disruption of learned or genetically determined behavioral patterns can be evoked by intra-cerebral administration of these peptides in microgram quantities[19,20,25,26]. The potency of the peptides to evoke these behavioral activities decreases with shortening of the C-terminal end of β-endorphin. The fact that specific opiate antagonists suppress these behavioral responses to β-LPH-like peptides is conso-nant with the notion that opiate receptors or opiate-sensitive structures in the brain are involved. Moreover, ACTH- and endorphin-like peptides may have a common denominator in their interactions with the central nervous system. Intracranial but not systemic administration of ACTH and related peptides induces excessive grooming behavior in the rat[27]. Similarly, β-endorphin evokes grooming behavior after intracerebroventricular administration. Like the opiate-like behavioral effects of endorphins, shortening the C-terminus of β-endorphin is accompanied by a reduction of these behavioral activities[28]. ACTH- and endorphin-induced grooming is suppressed by opiate antagonists and there exists an acute cross-tolerance in this respect between $ACTH_{1-24}$ and β-endorphin[27-29]. This indicates an interaction of both peptides with opiate receptors in the brain.

The effects of endorphins and of ACTH-related peptides on adaptive behavioral responses are, however, independent of opiate receptors. Opiate antagonists do not abolish the effect of α-endorphin or $ACTH_{4-10}$ on active avoidance extinction[21] or of β-endorphin on passive avoidance behavior. The influence of γ-endorphin on avoidance behavior is also independent of the opiate-like activity of this peptide. Removal of the N-terminal amino acid residue tyrosine, which eliminates opiate-like activity, resulted in a peptide that was much more potent in attenuating avoidance behavior than the parent molecule[24].

The present observations suggest multiple interactions between ACTH- and β-LPH-like peptides and central nervous mechanisms. Behavioral influences may be mediated through at least two putative receptor systems. One of these cannot be blocked by opiate antagonists and does not require the opioid properties of the peptides. The other receptor system seems to be the opioid system in the brain. Since ACTH-like peptides do not share the majority of opiate-like behavioral activities, these peptides may act as partial agonist–antagonists on opiate receptors. That ACTH- fragments are able to inhibit morphine-induced analgesia[30] and show affinity for both agonist and antagonist opiate receptor sites[31] provides further support for this notion. It is of special interest that peptide effects mediated by opiate receptors require much higher doses after exogenous administration than do opiate receptor-independent effects. Therefore it may well be that stimulation of seemingly high-affinity opiate receptors requires large amounts of exogenous peptides because of a limited access to receptors *in vivo*.

BEHAVIORALLY EFFECTIVE ACTH- AND β-LPH-LIKE NEUROPEPTIDES: PITUITARY OR BRAIN ORIGIN?

Since the blood–brain barrier is practically impermeable to large peptide molecules such as ACTH[32], ACTH- and β-LPH-related peptides which are present in the cerebrospinal fluid (CSF)[32,33] may originate either from the pituitary *via* retrograde transport, or in the brain. Evidence for retrograde transport of an ACTH-like peptide has been provided by the appearance of label in the brain after intrapituitary injection of $[^3H] Phe^7$-D-Lys^8-$ACTH_{4-9}$[34]. Intrapituitary injection resulted in regionally different uptake of the label in brain. The highest activity was found in the hypothalamus. Stalk section performed 24 h earlier decreased uptake in the hypothalamus, but not in other brain regions. Hypothalamic uptake was normal, however, 8 days after stalk section. It was suggested that transport to the hypothalamus is partly vascular *via* the stalk vessels. Transport to other areas may occur through the CSF. This finding is consonant with the observations of Oliver *et al.*[35] who found that several pituitary hormones, including ACTH and α-MSH, appear in the proximal end of stalk owing to vascular transport along the pituitary stalk.

The presence of bio-and immuno-reactive ACTH, α-MSH and endorphins in the brain even long after hypophysectomy[36-38] has been used as an argument that these neuropeptides are produced by the brain itself. Further, immunocyto-chemical studies have demonstrated ACTH, α-MSH, β-LPH/β-endorphin and enkephalin systems (cells and axons) in the brain[37,39-41]. It has been suggested that these systems may represent the neuromodulator/neurotransmitter function of neuropeptides of brain origin. As has been mentioned earlier, the removal of the pituitary results in impairments in adaptive behaviors[11-13] and the deficits can be corrected by exogenous peptide treatment[11,13,14]. Accordingly, ACTH, MSH and endorphins of brain origin cannot maintain adaptive behavior in the absence of the pituitary. Removal of the pituitary also blocks some of the effects of endogenous endorphins that are apparently dependent on the opiate receptor, such as acupuncture or stress-induced analgesia[42,43]. It is therefore likely that the pituitary is the source of ACTH- and endorphin-like peptides involved in behavioral modulation.

The functional significance of ACTH- and β-LPH-like peptides of brain origin thus remains unclear. Removal of the pituitary failed to affect the level of ACTH in the brain. Adrenalectomy, on the other hand, appeared to change selectively ACTH levels in the brain.[44]. ACTH levels in the hippocampus decreased, re-mained unaltered in the hypothalamus and in the anterior and posterior lobe of the pituitary, and increased in the plasma. Brain ACTH levels of adrenalectomized rats were not different from the controls 14 days after surgery. Accordingly, the absence of corticosterone caused a selective transient alteration in the hippo-campal ACTH level which was opposite to the changes observed in the plasma level of this peptide.

These observations indicate that brain ACTH levels are not completely inde-pendent of the endocrine state of the organism. It may be more than a coinci-dence that the concentration of ACTH was selectively changed in the hippocam-pus. The hippocampus represents the major receptor region for corticosterone in the brain[45]. Experiments are in progress to investigate the relationship between hippocampal ACTH and corticosterone receptors.

CORTICOSTERONE AND BEHAVIOR: HIPPOCAMPAL RECEPTORS ARE IMPLICATED.

Early behavioral experiments using ACTH suggested, at least from a classical endocrinological point of view, that corticosteroids are the primary candidates for the behavioral effects of ACTH. It appeared, however, that most of the effects of corticosteroids on behavioral responses are opposite to those of ACTH and related peptides[2]. It remained questionable, however, whether the behavioral effects of corticosteroids are physiologically significant. The major receptor system for corticosteroids has been located in the hippocampus and appears to be highly specific for corticosterone[45,46]. Such behavioral specificity was, however, absent when relatively high amounts of steroids were used[2,47,48].

Our recent observations clearly indicate that corticosterone is physiologically involved in the modulation of adaptive behavior in the rat and that hippocampal receptors are involved in its mechanism of action[49]. It was found that rats display impaired extinction behavior in a forced extinction paradigm 1 h after adrenalectomy. This behavioral deficit can be corrected by substitution of corticosterone in physiological amounts (30 μg per 100g). A similar or a ten-times higher dose of dexamethasone, 11-deoxycorticosterone, progesterone or pregnenolone failed to normalize behavior. Accordingly, corticosterone appeared to influence this form of behavior highly specifically. The ineffective steroids, however, showed antagonist properties. Dexamethasone and progesterone pretreatment attenuated the effect of corticosterone substitution of adrenalectomized rats. 11-Deoxycorticosterone could block the effect of low but not of a high (300 μg) dose of corticosterone. Antagonistic properties of dexamethasone, progesterone and 11-deoxycorticosterone are interpreted as the result of competition for cytosolic corticosterone binding sites in the hippocampus and consequent block of entry of corticosterone into the cell nuclei. The similarities between the specificity of the behavioral effect of corticosteroids and their properties in binding to soluble hippocampal cytosol receptors and transport to the cell nuclei indicate that the effect of corticosterone on extinction behavior is mediated through hippocampal receptors. At 1 h after adrenalectomy, when a behavioral deficit is already present, only 35 per cent of the binding sites are occupied by corticosterone in the hippocampus. Administration of a maintenance dose of corticosterone restored the occupation of receptors to the level observed in intact control rats. These observations further support our hypothesis.

Surgical removal of the hippocampus may result in a behavioral deficit in extinction behavior similar to that seen after adrenalectomy. It seems therefore that the removal of a site of action of corticosterone causes a deficit similar to that which follows deprivation of the hippocampal receptor system of endogenous corticosterone. One of the functions of the hippocampal complex is to adjust behavior to new requirements under circumstances of environmental uncertainty. By suppressing older memories, the hippocampal function allows new actions to be taken. Accordingly, corticosterone may play a role in these behavioral adjustment processes.

Competition experiments in the behavioral studies and in hippocampal nuclear uptake *in vitro* showed full parallelism. Competition for nuclear uptake *in vivo*, however, could not be demonstrated[46]. It is therefore questioned whether a classical genomic process is involved in this behavioral effect of corticosterone. Table I compares the agonistic and antagonistic properties of steroids in feedback, behavioral effects and hippocampal receptor interaction in the rat. It is noteworthy that the agonistic and antagonistic properties of steroids are strikingly parallel in three distinct systems: fast feedback as studied in hypothalamic tissue *in vitro*[50], in the behavioral effect during forced extinction, and in the hippocampal receptor binding and nuclear uptake[45,46]. Dexamethasone represents the only exception. This synthetic steroid behaves as an agonist in fast feedback *in vitro*[50] but not *in vivo*[51] and as an antagonist on forced extinction and hippocampal receptor interaction. The differences may be explained by the existence of multiple corticosteroid binding systems in the brain[52]. Preliminary observations suggest that binding characteristics of

Table I. Comparative agonistic (agon.) and antagonistic (antag.) properties of steroids in feedback and behavioral effects and hippocampal receptor interaction in the rat

STEROID:	FEEDBACK Fast[a] Agon.	Fast[a] Antag.	Delayed[a] Agon.	Delayed[a] Antag.	Med. em. implants	BEHAVIOR Forced ext. Agon.	Forced ext. Antag.	Extinct s.c. treatment	Retention Hippoc. implants	RECEPTOR[a] Hippocampal receptor binding and nucl. uptake Agon.	Antag.
Corticosterone	+	−	+	+	+	+	+	+	+	+	+
11-Deoxycorticosterone	−	+	+	n.d.	+	−	+	n.d.	−	(+)[b]	+
18-Hydroxycorticosterone	n.d.	+	n.d.	n.d.	n.d.	n.d.	n.d.	n.d.	n.d.	n.d.	n.d.
Progesterone	−	+	−	−	−	−	+	+	n.d.	(+)[b]	+
Pregnenolone	n.d.	n.d.	n.d.	n.d.	−	−	n.d.	+	n.d.	n.d.	n.d.
Cortisol	+	−	n.d.	n.d.	+	n.d.	n.d.	n.d.	+	+	+
11-Deoxycortisol	−	+	n.d.	+	−	n.d.	n.d.	n.d.	n.d.	n.d.	n.d.
Dexamethasone	+	n.d.	n.d.	n.d.	+	−	+	+	n.d.	(+)[b]	+
Reference	50		50		53	49		48	14	46	

a Studies *in vitro*.
b Parentheses denote cytostol binding only.
  n.d., Not determined.

corticosterone and dexamethasone in the hippocampus are distinctly different after adrenalectomy, whereas in the hypothalamus they are similar.

Agonistic properties of steroids in delayed feedback, as studied in the hypothalamus *in vitro*[50], in the suppression of ACTH release after implantation in the median eminence[53], in the effect on extinction behavior in intact rats at pharmacological dose levels[48] and in the attenuation of retention behavior after implantation in the hippocampus[54] are rather similar. It seems that these actions of steroids involve receptor system(s) that are distinctly different from the fast-feedback type or hippocampal corticosterone receptor system. The multiplicity of binding systems as mentioned above may be the clue to the differences in steroid action on the brain. Beside their multiplicity, corticosterone receptors may also be localized differentially in the brain[55,56].

CONCLUDING REMARKS

ACTH, β-endorphin and related peptides modulate adaptive behavior and induce behavioral responses resembling opiate-evoked reactions. These inter-actions with the central nervous system may involve at least two putative receptor systems. Our observations point to a role of these neuropeptides in homeostatic brain functions. Discrete changes in the generation of fragments of β-endorphin, as determined by the site of cleavage, may assure a well-balanced modulation of behavioral adaptation to environmental events. In contrast, an imbalance of the system may lead to disturbances in adaptive processes. It is not yet clear whether ACTH- and endorphin-like peptides modulate adaptive behavior through the same putative receptors. The $ACTH_{4-10}$ sequence also occurs in the N-terminal fragment of β-LPH (β-LPH_{47-53}). It thus seems that two active sequences present in the same molecule may modulate behavior in a synergistic way. On the other hand, the $ACTH_{7-16}$ sequence, which only occurs in the ACTH molecule, appears to be as potent as $ACTH_{4-10}$ and can be highly potentiated by structural modifications[57]. Comparison of the behavioral profile of ACTH- and endorphin-like peptides does not yet allow the conclusion that different behavioral processes are affected by the two types of neuropeptides.

Very recently Jacquet[58] proposed the existence of two putative receptor systems in the periaqueductal grey in the brain. One is a stereospecific endorphin receptor system which is sensitive to opiate antagonists; the other is non-stereo-specific, and insensitive to opiate antagonists; ACTH may be the endogenous ligand for the latter receptors. The number of differences in the characteristics of this type of ACTH receptor (e.g. shortening of chain length decreases the potency) and of those described by us raised the possibility of the existence of multiple ACTH receptor systems in the brain. Whether the endogenous ligands (ACTH- and β-LPH-like peptides) for these multiple receptors originate separately in the pituitary and the brain (brain-born ACTH, α-MSH and endorphins) remains a question to be answered.

The pituitary–adrenal system *per se* through corticosteroid action on brain also serves as a modulator of adaptive behavior. Although corticosterone frequently affects behavior in a way opposite to that of neuropeptides, the physiological role of this system is primarily to ensure the elimination of non-relevant behavioral responses. Accordingly, interactions between the different modulator systems of brain homeostatic processes through agonistic and antagonistic mechanisms ensure endocrine regulation of behavioral adaptation.

REFERENCES

1.   De Wied, D. (1969). *In* "Frontiers in Neuroendocrinology" (Ganong, W. F. and Martini, L. eds.), pp. 97–140, Oxford University Press, New York.
2.   Bohus, B. (1970). *In* "Pituitary, Adrenal and the Brain, Progress in Brain Research", (de Wied, D. and Weijnen, J. A. W. M. eds.), Vol. 32, pp. 171–184, Elsevier, Amsterdam.
3.   De Wied, D. (1977). *Life Sci.* **20**, 195.
4.   Barchas, J. D. *et al.* (1978). *Science* **200**, 964.
5.   Bloom, F. *et al.* (1976). *Science* **194**, 630.
6.   Jacquet, Y. F. and Marks, N. (1976). *Science* **194**, 632.
7.   De Wied, D. (1978). *In* "Characteristics and Function of Opioids", (van Ree, J. M. and Terenius, L. eds.), pp. 113–122, Elsevier, Amsterdam.
8.   Gold, P. W. *et al.* (197). *Lancet* i, 1233.
9.   Orth, D. N. and Nicholson, W. E. (1977). *Ann. N.Y. Acad. Sci.* **297**, 27.
10.   Guillemin, R. *et al.* (1978). *Science* **197**, 1367.
11.   De Wied, D. (1964). *Am. J. Physiol.* **207**, 255.
12.   Lissak, K. and Bohus, B. (1972). *Int. J. Psychobiol.* **2**, 103.
13.   Gold, P. E. *et al.* (1977). *Horm. Behav.* **8**, 363.
14.   Bohus, B. *et al.* (1973). *Neuroendocrinol.* **11**, 137.
15.   Bohus, B. *et al.* (1968). *Int. J. Neuropharmacol.* **7**, 307.
16.   Bohus, B. (1978). *Pharmacology (in press).*
17.   De Wied, D. *et al.* (1970). *In* "Pituitary, Adrenal and the Brain, Progress in Brain Research", (De Wied, D. and Weijnen, J. A. eds.), Vol. 32, pp. 213–218 Elsevier, Amsterdam.
18.   Lande, S. *et al.* (1973). *In* "Drug Effects on Neuroendocrine Regulation, Progress in Brain Research", (Zimmermann, E. *et al.* eds.), Vol. 39, pp. 421–427, Elsevier, Amsterdam.
19.   Guillemin, R. *et al.* (1977). *Ann. N.Y. Acad. Sci.* **297**, 131.
20.   Gispen, W. H. *et al.* (1977). *Int. Rev. Neurobiol.* **20**, 209.
21.   De Wied, D. *et al.* (1978). *J. Pharm. Exp. Ther.* **204**, 570.
22.   Lissitzky, J. C. *et al.* (1978). *Life Sci.* **22**, 1715.
23.   Austen, B. M. *et al.* (1977). *Nature, London* **269**, 619.
24.   De Wied, D. *et al.* (1978). *Eur. J. Pharmacol.* **49**, 427.
25.   Loh, H. H. and Li C. H. (1977). *Ann. N.Y. Acad. Sci.* **297**, 115.
26.   Bohus, B. and Gispen, W. H. (1978). *In* "Characteristics and Function of Opioids" (van Ree, J. M. and Terenius, L. eds.), pp. 367–376, Elsevier, Amsterdam.
27.   Gispen, W. H. *et al.* (1975). *Life Sci.* **17**, 645.
28.   Gispen, W. H. *et al.* (1976). *Nature, London* **264**, 794.
29.   Wiegant, V. M., Jolles, J. and Gispen, W. H. (1978). *(in press).*
30.   Gispen, W. H. *et al.* (1976). *Eur. J. Pharmacol.* **39**, 397.
31.   Terenius, L. (1976). *Eur. J. Pharmacol.* **38**, 211.
32.   Allen, J. P. *et al.* (1974). *J. Clin. Endocrinol. Metab.* **38**, 586.
33.   Jeffecote, W. J. *et al.* (1978). *Lancet* ii, 119.
34.   Mezey, E. *et al.* (1978). *Life Sci.* **22**, 831.

35. Oliver, C. *et al.* (1977). *Endocrinology* **101**, 598.
36. Krieger, D. T. *et al.* (1977). *Brain Res.* **128**, 575.
37. Bloom, F. E. *et al.* (1978). *Adv. Biochem. Psychopharm.* **18**, 89.
38. Kobayashi, R. M. *et al.* (1978). *Life Sci.* **22**, 527.
39. Watson, S. J. *et al.* (1978). *Science* **200**, 1180.
40. Watson, S. J. *et al.* (1978). *Nature, London* **275**, 226.
41. Pelletier, G. and Dube, D. (1977). *Am. J. Anat.* **150**, 201.
42. Pomeranz, B. *et al.* (1977). *Exp. Neurol.* **54**, 172.
43. Amir, S. and Amiti, Z. (1978). *Life Sci.* **23**, 1143.
44. Dijk, A.M.A. van *et al.* (1979). *J. Endocrinol.* **80**, 60P.
45. McEwen, B. S. *et al.* (1975). *In* "The Hippocampus", (Isaacson, R. L. and Pribram, K. H. eds.), pp. 285–322, Plenum Press, New York.
46. de Kloet, E. R. and McEwen, B. S. (1976). *In* "Molecular and Functional Neurobiology", (Gispen, W. H. ed.), pp. 257–307, Elsevier, Amsterdam.
47. Bohus, B. (1975). *In* "The Hippocampus", (Isaacson, R. L. and Pribram, K. H. eds.), pp. 323–353, Plenum Press, New York.
48. van Wimersma Greidanus, Tj. B. (1970). *In* "Pituitary, Adrenal and the Brain, Progress in Brain Research", (de Wied, D. and Weijnen, J. A. W. M. eds.), Vol. 32. pp. 185–191, Elsevier, Amsterdam.
49. Bohus, B. and de Kloet, E. R. (1977). *J. Endocrinol.* **12**, 64P.
50. Jones, M. T. *et al.* (1977). *J. Endocrinol.* **74**, 415.
51. Abe, K. and Critchlow, V. (1977). *Endocrinology* **101**, 498.
52. de Kloet, E. R. (1977). *In* "Multiple Molecular Forms of Steroid Hormone Receptors", (Agarwal, M. K. ed.), pp. 65–79, Elsevier/North Holland, Amsterdam.
53. Bohus, B. and Strashimirov, D. (1970). *Neuroendocrinol.* **6**, 197.
54. Bohus, B. (1973). *In* "Drug Effects on Neuroendocrine Regulation, Progress in Brain Research", (Zimmermann, E. *et al.* eds.), Vol. 32, pp. 407–420, Elsevier, Amsterdam.
55. Stumpf, W. E. and Sar, M. (1975). *In* "Anatomical Neuroendocrinology", (Stumpf, W. E. and Grant, L. D. eds.), pp. 254–261, Karger, Basel.
56. Rees, H. D. *et al.* (1975). *In* "Anatomical Neuroendocrinology", (Stumpf, W. E. and Grant, L. D. eds.), pp. 262–269, Karger, Basel.
57. Greven, H. M. and de Wied, D. (1977). *Front. Horm. Res.* **4**, 150.
58. Jacquet, Y. F. (1978). *Science* **201**, 1032.

3

REGULATION OF CORTICOTROPIN-RELATED PEPTIDES IN THE INTERMEDIATE LOBE AND THEIR POSSIBLE RELATION TO OBESITY

J. A. Edwardson and Amanda Donaldson

Department of Physiology, St. George's Hospital Medical School, London SW17 0QT, U.K

INTRODUCTION

In species ranging from elasmobranch fishes to rodents, the pituitary intermediate lobe has been shown to contain two peptides which exhibit complete homology of structure with regions of the corticotropin (ACTH) molecule[1]. One of these is melanotropin (α-MSH) which possesses the NH_2-terminal 1-13 sequence of ACTH and which exhibits a wide spectrum of biological activity including effects on pigmentation, sebum production, foetal development and behaviour (for reviews see other chapters in ref. 1). The other is corticotropin-like intermediate lobe peptide (CLIP), the free 18–39 COOH-terminal fragment of ACTH. In contrast to α-MSH, little is known about the biological significance of CLIP or the mechanism of its hypothalamic control. In this respect, the genetically obese *(ob/ob)* mouse is of considerable interest since the pars intermedia of this species secrete considerable quantities of CLIP and α-MSH. Also, the pars distalis of the *ob/ob* mouse contains increased levels of ACTH, suggesting some common element in the control of these structurally related peptides by the two lobes of the adenohypophysis.

The *ob* gene arose spontaneously at the Jackson Laboratories, Bar Harbour[2], and has been incorporated into mice of many different genetic backgrounds over the last three decades. It is a recessive gene, the heterozygous *(ob/+)* carriers being lean whereas the homozygous *(ob/ob)* animals exhibit marked obesity accompanied by a constellation of metabolic, physiological and endocrine defects.

17

Table I.   Metabolic, endocrine and physiological abnormalities in the genetically obese *(ob/ob)* mouse.

---

1.   Hyperphagia

2.   Obesity — an increase in both the amount and proportion of body fat, even when pair-fed with lean littermate controls

3.   Hyperglycaemia and hyperlipidaemia in the presence of abnormally high insulin levels and insulin resistance

4.   Hypogonadism and infertility

5.   Adrenocortical hypertrophy and increased corticosterone secretion

6.   Impaired thermoregulation in cold environment

For details of above see reviews[2,3,4].

These abnormalities have been reviewed extensively[3,4] and some of the most conspicuous are listed in Table I. A hypothalamic origin for these defects has been proposed by several groups and evidence for a widespread impairment involving monoamine neurotransmitters, hypophysiotropic peptides and feedback regulation by steroid hormones has been described elsewhere[5].

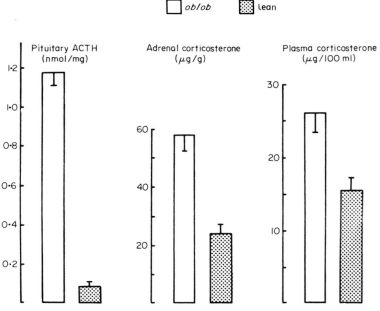

Fig. 1.   Concentrations of adrenal corticosterone, plasma corticosterone and immunoreactive ACTH in the anterior pituitary of 16-week-old genetically obese *(ob/ob)* mice and lean littermate controls. ACTH was measured with an antiserum raised against synthetic 1–24 ACTH. For other experimental details see ref. 6.

THE HYPOTHALAMO-PITUITARY-ADRENOCORTICAL SYSTEM
OF THE *ob/ob* MOUSE

The adult *ob/ob* mouse shows a striking increase in both the adrenal content and plasma concentration of corticosterone, whereas the adenohypophysis contains approximately 2–3 nmol of ACTH, a 14-fold elevation compared with lean littermate controls (Fig. 1). By using a superfusion system *in vitro*, we have shown[6] that adenohypophyses isolated from *ob/ob* mice released considerably more ACTH than those of lean controls. Although this could simply be due to the increased content of the *ob/ob* gland, it seems more likely to reflect increased stimulation by corticotropin-releasing factor (CRF; corticoliberin) *in vivo*, since an increased rate of release is also obtained with glands taken from *ob/ob* mice on a restricted diet where the ACTH content resembles that of lean controls (Fig. 2).

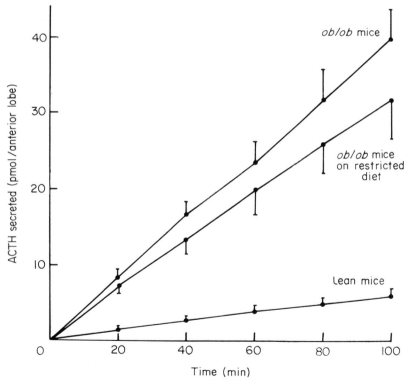

Fig. 2. ACTH secretion by isolated, superfused pituitary glands from 16-week-old lean mice, *ob/ob* mice, and *ob/ob* mice placed on a restricted diet. A preliminary period of 30 min superfusion was carried out and only the steady rates of secretion in the subsequent 100 min are shown. The pituitary ACTH content in the restricted-diet *ob/ob* mice and lean controls was not significantly different. For other experimental details see ref. 6.

The hypothalamic content of CRF in *ob/ob* mice does not appear to be greater than that in lean animals[6] although this finding does not exclude the possibility of an increased turnover and release of CRF. Rather more difficult to explain is the finding of no difference between *ob/ob* and lean mice in either the basal or stress-induced levels of immunoreactive ACTH in plasma[6]. However, the studies *in vitro* described above and the increased levels of adrenal, plasma and free urinary corticosterone strongly suggest that under some circumstances the release of ACTH is elevated in *ob/ob* animals. This conclusion led us to ask whether ACTH could contribute to the hyperinsulinaemia of the *ob/ob* mouse since there are several reports of a direct insulin-releasing action of corticotropin in rodent species (for references, see 7). To test this hypothesis, isolated pituitary glands were superfused in series with microdissected pancreatic islets from lean mice and it was shown that whereas the superfusate from *ob/ob* glands rapidly stimulated insulin release, that from lean pituitaries was ineffective[7].

THE NATURE OF THE PITUITARY INSULIN SECRETAGOGUE

In further attempts to identify the insulin-releasing factor in the superfusate from *ob/ob* pituitaries, purified porcine ACTH was tested for its effect on isolated pancreatic islets. Although a consistent increase in insulin release was obtained[8,9], the response was much smaller than that observed with the *ob/ob* pituitary superfusate. In the same series of experiments Synacthen, the synthetic NH_2-terminal 1–24 fragment of ACTH, was also tested and shown to be ineffective. These results indicated that the insulin-releasing effect may be a function of the COOH-terminal sequence of ACTH and even that CLIP itself might be the active factor. In the absence of adequate supplies of purified CLIP, the synthetic 17–39 fragment of human ACTH was tested. In 33 experiments, 15 islet preparations responded with an increase in insulin release of more than 50% above basal levels and the mean response of this group for the peak of insulin release was 191 ± 36% (mean ± S.E.) above control values[10]. Despite the variation in these responses, increased release of insulin has not been observed in similar experiments with other purified anterior or posterior pituitary hormones. Further, it should be noted that although the steroidogenic, NH_2-terminal 1–24 sequence of ACTH is common to all mammals, there is species variation in the COOH-terminal sequence which could partly explain the diminished response to $17–39_h$ ACTH.

Two further pieces of evidence support the idea that CLIP or a closely related peptide may be the insulin secretagogue released from the *ob/ob* pituitary. First, experiments with the dissected pituitary have shown that the isolated adenohypophysis which releases ACTH is without effect, although the isolated neurointermediate lobe is as active as the whole pituitary (Fig. 3). Secondly, incubation of superfusate from *ob/ob* pituitaries with an antiserum raised against $17–39_h$ ACTH has been shown to abolish the insulin-releasing effect. The mean peak of insulin release from microdissected islets was 46.2 ± 23.6% (mean ± S.E., $n = 6$) above basal levels, whereas the response from *ob/ob* pituitary superfusate incubated under identical conditions with control rabbit serum was 311.0 ± 40.6%.

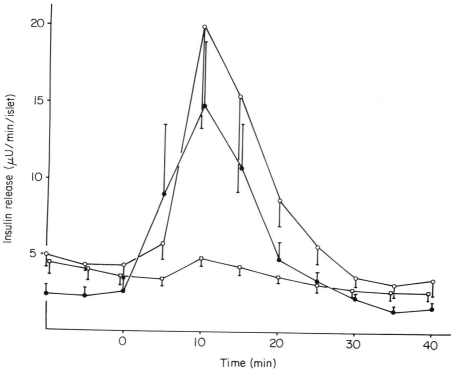

Fig. 3. Effect of the whole *ob/ob* pituitary gland (*n* = 8) *ob/ob* neurointermediate lobe (*n* = 12) and *ob/ob* pars distalis of anterior pituitary (*n* = 14) on insulin release from isolated, pancreatic islets of lean mice. For experimental details see ref. 7. Values show mean (± S.E.M.).

SECRETION OF CORTICOTROPIN-RELATED PEPTIDES BY THE PARS INTERMEDIA OF *ob/ob* MICE

Superfusate from the pituitary glands of lean *(+/+)* mice does not exhibit insulin-releasing activity. If the active factor were CLIP or a related peptide, it follows therefore that the pars intermedia of *ob/ob* animals should contain or release increased amounts of a COOH-terminal fragment of ACTH. Fig. 4 shows the content of immunoreactive NH_2-terminal 'ACTH', COOH-terminal 'ACTH' and α-MSH in extracts of the intermediate lobe from *ob/ob* and lean *(+/+)* mice. The considerable excess of COOH-terminal activity has been found by gel filtration to have chromatographic properties similar to $17–39_h$ ACTH and is presumably CLIP. There is a striking increase in the content of this peptide in *ob/ob* glands compared with the lean controls. In both the obese and lean animal the proportion of immunoreactive NH_2-terminal ACTH is less than 2% of the total corticotropin-related peptides, suggesting that ACTH is not a major storage form of CLIP and α-MSH. The difference in the molar ratios of CLIP to α-MSH in the intermediate lobes of *ob/ob* and lean mice indicates that there must be indepen-

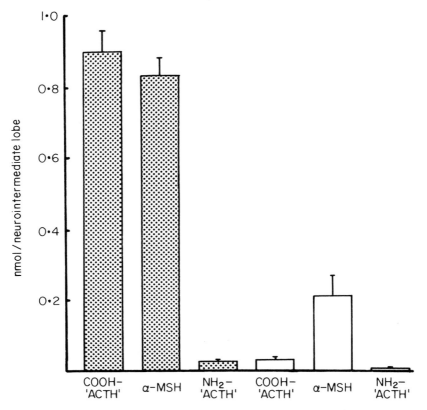

Fig. 4. Content of immunoreactive corticotropin-related peptides in neutralized 0.1 M HCl extracts of neurointermediate lobes from *ob/ob* (▨) and lean (+/+) (☐) mice. NH₂- and COOH-terminal 'ACTH' immunoreactivity was measured with antisera raised against synthetic 1–24 ACTH and 17–39ₕ ACTH respectively. Means (± S.E.M') of values from six neurointermediate lobes in each group are shown.

dent mechanisms for either the post-ribosomal processing, or release of these peptides.

Studies with the superfused neurointermediate lobe show that CLIP and α-MSH are also released in different molar ratios from obese and lean glands (Fig. 5). The ability of the pars intermedia to both store and release CLIP in different ratios from α-MSH strongly suggests a hormonal function for the former.

THE REGULATION OF CLIP RELEASE FROM THE INTERMEDIATE LOBE

Two important questions raised by the hypothesis that CLIP may be a hormone concern the mechanism of its hypothalamic regulation and the nature of stimuli that elicit its release. Elsewhere in this volume Smelik has described

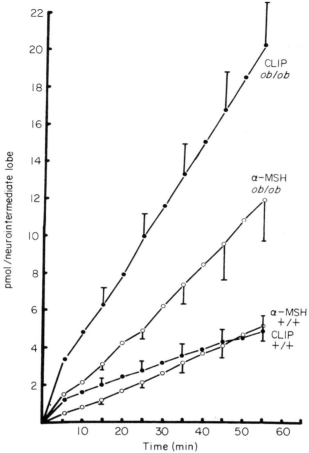

Fig. 5.   Release of immunoreactive COOH-terminal ACTH-like activity (−•−•−) and
α-MSH (−○−○−) from superfused neurointermediate lobes of *ob/ob* and lean *(+/+)* mice.
Results are expressed as a cumulative plot (pmol/lobe) of peptide released in 60 min superfusion. NH_2-terminal ACTH-like activity was not detectable (10pg/ml) in the superfusate.
Values represent means ± S.E.M., n = 5 or 6.

evidence that the release of α-MSH is under inhibitory control via a dopaminergic
secretomotor innervation of the pars intermedia. We have tested neurotransmitters and other substances on the superfused neurointermediate lobe of
normal lean control mice to determine whether such factors may be involved in
the regulation of CLIP release. Dopamine, noradrenaline, serotonin (5-hydroxy-
tryptamine) and acetylcholine failed to have an effect on CLIP release at
concentrations ranging from 1 mM to 1 μM. Vasopressin was also inactive.
However, when the superfused lobe was exposed to a neutralized HC1 extract
of the hypothalamus for 5 min, there was an immediate increase in CLIP release
which was sustained for a period of between 20 and 30 min (Fig. 6). Although

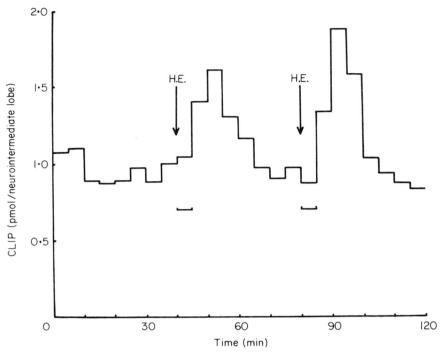

Fig. 6. Response of superfused neurointermediate lobes from lean mice to HCl extract of lean mouse hypothalamus. Extract (1 hypothalamic equivalent; HE) was added during 5 min superfusion and levels of immunoreactive COOH-terminal ACTH in the superfusate are shown. Values represent the mean of six experiments and the S.E.M., which is less than 10% in all cases, is not shown.

there was a consistent release of CLIP under these conditions, the effect on release of α-MSH was variable with inhibition occurring in some cases and no response observed in others. These results indicate that the secretion of CLIP is under the excitatory control of the hypothalamus, perhaps via a humoral releasing factor, although the possibility that the active substance may be delivered locally by peptidergic or other secretomotor innervation of the pars intermedia remains open.

The evidence that CLIP may be one of the multiple factors involved in the regulation of insulin secretion prompted experiments to determine whether glucose or other blood nutrient levels may provide a stimulus for the release of CLIP. The effects of normal (5mM) and high (20mM) glucose levels on either the isolated neurointermediate lobe or co-incubates of the neurointermediate lobe with the isolated mediobasal hypothalamus were tested. Although increased glucose levels had no effect on CLIP release from the neurointermediate lobe incubated alone, in some co-incubates with the hypothalamus fragments, a marked increase in CLIP release was observed. However, this response was extremely variable. An explanation for this inconsistent response is suggested by the recent report of Beloff-Chain et al.[11] showing that the release of the insulin secretagogue from superfused pituitaries is altered according to the previous nutritional status of the donor animal. Overnight starvation (18 h) of the *ob/ob* mouse decreased the insulin-releasing effects of such superfusates and 48 h starvation abolished the activity. In contrast, with glands from lean animals, which do not normally stimulate insulin release, a significant stimulatory effect was observed when the animals were starved and then re-fed or administered a glucose dose.

Further evidence that CLIP secretion may be determined by the nutritional status of the animal is presented in Table II, which shows levels of CLIP and

Table II. Amounts of COOH-terminal 'ACTH' (CLIP) and α-MSH in the neurointermediate lobes of gold thioglucose- and high-fat diet-treated mice and age-matched controls.
Groups are untreated controls, mice receiving a single injection of gold thioglucose (1g/kg) or maintained on a diet of standard pellet crushed and mixed with an equal weight of butter. Values show mean ± S.E.M. for groups of six to nine mice. Over 90 days, the body weights increased from 23 ± 1g (all groups) to 43 ± 2 (controls), 67 ± 4 (gold thioglucose) and 57 ± 1 (high-fat diet).

Day of treatment	Controls	Gold thioglucose (pmol of CLIP/lobe)	High-fat diet
1	58 ± 9	66 ± 17	57 ± 9
4	43 ± 7	10 ± 3	56 ± 10
7	31 ± 6	38 ± 9	58 ± 12
14	34 ± 6	45 ± 12	99 ± 16
28	44 ± 6	78 ± 11	127 ± 20
90	100 ± 66	383 ± 40	431 ± 114
		(pmol of α-MSH/lobe)	
1	220 ± 46	205 ± 27	195 ± 27
4	145 ± 15	145 ± 26	170 ± 50
7	303 ± 50	142 ± 32	214 ± 24
14	185 ± 22	236 ± 42	464 ± 84
28	317 ± 62	711 ± 96	542 ± 56
90	316 ± 42	925 ± 315	768 ± 90

α-MSH in the intermediate lobes of mice placed on either a high-fat diet or made obese by treatment with gold thioglucose. With the high-fat diet, a significant increase in both CLIP and α-MSH is evident after 14 days and the content of both peptides continues to rise slowly. After treatment with gold thioglucose, which is supposed to be taken up by and to destroy the ventromedial hypothalamic satiety centre, a massive fall in CLIP and a smaller decrease in α-MSH is evident after 4 days. At this stage appetite is almost completely suppressed. As feeding is restored, an increase in the levels of CLIP and α-MSH is observed and at 28 days α-MSH is significantly elevated but levels of CLIP are restored to normal. In both gold thioglucose- and high-fat diet-treated animals after 3 months there is a 4-fold increase in levels of CLIP and a 2–3-fold increase in levels of α-MSH.

DISCUSSION AND CONCLUSIONS

In the adult genetically obese mouse there are large, concomitant increases in the content of ACTH in the pars distalis and both CLIP and α-MSH in the pars intermedia. Recently Margules *et al.*[12] reported elevated concentrations of the endogenous opioid peptide β-endorphin in the pituitaries of *ob/ob* mice and fatty *(fa/fa)* rats. There is evidence that the whole family of corticotropin- and lipotropin-related peptides is derived from a single macromolecular precursor[13] and our studies suggest that in addition to this prohormone there may be some common element in the mechanisms that control their secretion, since they are elevated together.

The ability of the pars intermedia both to store and to release α-MSH and CLIP in different ratios under different physiological circumstances points to separate and independent mechanisms in the control of their secretion. Although in the case of α-MSH this control may be mediated through the dopamine-containing neurons that arise in the arcuate nucleus, it seems that in the case of CLIP some other mechanism may operate since both monoamines and acetyl-choline were without effect on the release of this peptide *in vitro*.

Although it remains to be shown definitively that the insulin-releasing factor secreted by the pituitaries of *ob/ob* mice is CLIP, the circumstantial evidence is very strong. Thus (a) the secretagogue is released from the neurointermediate lobe but not the pars distalis, (b) the insulin-releasing activity is neutralized by an antiserum raised against $17–39_h$ ACTH, (c) although the steroidogenic NH_2 1–24 sequence of ACTH is inactive, peptides having the COOH-terminal 17–39 sequence are active and (d) levels of both CLIP and the insulin secretagogue are raised in *ob/ob* animals. However, the intermediate lobe contains a variety of peptides[14], several of which show immunological similarities with corticotropin- and lipotropin-related fragments, and it is possible that the insulin secretagogue may be one of these peptides rather than CLIP itself. Whatever the true identity of the insulin secretagogue, the insulin-releasing activity of synthetic $17–39_h$ ACTH *in vitro* is the first demonstration of a biological effect for the COOH-terminal region of the ACTH molecule. This finding raises the possibility that some of the many other extra-adrenal effects of ACTH (for review, see 15) are also attributable to the non-steroidogenic portion of the molecule.

Several lines of evidence point to a role for the pituitary gland in the acute regulation of insulin secretion. The effect of cyproheptadine, which depletes pancreatic insulin in the rat[16], is eliminated by hypophysectomy[17]. Chieri *et al.*[18] have reported that glucose infusion *via* the carotid artery in dogs stimulates insulin release in the presence of normal peripheral plasma glucose levels. This effect was also abolished by hypophysectomy. The elevated concentrations of corticotropin- and lipotropin-related peptides in the pituitaries of *ob/ob* mice and *fa/fa* rats suggests that one or more of these hormones may be the putative insulin secretagogue and may contribute to the hyperinsulinaemia of obesity. Further, the increased content of α-MSH and CLIP in the intermediate lobes of normal animals made fat by gold thioglucose or a high-fat diet suggests that these peptides may be involved in non-genetic forms of obesity. The extreme conservation of structure of α-MSH and CLIP in vertebrate species points to an important biological role. It seems likely that the precise functions for these hormones in mammals may be in relation to the complex neuroendocrine mechanisms that regulate and synchronize feeding behaviour, blood fuel homoeostasis and metabolic control.

ACKNOWLEDGEMENTS

We gratefully acknowledge our collaboration with Dr. Anne Beloff-Chain and members of her group who have carried out the studies on insulin release reported here. This work was supported by research grants from the Medical Research Council and Wellcome Trust. A. Donaldson was supported by a SRC studentship in cooperation with Imperial Chemical Industries Ltd. We thank Dr. D. Stribling (I.C.I. Ltd.) for advice and collaborative support and Mrs. J. Pennington for valuable technical assistance. Ciba-Geigy Ltd. provided generous gifts of corticotropin-related peptides.

REFERENCES

1. Lowry, P. J. and Scott, A. P. (1977). *Front. Horm. Res.* **4**, 11.
2. Ingalls, A. M. *et al.* (1950). *J. Hered.* **41**, 317.
3. Bray, G. A. and York, D. A. (1971). *Physiol. Rev.* **51**, 598.
4. Herberg, L. and Coleman, D. L. (1977). *Metabolism* **26**, 59.
5. Edwardson, J. A. and Donaldson, A. (1979). *In* "Genetic Models of Obesity in Laboratory Animals" (Festling, M. ed.), MacMillan, London.
6. Edwardson, J. A. and Hough, C. A. M. (1975). *J. Endocrinol.* **65**, 99.
7. Beloff-Chain, A. *et al.* (1975). *J. Endocrinol.* **65**, 109.
8. Hawthorn, J. (1976). Ph. D. Thesis, University of London.
9. Beloff-Chain, A. *et al.* (1977). *J. Endocrinol.* **73**, 28P.
10. Beevor, S. *et al.* (1979). *In preparation.*
11. Beloff-Chain, A. *et al.* (1979). *J. Endocrinol. (in press).*
12. Margules, D. L. *et al.* (1978). *Science* **202**, 988.
13. Mains, R. *et al.* (1977). *Proc. Natl. Acad. Sci. USA* **74**, 3014.
14. Scott, A. P. *et al.* (1976). *J. Endocrinol.* **70**, 197.
15. Lebovitz, H. E. (1973). *In* "Methods in Investigative and Diagnostic Endocrinology" (Berson, S. A. and Yalow, R. S., eds.), Vol. 2A, North Holland, Amsterdam.
16. Longnecker, D. S. *et al.* (1972). *Diabetes* **21**, 71.
17. Richardson, B. P. (1974). *Diabetalogia* **10**, 479.
18. Chieri, R. A. *et al.* (1976). *Horm. Metab. Res.* **8**, 329.

4

DIFFERENTIAL CONTROL OF ANTERIOR LOBE AND INTERMEDIATE LOBE CORTICOTROPIN (ACTH) SECRETION IN THE RAT

P. G. Smelik and F. J. H. Tilders

Department of Pharmacology, Medical Faculty, Free University,
1007 MC Amsterdam, The Netherlands.

EXISTENCE OF CORTICOTROPIN (ACTH) IN THE INTERMEDIATE LOBE

Since the original observation of Mialhe-Voloss[1], the presence of ACTH in the neurointermediate lobe complex of mammals has been confirmed repeatedly by a variety of assay systems. Pronounced differences in corticotropic activity in rat neurointermediate lobe have been reported, ranging from about 20 mU[2] to 400 mU[3] per lobe. Possibly, differences in assay procedures, extraction methods, rat strains, sex, etc., play an important role since parallel variations were reported in anterior lobe ACTH content. With one exception[3], the reports indicate that between 2.5 and 7% of total pituitary ACTH activity originates from the neuro-intermediate lobe[2,4,5-9].

Scott and colleagues[9] have suggested that the corticotropic substance from the neurointermediate lobe is identical to anterior lobe $ACTH_{1-39}$, which fits well with current concepts of biosynthesis of intermediate lobe peptides[10]. Accordingly, by using the dispersed adrenal cell assay of Sayers[11], anterior lobe extracts and neurointermediate lobe extracts had activities (slope, maximum) identical with $ACTH_{1-39}$. However, since conflicting data have recently been reported[12], the exact nature of neurointermediate lobe ACTH remains to be established.

Quantitation of neurointermediate lobe ACTH by radiommunoassays (RIAs) generates specific problems because of the presence of both N-terminal (melano-tropin, α-MSH) and C-terminal (corticotropin-like intermediate lobe peptide,

CLIP) fragments of ACTH which do not show corticotropic activity (see Table I). Many RIAs used for the determination of ACTH in tissue extracts and plasma are useless in studies on neurointermediate lobe ACTH, unless performed in combination with separation techniques, because of cross-reaction with these ACTH fragments[6,9,10]. For example, the ACTH antiserum of Dr. C. D. West (supplied by the National Pituitary Agency, NIAMDD) gave excellent results in our studies with anterior lobes *in vitro*, and these corresponded nicely to bio-assay data. However, neurointermediate lobe extracts and $ACTH_{1-39}$ gave non-parallel displacement of labelled $ACTH_{1-39}$ as did purified CLIP (gift from Dr. P. J. Lowry). Thus because of the relative abundance of α-MSH and CLIP (Table I) ACTH-RIAs used in studies on the neurointermediate lobe should exhibit extremely low cross-reactivity with these two intermediate lobe peptides [9,13]. The exact origin and cellular localization of "posterior pituitary ACTH" has been a subject of speculation[4,5,14,15]. Determination of corticotropic activity in extracts of carefully separated neural and intermediate lobes showed that "posterior pituitary ACTH" is present in the intermediate lobe rather than in the neural lobe[3]. In addition, intermediate-lobe cell suspensions were found to contain and secrete $ACTH$[16].

This is further supported by the results of immunolocalization studies suggesting the presence of ACTH in all endocrine cells of the pars intermedia[17,18]. However, since the specificity of the methods used remains questionable, evaluation of these results is difficult. In the earlier studies, one was mainly concerned with cross-reaction with α-MSH. To avoid any possible cross-reaction with this peptide, antibodies against $ACTH_{17-39}$ have been introduced and many workers have concluded that a positive reaction with such antibodies is evidence for the presence of $ACTH_{1-39}$ [17,18]. In view of the occurrence of relatively high concentrations of $ACTH_{18-39}$ in the neurointermediate lobe of rats and other vertebrates[10] these data could be interpreted primarily as evidence for the co-existence of α-MSH and CLIP within the same cells of the pars intermedia.

INTERMEDIATE LOBE ACTH: PRECURSOR OR HORMONE?

The intermediate lobe has long been known as the source of melanocyte-stimulating hormones. In the rat, α-MSH is the predominant melanotropic peptide, which according to its amino acid sequence, can be considered as an *N*-terminal fragment of ACTH (see Table I).

In addition to α-MSH, a peptide identical to $ACTH_{18-39}$ was identified from rat, pig and dogfish pituitaries[9,10,19,20] and this *C*-terminal fragment of ACTH appeared to be localized mainly in the intermediate lobe[9]. Consequently, it was named CLIP, an acronym for corticotropin-like intermediate lobe peptide. CLIP and α-MSH are present in roughly equimolar amounts[9]. Further, neurointermediate lobes were found to secrete both α-MSH and CLIP *in vitro*[9], which is in agreement with the co-existence of α-MSH and CLIP in the secretory granules of intermediate lobe cells[18].

In accordance with these and other observations, it was postulated that intermediate lobe ACTH serves as a precursor mulecule ('prohormone') for the biosynthesis of α-MSH and CLIP[10,19,20].

In view of this hypothesis, there are obvious parallels with other endocrine systems:

a. The concept of biosynthesis of peptide hormones via cleavage of large molecular prohormones is well documented.

b. Cleavage of prohormones is reported to occur at sites marked by the presence of sets of basic amino acids as found in ACTH at positions 15–18.

c. As shown for instance for insulin, secretion of the actual hormone may be accompanied by secretion of other precursor fragments ('connecting peptide') and sometimes by small amounts of intact prohormone (proinsulin).

d. Prohormones show only low biological activity (if any) when compared to the 'final hormone'. If we consider α-MSH to be the 'final hormone' of the intermediate lobe, the relatively low melanotropic activity of $ACTH_{1-39}$ (about 100 times less than that of α-MSH) is in accordance with this. Although CLIP was initially suggested to be a biologically inactive fragment since it did not show melanotropic or corticotropic activity, it was recently shown to stimulate insulin release[21]. Once again, $ACTH_{1-39}$ appeared to be less active in releasing insulin than CLIP.

In addition to these ACTH-related peptides, the intermediate lobe is known to produce various other peptides (e.g. β-MSH) which can be considered as fragments of β-LPH (lipotropin)[10,20]. Recently, large quantities of endorphins (C-terminal LPH fragments) such as β-endorphin, were found in the intermediate lobe of rats and again this peptide is not biologically inactive, but shows pronounced opiate-like activity[22-24]. Evidence is rapidly accumulating suggesting that peptides like α-MSH, CLIP, ACTH, LPH, β-MSH, β-endorphin, etc., can be produced simultaneously within the same pars intermedia cells[25-27]. With regard to the peptides that are present in the rat intermediate lobe in roughly equal amounts, α-MSH, CLIP and β-endorphin, it is surprising that although many effects have been ascribed to these peptides, very little is known about their physiological role(s). As a consequence, one might question whether any of these peptides meet the criteria for being considered true hormones in mammals.

In fact, ACTH is the only peptide of all of the peptides found in the intermediate lobe with a well-established physiological effect. However, since only a small part of total pituitary ACTH is located in the intermediate lobe, we must consider whether ACTH from this particular source plays a physiological role as a corticotropic hormone.

According to early workers in the field of the stress response, noxious stimuli can be divided into two classes: *neurogenic* or emotional, and *systemic* or somatic[28].

Mialhe-Voloss[1,15] reported that emotional stimuli induced a decrease in intermediate lobe ACTH, without affecting anterior lobe ACTH content, whereas ACTH in the anterior lobe was selectively affected by systemic stimuli. Although these observations were confirmed by several workers[4,18,29] conflicting results have been presented as well[7].

Adrenocortical activation in response to neurogenic stress was greatly decreased after extirpation of the neurointermediate lobe, whereas the response to systemic stimuli remained unaffected[14,29-32]. These data suggest that ACTH is released from the intermediate lobe during neurogenic stress and might play a direct role in the adrenocortical response; however, alternative explanations have also been postulated[33,34]. Although many controversial results have been generated, there is general agreement that the intermediate lobe, in the absence of the anterior lobe, is unable to maintain adrenal weight and to evoke stress-induced stimulation of the adrenal cortex[30,31].

STUDIES *IN VITRO* ON THE RELEASE OF ACTH FROM THE INTERMEDIATE LOBE

Since results of experiments *in vivo* have not clarified the role of intermediate lobe ACTH, we have performed studies *in vitro* to find answers to the following questions:

a. Can ACTH be released from the intermediate lobe?
b. If so, which factors affect the release of intermediate lobe ACTH?
c. Is the release from intermediate and anterior lobes influenced by different mechanisms?

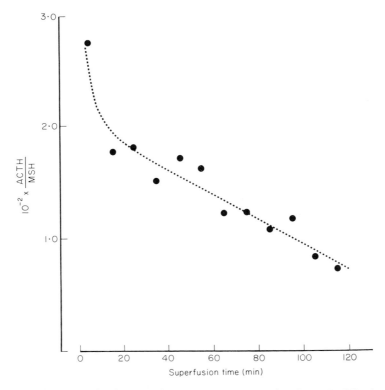

Fig. 1.   The relationship between the spontaneous release of ACTH and α-MSH from rat neurointermediate lobes superfused with Krebs–Ringer bicarbonate medium. ACTH was measured by bioassay[11] and α-MSH was determined by RIA[35]. The ordinate shows the ratio of pg of $ACTH_{1-39}$ to pg of α-MSH.

d. Does a strict correlation exist between release of ACTH and α-MSH from the intermediate lobe?

We used freshly prepared neurointermediate lobes and anterior lobe fragments from adult female rats. Groups of 10–15 neurointermediate lobes or quarters of two anterior lobes were superfused with a Krebs–Ringer bicarbonate buffer as described earlier[36]. Effluent medium was collected at 5 min intervals and was assayed for ACTH by using the adrenal cell suspension method[11,37] and for α-MSH by RIA[35].

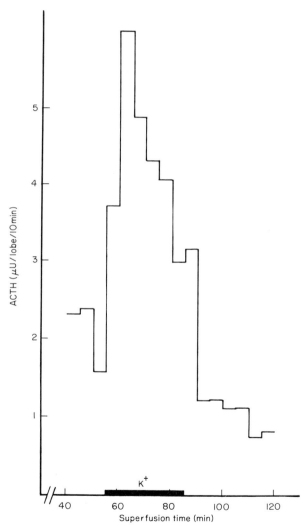

Fig. 2.   Effect of high potassium concentration on the release of ACTH from rat neurointermediate lobes *in vitro*. K$^+$ indicates the period of superfusion with medium containing 45 mM KCl.

34 P. G. Smelik and F. J. H. Tilders

During superfusion, the release rate of ACTH is initially high but falls off rapidly during the first 20–30 min. A similar change is observed in the efflux rate of α-MSH[36,38]. In contrast to α-MSH, however, the release rate of ACTH did not stabilize but showed a progressive decline. As a consequence, the ratio of ACTH/MSH released by neurointermediate lobes is not constant (Fig. 1). This might indicate that these peptides are released from different cellular or subcellular pools[18].

We have reported previously, that superfusion of neurointermediate lobes with a membrane-depolarizing medium, resulted in inhibition of the release of α-MSH as determined by bioassay[36,39] and RIA[40]. During superfusion with 45 mM K$^+$, complete dissociation was observed between the release of α-MSH and ACTH since inhibition of α-MSH release was associated with stimulation of ACTH release (Fig. 2.). Since membrane depolarization has been reported not to affect ACTH release from isolated pars intermedia cell suspensions[41], the results might represent an indirect effect mediated by release of some neurogenic factor in the preparation.

As described earlier[36,39], the effect of K$^+$ on α-MSH release is mediated by depolarization-induced release of dopamine from nerve terminals in this preparation. In accordance with this hypothesis, the effect of K$^+$ on α-MSH release could be mimicked by superfusion with a dopamine-containing medium (Fig. 3).

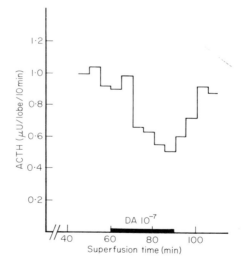

Fig. 3. Effect of dopamine on the release of ACTH from rat neurointermediate lobes *in vitro. DA* indicates the period of superfusion with medium containing 0.1 μM of dopamine.

We have recently repeated these experiments and found that superfusion of neurointermediate lobes with dopamine (0.1–1 μM) resulted in a parallel inhibition of α-MSH and ACTH release[40]. No effects of dopamine were found on the release of ACTH from the anterior lobe. Isoprenaline was recently found to stimulate the release of α-MSH from rat neurointermediate lobes[40] which agrees with observations on lower vertebrates[42]. We therefore studied the effect of β-adrenergic stimulation (isoprenaline, 1–100nM) and found a parallel, dose-related stimulation of the release of both α-MSH and ACTH (see Fig. 4).

Consequently, the effects of naturally occuring catecholamines were subsequently tested and we observed that adrenaline also induces isoprenaline-like stimulation of both α-MSH and ACTH release at concentrations down to 1–100nM. Once again, ACTH release from anterior lobe fragments was not affected.

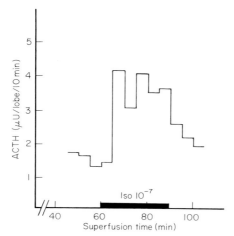

Fig. 4.   Effect of isoprenaline on the release of ACTH from rat neurointermediate lobes *in vitro*. Iso indicates the period of superfusion with medium containing 0.1μM of isoprenaline.

As shown by others[41,43], the release of ACTH from the intermediate and anterior lobes can be stimulated by hypothalamic extracts. However, a partially purified corticoliberin (CRF) preparation that was active on the anterior lobe did not affect intermediate lobe ACTH secretion[16,41].

So far, some of the questions formulated above can be answered. The results clearly show that ACTH can be released from the intermediate lobe cells. Although, in our hands, catecholamines induced parallel changes in the release of α-MSH and ACTH, release of both peptides is not necessarily correlated. Further, there is a clear dissociation in response of anterior and intermediate lobe ACTH release and our present results indicate that β-adrenergic stimulation results in release of ACTH from the intermediate lobe without affecting the secretion of ACTH from the anterior lobe.

STUDIES *IN VIVO*

The observation that isoprenaline releases ACTH from the intermediate lobe, but not from the anterior lobe *in vitro* poses the question whether this is the case *in vivo*, and whether the plasma ACTH levels achieved would be sufficiently high to stimulate the adrenal cortex.

Accordingly, intravenous infusions of small amounts of isoprenaline were given to rats anesthetized with Nembutal^R, and plasma corticosterone levels were determined after several time intervals. Simultaneously, plasma α-MSH levels were measured to check whether the intermediate lobe cells were activated by the isoprenaline infusion. As shown in Table I amounts of 100 ng of isoprenaline/min/kg body weight were capable of inducing an appreciable increase in circulating corticosterone and α-MSH levels. Such experiments indicate that isoprenaline infusions induce ACTH release *in vivo*, but do not indicate the exact site of action. To rule out any 'non-specific' action of isoprenaline resulting in CRF release, similar experiments were conducted in rats with hypothalamic lesions.

Electrothermic lesions to destroy the ventromedial part of the hypothalamus, including the arcuate nucleus and the median eminence, were made 10 days before the experiment, as described elsewhere[44]. From results of these experiments (see Fig. 5), it is clear that destruction of the hypothalamic input to the

Table I.   Effect of isoprenaline on plasma α-MSH and corticosterone levels in female rats anaesthetized with Nembutal^R (40mg/kg, i.p., 30 min before infusion). Isoprenaline was infused *via* the tail vein at a rate of 0.4 μg/min/kg body weight. n is the number of animals. Data represent means ± S.E.M. Values were compared to vehicle-infused controls by Student's *t*-test. n.s., Not significant.

Infusion	n	Period (min)	Plasma corticosterone (μg/100 ml)	Plasma α-MSH (pg/ml)
Vehicle	6	10	7.4 ± 1.9	174 ± 15
Isoprenaline	7	5	10.4 ± 1.5 ns	284 ± 24[b]
Isoprenaline	8	10	24.6 ± 6.8[b]	240 ± 15[a]
Isoprenaline	7	20	43.9 ± 2.7[b]	358 ± 16[a]

[a] $p < 0.01$
[b] $p < 0.001$

pituitary does not prevent isoprenaline-induced stimulation of ACTH release. This strongly suggests that isoprenaline acts directly on the pituitary.

Further, Fig. 6 shows that the effect of isoprenaline is indeed mediated by β-adrenergic receptors, since the rise in plasma corticosterone levels induced by isoprenaline is completely prevented by propranolol. Since it had been shown *in vitro* that the intermediate lobe, but not the anterior lobe, is sensitive to β-adrenergic stimulation, this experiment again suggests that the action of isoprenaline is on intermediate lobe cells.

Final evidence for this site of action of isoprenaline should be derived from experiments with rats in which either the anterior lobe or the intermediate lobe had been removed. Such a preparation demands considerable technical and surgical skill. However, early observations in rats in which the neurointermediate lobes had been removed, appear to be in perfect accordance with our hypothesis. Smelik[14] has shown that an intravenous infusion of a total amount of 600 ng

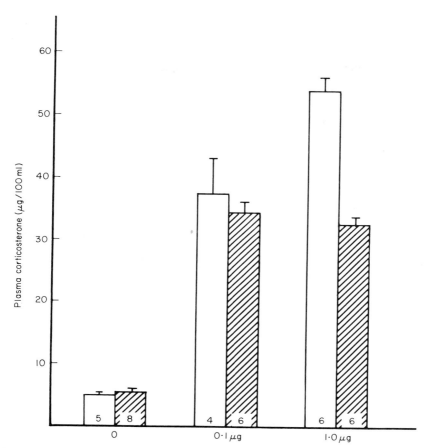

Fig. 5. Effects of isoprenaline on plasma corticosterone levels of adult female rats. Rats were anaesthetized with Nembutal[R] (40 mg/kg i.p., 15 min before infusion). An infusion was given with vehicle (0) or isoprenaline at a rate of 0.1 or 1.0 μg/min/kg for 20 min *via* a lateral tail vein. Subsequently, rats were decapitated and trunk blood was collected. Open bars, intact controls; hatched bars, rats bearing electrothermic lesions in the mediobasal hypothalamus for 10 days.

of adrenaline over 1 h induced an appreciable release of ACTH (as judged by ascorbic acid-depletion in the adrenal) in intact rats but had no effect at all in neurointermediate-lobectomized rats.

In view of our results we would like to propose that catecholamines, in concentrations that approach circulating levels, are capable of releasing ACTH from the intermediate lobe in quantities sufficient to activate the adrenal cortex. This would mean that possibly, apart from the hypothalamic control of anterior lobe ACTH, a peripheral control of intermediate lobe ACTH may play a role in certain conditions. It may be suggested here that this peripheral control is exerted *via* the sympathetic nervous system, as has been proposed in early studies on the stress response[45-47].

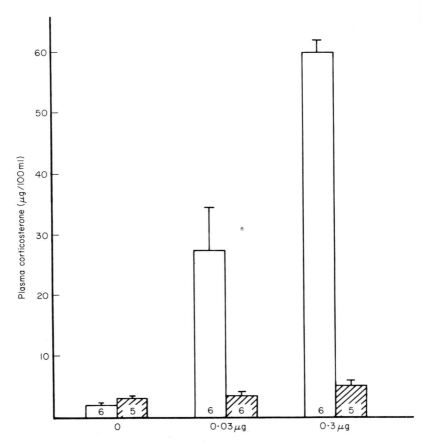

Fig. 6. Effects of propranolol on isoprenaline-induced increase in plasma corticosterone levels in intact female rats anaesthetized with Nembutal^R (40 mg/kg i.p., 15 min before infusion). An infusion was given with vehicle (0) or isoprenaline at a rate of 0.03 or 0.3 μg/min/kg for 20 min, *via* a lateral tail vein. Open bars, saline-injected controls; hatched bars, rats treated with propranolol (2.5 mg/kg i.p. 30 min before the infusion).

REFERENCES

1. Mialhe-Voloss, C. J. (1955). *Pysiol. (Paris)* **47** 251.
2. Mialhe C. and Briaud, B. (1977). *Front. Horm. Res.* **4**, 193.
3. Kraicer J. *et al.* (1973). *Neuroendocrinol.* **11**, 156.
4. Rochefort, G. J. *et al.* (1959). *J. Physiol. (Lond.)* **146**, 105.
5. Itoh, S. (1964). *Gunma Symp. Endocr.* **1**, 143.
6. Moriarty, C. M. and Moriarty, G. C. (1975). *Endocrinology* **96**, 1419.
7. Kraicer, J. *et al.* (1977). *Neuroendocrinol.* **23**, 352.
8. Tilders, F. J. H. and Smelik, P. G. *(to be published)*.
9. Scott, A. P. *et al.* (1974). *J. Endocrinol.* **61**, 355.

10. Lowry, P. J. and Scott A. P. (1977). *Front. Horm. Res.* **4**, 11.
11. Swallow, R. L. and Sayers, G. (1969). *Proc. Soc. Exp. Biol. Med.* **131**, 1.
12. Zimmerman, A. E. & Kraicer, J. (1978). *60th annual meeting Endocrine Soc. Abst.* 537.
13. Usategui, R. *et al.* (1976). *Endocrinology* **98**, 189.
14. Smelik, P. G. (1960). *Acta Endocr.* **33**, 437.
15. Mialhe-Voloss, C. (1958). *Acta Endocr. Copenh. suppl.* 35.
16. Kraicer, J. (1977) *Front. Horm. Res.* **4**, 200.
17. Naik, D. V., (1976). *In* 'Cellular and Molecular bases of Neuroendocrine Processes" (Endroczi ed.), pp. 431–450, Akademiai, Kiądo Budapest.
18. Moriarty, G. C. and Garner, L. L. (1977). *Front. Horm. Res.* **4**, 26.
19. Scott, A. P. *et al.* (1973). *Nature New Biol.* **244**, 65.
20. Lowry, P. J. *et al.* (1977). *Ann. N.Y. Acad. Sci.* **297**, 49.
21. Beloff-Chain, A. *et al.* (1977). *J. Endocrinol.* **73**, 28P.
22. Li, C. H. *et al.* (1977). *Ann. N.Y. Acad. Sci.* **297**, 158.
23. Ross, M. *et al.* (1977). *Brain Res.* **124**, 523.
24. Snyder, S. H. and Simantov, R. (1977). *J. Neurochem.* **28**, 13.
25. Eipper, B. A. and Mains, R. E. (1978). *J. Biol. Chem.* **253**, 5732.
26. Pelletier, G. *et al.* (1977). *Endocrinology* **100**, 770.
27. Bloom, F. *et al.* (1977). *Life Sci.* **20**, 43.
28. Mialhe, C. and Briaud, B. (1977). *Front. Horm. Res.* **4**, 193.
29. Smelik, P. G. *et al.* (1962). *Acta Physiol. Pharmacol. Neerl.* **11**, 20.
30. Greer, M. A. *et al.* (1975). *Endocrinology* **96**, 718.
31. Kraicer, J. (197). *Can. J. Physiol. Pharmacol.* **54**, 809.
32. Arimura, A. *et al.* (1965). *J. Physiol. (London).* **15**, 278.
33. De Wied, D. (1961). *Endocrinology* **68**, 956.
34. De Wied, D. (1968). *Neuroendocrinol.* **3**, 129.
35. Penny, R. J. and Thody, A. J. (1978). *Neuroendocrinol.* **25**, 193.
36. Tilders, F. J. H. *et al.* (1975). *Neuroendocrinol.* **18**, 125.
37. Mulder, G. H. & Smelik, P. G. (1977). *Endocrinology* **100**, 1143.
38. Tilders, F. J. H., van der Woude, H. A., Swaab, D. F. and Mulder, A. H. *Brain Res. (in press).*
39. Tilders, F. J. H. and Smelik, P. G. (1977). *Front. Horm. Res.* **4**, 80.
40. Tilders, F. J. H. *J. Endocrinol. (in press).*
41. Kraicer, J. and Morris, A. R. (1976). *Neuroendocrinol.* **20**, 70.
42. Bower, A. *et al.* (1974). *Science* **184**, 70.
43. Briaud, B. *et al.* (1978). *Neuroendocrinol.* **25**, 47.
44. Tilders, F. J. H. and Smelik, P. G. (1978). *Neuroendocrinol.* **25**, 275.
45. Long, C. N. H. (1947). *Fed. Proc.* **6**, 461.
46. McDermott, W. V. *et al.* (1950). *Yale J. Biol. Med.* **23**, 52.
47. Gordon, M. L. (1950). *Endocrinology* **47**, 347.
48. Tilders, F. J. H. *et al.* (1975). *J. Endocrinol.* **66**, 165.

5

PERSPECTIVES ON CORTICOTROPIN-RELEASING HORMONE (CRH)

B. Gillham, R. L. Insall and M. T. Jones*

Department of Biochemistry and Sherrington School of Physiology,
St. Thomas's Hospital Medical School, London SE1 7EH, U.K.*

ONE CRH MOLECULE OR SEVERAL?

One conclusion that may be drawn with some certainty from the experimental data of the past 30 years is that a wide range of compounds are capable of acting as corticotropin-releasing factors (CRFs; corticoliberin). That is to say molecules as diverse as vasopressin, bromocriptine and ammonium ions have been shown (or inferred) to be capable of causing the secretion of corticotropin (ACTH) from the corticotroph cells of the adenohypophysis. It is equally true that none of these compounds has been shown to meet all of the criteria required to establish that it is the corticotropin-releasing hormone (CRH)[1]. However, the underlying assumption behind much of the work on CRH has been that although CRF molecules proliferate, there is but one CRH molecule, as there is just one gonado-tropin-releasing hormone (gonadoliberin) and one thyrotropin-releasing hormone (thyroliberin).

Recently the findings of several groups of workers have caused this assumption to be questioned[2]. It has been suggested that since ACTH secretion is affected by diverse physiological factors, it may be that multiple CRHs exist, each relevant to particular regulatory circumstances. This view seems to find support in the work of several groups who have shown that hypothalami contain several compounds that affect ACTH secretion[3,4,5]. Strictly speaking, however, what has been shown is that acid extracts of either stalk median eminences or whole hypothalami contain such activities. It is arguable therefore that the smaller entities with activity are merely degradation products of a larger CRH molecule, since peptidases with acid pH optima have been characterized in the hypothalamus. The results of alternative experimental approaches to the isolation of CRH will be of particular interest in resolving this problem of multiple CRHs.

One such alternative approach has been to allow the tissue to perform the initial purification of the molecule(s). This has been achieved by incubating the isolated rat hypothalamus *in vitro* and stimulating it to release CRH by the addition to the incubation medium of either acetylcholine or serotonin (5-HT; 5-hydroxytryptamine)[6]. Such preparations were acidified to pH 4, passed through a Millipore filter and concentrated by freeze-drying. The concentrate was then passed through a column of Sephadex G-25 (fine grade) equilibrated with 10mM acetic acid. (This contrasts with earlier published work[6] in that the column material was then equilibrated with 0.9% (w/v) NaCl adjusted to pH 3 with hydrochloric acid.) Figs. 1 and 2 show the profiles of activity obtained when

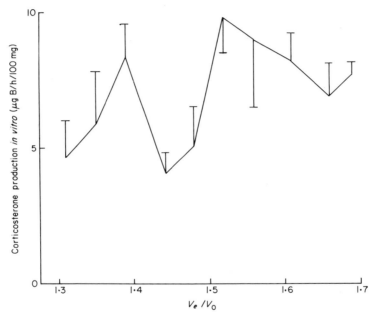

Fig. 1. Chromatography of CRH on a column (2.5cm × 80cm) of Sephadex G-25 (fine grade). The CRH was obtained by repeated stimulation *in vitro* of 120 hypothalami taken from rats adrenalectomized at least 7 days before. The stimulation was with acetylcholine (3pg/ml) and the column was equilibrated with acetic acid (10mM). V_e, Elution volume; V_0, void volume.

the CRH was obtained by repeated stimulation (13 × 5min periods in 3 h) of hypothalami taken from 120 rats that had been adrenalectomized at least 7 days before. The results for both neurotransmitters are expressed in terms of the *in vivo/in vitro* assay[7] where the end-point is the production of corticosterone by adrenals incubated *in vitro*. Two major peaks of activity are seen and these appear to correspond to the CRHs A and B already reported[8]. In addition, a small peak positioned between A and B is suggested once more and it is possible that the larger column now used may have also resolved peak B into more than one activity. This is seen most clearly in the experiments in which stimulation was by 5-HT.

When 5-HT stimulation was used, the column separation was followed by high-voltage paper electrophoresis of each of the two broad regions corresponding to CRH A and B. The resulting electrophoretograms were cut into strips and the fractions were eluted. The CRH content of each eluted fraction was determined by the cytochemical assay[9] as adapted for CRH[10]. After electrophoresis of the CRH A fraction at pH 6.5 (58V/cm for 0.75h), two bands of bioactivity were

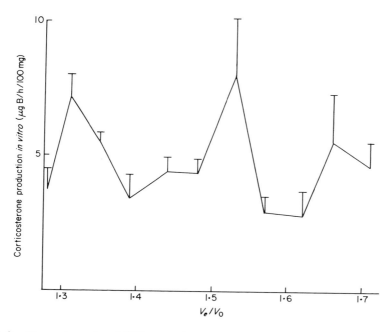

Fig. 2. Chromatography of CRH on a column (2.5cm × 80cm) of Sephadex G-25 (fine grade). The CRH was obtained by repeated stimulation *in vitro* of 120 hypothalami taken from rats adrenalectomized at least 7 days before. The stimulation was with 5-HT (10ng/ml) and the column was equilibrated with acetic acid (10mM).

eluted from the paper (Fig. 3). These bands had mobilities (m) of 0.05–0.08 and 0.75 (relative to aspartic acid at −1). Elution of the biological activity (m = 0.05–0.08) followed by a second longer (3h) electrophoresis at pH 6.5, which was designed to move CRH A away from the neutral band and to expose any heterogeneity, gave rise to only one major band of activity. To correspond to a molecular weight of 3000–4000, a molecule of this mobility would have to carry one net positive charge. The peptide nature of this CRH A was examined in several ways. Its biological activity was destroyed by brief acetylation (< 1 min at 0°C) with methanol/acetic anhydride (4:1, v/v), by exposure to performic

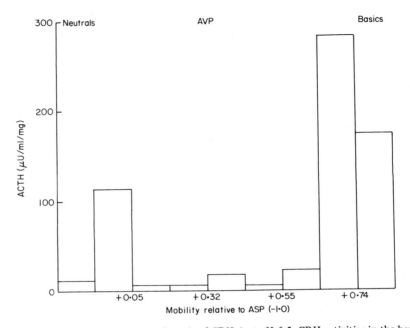

Fig. 3.   High-voltage paper electrophoresis of CRH A at pH 6.5. CRH activities in the bands are expressed in terms of the ability to cause the release of ACTH from pituitary fragments, as assessed by the cytochemical assay. 'Neutrals', 'basics' and AVP refer respectively to the positions of the neutral and basic amino acids and arginine vasopressin on the electrophoretogram.

acid, or to leucine aminopeptidase, or to trypsin or to pH 2.1 buffer. The bioactivity of this CRH A was unaffected by carboxypeptidase A or B. These data suggest therefore that CRH A/m = 0.05–0.08 is a peptide with a free *N*-terminus and a blocked *C*-terminus.

Electrophoresis of CRH B at pH 6.5 gave three bands of bioactivity which were eluted from the paper (Fig. 4). The mobilities of these bands relative to aspartic acid (-1) were 0.05, 0.55 and 0.75, varying slightly with conditions. Re-electophoresis of the CRH B/m = 0.55 at pH 2.1 gave rise to several bands of activity with mobilities relative to serine $(+1)$ of 0.4, 0.7, 1.0 and 1.2 (Fig. 5). At this pH value the mobilities of arginine vasopressin (AVP), lysine vasopressin (LVP) and arginine vasotocin (AVT) were 0.9, 0.9 and 0.95 respectively and were distinctly separated from CRH B/m = 1.0. Re-electrophoresis of this m = 1.0 band at pH 6.5 gave activity in the original position, i.e. m = 0.55. AVP, LVP and AVT also ran behind this band at this pH value. Enzyme and chemical studies on the pH 6.5/m = 0.55 band of CRH B suggested a peptide with a blocked *N*-terminus and a free *C*-terminus. For the observed mobility the peptide might possess either a net charge of +1 and a molecular weight of about 500 or a charge of +2 and a molecular weight of about 1000.

Attempts to determine whether cysteine is present in either CRH A/m = 0.05–0.08 or CRH B/m = 0.55 by treatment with 2-mercaptoethanol followed by

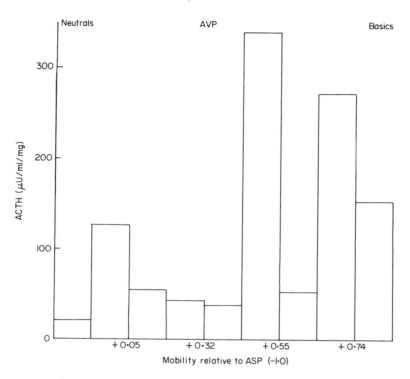

Fig. 4. High-voltage paper electrophoresis of CRH B at pH 6.5. CRH activities in the bands are expressed in terms of the ability to cause the release of ACTH from pituitary fragments, as assessed by the cytochemical assay. 'Neutrals', 'basics' and AVP refer respectively to the positions of the neutrals and basic amino acids and arginine vasopressin on the electrophoretogram.

iodo [^{14}C] acetic acid produced negative results. This suggests, but does not prove, that cyst(e)ine is absent from both of these CRH molecules.

At face value these data seem to argue that CRH A/m = 0.05–0.08 and CRH B/m = 0.55 cannot be related in any simple way. CRH A is the larger molecule and if any relation were to exist, this compound would have to be the precursor of the smaller CRH B. However, it is difficult to see how, in a simple way, a peptide blocked in the *C*-terminus and free in the *N*-terminus could be the precursor of a smaller peptide in which the reverse situation obtains. Set against this is the finding that CRH B/m = 0.55, when re-electrophoresed at pH 2.1 gave four bands of activity. It is just possible that the original band concealed the four activities, but it seems more likely that at low pH values chemical changes are induced in the molecule.

In summary, the data are certainly compatible with the existence of at least two CRH molecules with the reservation that the conditions used for the purification may lead to the generation of some (maybe all) of the forms.

It does seem that for CRH the sentiments of Martin *et al.*[11] on the release

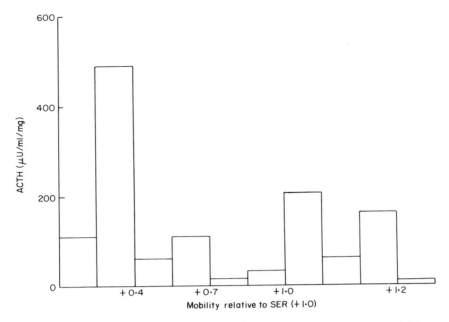

Fig. 5.   High-voltage paper electrophoresis of CRH B/m = 0.55 at pH 2.1. CRH activities in the bands are expressed in terms of the ability to cause the release of ACTH from pituitary fragments, as assessed by the cytochemical assay.

of growth hormone may be echoed. They concluded "These results are an embarrassment of riches. It is apparent that a host of molecules of various sizes and structures . . . are effective in causing GH secretion".

CRH AND VASOPRESSIN

Ever since CRH has been sought there have been investigators to support the view that such a search is pointless because the molecule has already been characterized as vasopressin. The most recent and challenging indication of a role for vasopressin in the control of ACTH secretion is reported in the present volume[12]. In this elegant study it is shown that acid extracts of stalk median eminence contain an unstable molecule which in the presence of vasopressin becomes a potent CRF, as attested by the response of a column of isolated anterior pituitary cells.

As was demonstrated in the previous section of this chapter all of the CRHs released by the hypothalamus *in vitro* are separable from vasopressin. Therefore these molecules would appear to be those that are potentiated by vasopressin. It is possible that this is the case because the assays used to monitor CRH have not been shown to be vasopressin-free, indeed the adenohypophyses used in the cytochemical assay are primed with vasopressin just before their exposure to

CRH[10]. Against this is the observation that the neurotransmitter-evoked
CRHs are relatively stable in the absence of reducing agents, whereas the factor(s)
that are potentiated by vasopressin appear particularly unstable[12].

Attempts to correlate experimental data in this way are hazardous but it does
seem likely that the major molecules with CRH activity, which are released from
hypothalami *in vitro* in response to stimulation by 5-HT, have an inherent
activity that is independent of vasopressin.

THE BIOSYNTHESIS OF CRH

Reference to recent work on the biosynthesis of releasing hormones[13]
would suggest that, in view of the problems associated with these studies, such
investigations on CRH are certainly premature. However, the absence of fully
characterized CRH does mean that bioassays have to be used in the study rather

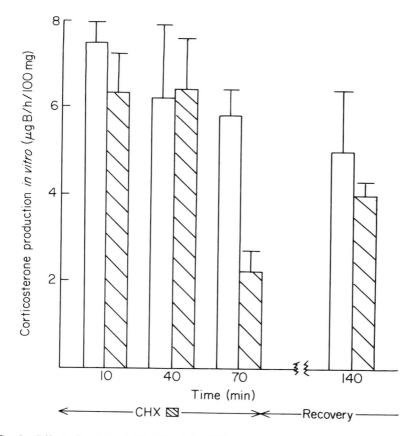

Fig. 6.   Effect of cycloheximide (10μg/ml; CHX) on the 5-HT-evoked release of CRH from
the rat hypothalamus *in vitro*.

than radioimmunoassays and hence spurious results due to cross-reactivity of antisera are eliminated.

The isolated hypothalamus incubated *in vitro* is a useful preparation for such studies, for there is a large body of data on the effects of neurotransmitters and steroids, their agonists and antagonists on the synthesis and release of CRH[14,15]. Therefore if any newly synthesized peptide does appear to be CRH the effects of these agonists and antagonists should be diagnostic. Thus if a radioactively labelled amino acid is incorporated into a molecule that appears to share the chemical characteristics of CRH, the release evoked by acetylcholine or 5-HT should be reduced by noradrenaline, by γ-aminobutyrate, or by corticosterone.

As a preliminary to studies on the incorporation of labelled amino acids into CRH, the effect of the protein synthesis inhibitor cycloheximide on the formation and release of CRH was investigated. In an initial experiment groups of three hypothalami (taken from rats adrenalectomized 7 days before) were incubated in the presence or absence of cycloheximide ($10\mu g/ml$). The tissues were challenged with 5-HT ($10ng/ml$) for 10 min followed by a 20 min rest period on three occasions in the course of 70 min. Fig. 6. shows that after the third stimulation, the response of the cycloheximide-treated tissues was significantly reduced ($p < 0.01$) as assessed by the *in vivo/in vitro* assay[7]. That the effect was not due to death of the tissue caused by the inhibitor was indicated by the recovery of the responsiveness of the treated tissues when the cycloheximide was removed from the incubation medium. These data suggest that a cycloheximide-sensitive step is necessary to allow CRH to be secreted, but they do not show that this step is the synthesis of CRH (or a precursor) on ribosomes.

A closer approach to the problem may be made if both the release and the tissue content of CRH are monitored throughout the experiment. In such an experiment (Fig. 7) the tissues were preincubated for 1 h with or without cycloheximide ($10\mu g/ml$) but always without stimulation. After 1 h, stimulations with 5-HT was instituted and the release and content (extractable with $0.1M$ HCl) of CRH were determined after stimulation. Once more, despite the 1 h preincubation with cycloheximide, the inhibition of release was significant ($p < 0.01$) only after three stimulations and at this time no effect was seen on the hypothalamic content of CRH. The content began to decline only after 3 h *in vitro* and this may well have derived from tissue death, since the release of CRH seemed to increase at that time.

There are several ways of viewing these data. The cycloheximide may inhibit the formation or action of a protein essential for CRH release and hence release is inhibited but preformed CRH remains in the tissue. Or, as cycloheximide might be expected to chelate metal ions, it may interfere with Ca^{2+} in their role in the secretion of CRH (however, the concentrations of cycloheximide and Ca^{2+} are $35\mu M$ and $1.45mM$ respectively). But in both cases why are these inhibitory events 5-HT-dependent? Another possibility is that, in common with neurotransmitters, there are two pools of CRH, one a small pool with a high turnover rate and the other a larger, more metabolically inert one.

From these studies it may be concluded that protein synthesis seems to be required to maintain the release of CRH from the hypothalamus *in vitro*. However, it is more difficult to associate the effect directly with an inhibition of ribosomal synthesis of CRH or a possible larger precursor molecule.

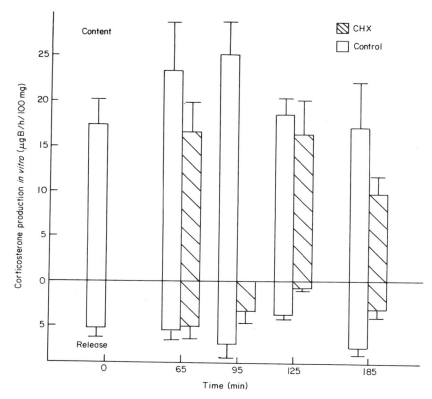

Fig. 7.   Effect of cycloheximide (10μg/ml; CHX) on the 5-HT-evoked release of CRH from the rat hypothalamus *in vitro* and the effect of stimulation on the hypothalamic content of CRH.

ACKNOWLEDGEMENTS

We gratefully acknowledge the collaborative work of H. R. Morris and Graham Taylor who performed the HVPE and peptide studies on CRH, and that of Julia C. Buckingham who carried out the cytochemical determinations of CRH. The work reported was carried out on a grant from the St. Thomas' Hospital Research (Endowment) Committee.

REFERENCES

1.   Donovan, B. T. (1970). Mammalian Neuroendocrinology, McGraw-Hill, London.
2.   Saffran, M. and Schally, A. V. (1977). *Neuroendocrinol.* **24**, 359.
3.   Vale, W. and Rivier, C. (1977). *Fed. Proc.* **36**, 2094.
4.   Seelig, S. and Sayers, G. (1977). *Fed. Proc.* **36**, 2100.
5.   Schally, A. V. *et al.* (1978). *Biochem. Biophys. Res. Com.* **82**, 582.

6.   Gillham, B. *et al.* (1975). *J. Endocrinol.* **65**, 12*P*.
7.   Bradbury, M. W. B. *et al.* (1974). *J. Physiol.* **239**, 269.
8.   Jones, M. T. *et al.* (1977). *Fed. Proc.* **36**, 2104.
9.   Daly, J. R. *et al.* (1974). *Clin. Endocrinol.* **3**, 311.
10. Buckingham, J. C. and Hodges, J. R. (1977). *J. Endocrinol.* **72**, 187.
11. Martin, J. B. *et al.* (1978). *In* 'The Hypothalamus', (Reichlin, S. *et al.* eds.), Raven Press, New York.
12. Gillies, G. and Lowry, P. J. (1979). This volume.
13. McKelvey, J. F. and Epelbaum, J. (1978). *In* 'The Hypothalamus', (Reichlin, S. *et al.* eds.), Raven Press, New York.
14. Jones, M. T. *et al.* (1979). This volume.
15. Buckingham, J. C. and Hodges, J. R. (1979). This volume.

6

THE RELATIONSHIP BETWEEN VASOPRESSIN AND CORTICOTROPIN-RELEASING FACTOR

Glenda Gillies and P. J. Lowry

*Pituitary Hormone Laboratory, St. Bartholomew's Hospital,
London EC1A 7BE, U.K.*

INTRODUCTION

The neurohumoral concept for the control of the anterior pituitary gland gained general acceptance after it had been so well summarized by Harris in 1948[1]. Corticotropin-releasing factor (CRF; corticoliberin) was the first of these postulated hypothalamic factors to be demonstrated in 1955[2,3]. The existence of other releasing factors in hypothalamic tissue was demonstrated in the early 1960's with the subsequent purification, isolation, chemical characterization and synthesis of thyrotropin-releasing hormone (TRH; thyroliberin), a tripeptide, luteinizing hormone-releasing hormone (LHRH; luliberin), a deca-peptide[4,5] and somatostatin (GHRIH), a tetradecapeptide[6]. Despite these accomplishments, the nature of CRF remains an enigma. Many authors have reported that CRF bioactivity appears to be due to a peptide[4,7-10]. However, it does not run chromatographically as a single simple peptide, such as TRH and LHRH, and it has often been reported that the majority of CRF bioactivity is lost after purification procedures[4,6,11-14]. This contrasts greatly to TRH, for example, where virtually 100% recovery of activity after chromatography of many thousands of hypothalami has been reported[15].

As early as 1954 Scharrer and Scharrer[59] proposed that neurosecretion of vasopressin into separate vascular channels may have a simultaneous effect on the kidneys to produce antidiuresis and on the anterior lobe of the pituitary to cause the secretion of corticotropin (adrenocorticotrophic hormone; ACTH). Also in 1954 McCann and Brobeck[16] noted a correlation between increasing diabetes insipidus produced by hypothalamic lesions and lack of anterior pituitary responsiveness to stress. They concluded that the supraopticohypophyseal tract may play a role in the regulation of ACTH secretion and that an antidiuretic hormone that was probably secreted directly into those capillaries that ultimately coalesced to form the portal vessels in the median eminence. It was known that arginine vasopressin (AVP) and lysine vasopressin (LVP) increase plasma hydroxycorticosteroids in man[17] and that they also cause the release of ACTH from pituitaries in a variety of systems both *in vitro* and *in vivo*[18-23]. However, the idea that vasopressin (VP) is CRF did not remain popular. For example, Nichols[24] objected that doses of VP necessary to stimulate ACTH release when given peripherally *in vivo* were unphysiological and the release of ACTH was not always paralleled by the release of VP into the peripheral circulation. However, Martini[25] argued that experimental results presented in support of the idea that CRF is distinct from vasopressin are always open to alternative interpretations. Further, Goldman and Lindner[26] have calculated that low peripheral and high hypophyseal portal blood concentrations of VP are not mutually exclusive and Zimmerman[27] has reported a concentration of 13.5ng/ml of immunoactive VP in monkey portal blood (1000 times greater than that found in peripheral blood). Investigations using neurohypophysectomized animals[28,29] and the Brattleboro strain of rats, which have diabetes insipidus and no VP, have resulted in conflicting conclusions as to the importance of VP in the stress response. Some chromatographic work has suggested that a CRF structurally related to VP may exist[12] but other work suggests that this is not the case[8,35,36]. Within the last 3 years several CRF's of molecular weights ranging from 500–5000 or more have been reported[37-41]. Thus the picture appears to be getting more complicated rather than clearer, and after more than 25 years of considerable work the nature and structure of CRF, and the role, if any, of VP in the hypothalamo–pituitary–adrenocortical axis is still unknown.

The identification of CRF has been complicated by several factors. First, its presence has been demonstrated in the posterior lobe of the pituitary as well as the hypothalamus, and both of these tissues have been used as a starting material for the purification of CRF[12,42] without success. Secondly, the difficulty incurred because of the great loss of CRF activity during fractionation procedures was enhanced by the insensitivity of the early CRF bioassays. Finally, VP is present in both the hypothalamus and posterior lobe in concentrations that are capable of directly stimulating ACTH release and it therefore greatly interferes in many CRF bioassays.

In the studies described here we used the perfused rat isolated anterior pituitary cell column, coupled with ACTH radioimmunoassay (RIA) as a simple, sensitive, specific bioassay for CRF[43,44].

IMMUNOLOGICAL CHARACTERIZATION OF VASOPRESSIN AND CRF IN THE RAT HYPOTHALAMUS

We have previously reported that AVP at concentrations as low as 100pg/ml[44] releases ACTH. The log dose–response curve for AVP was less steep and significantly non-parallel to the curve for our crude rat stalk-median eminence extract (SME), which was also the case for LVP, arginine vasotocin (AVT) and oxytocin

(OT). This non-parallelism has been reported in a number of assays *in vitro*[19,20, 34,45] and is a means whereby VP may be distinguished from SME in these systems. The crude extract contained an average of 10.83ng (7.7-14.3ng, n = 12) of immunoactive VP per SME, which could be characterized as AVP, not LVP, AVT or OT, using three VP antisera of differing specificities[46].

This amount of VP in our SME could account for no more than 30% of the CRF activity of the extract. However, we have also shown that preincubation of crude SME at 4°C for 24 h with specific VP antisera totally and specifically quenched the CRF activity of the extract, suggesting that all CRF activity was due to a VP-like molecule[46]. The CRF bioactivity of VP can be similarly quenched with various VP antisera. The idea that VP may play a role in the control of ACTH release has been re-awakened by some recent results from immunological and immunocytochemical studies. In 1974, Watkins *et al.*[58] proposed the presence of a CRF-associated neurophysin (NP) in the external zone of the median eminence and later Zimmerman and his co-workers[27,47] demonstrated a direct axonal pathway to the hypophyseal portal system containing VP and NP, which is regulated by the adrenal cortex, unlike the VP pathways to the posterior lobe.

CRF IN THE POSTERIOR PITUITARY

Most of the early work on purification of CRF was done with commercial preparations of posterior lobe extracts such as protopituitrin and pitressin[48,49]. The reasons for this were twofold. First, it was thought that the posterior pituitary contained a CRF distinct from VP and this is still a controversial point today[21,45,50-52]. Secondly, the commercial powders were much more readily available than large numbers of hypothalami.

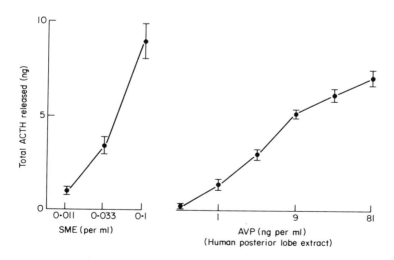

Fig. 1.   Comparison of CRF bioactivity of a crude SME extract and an extract of human posterior lobe.

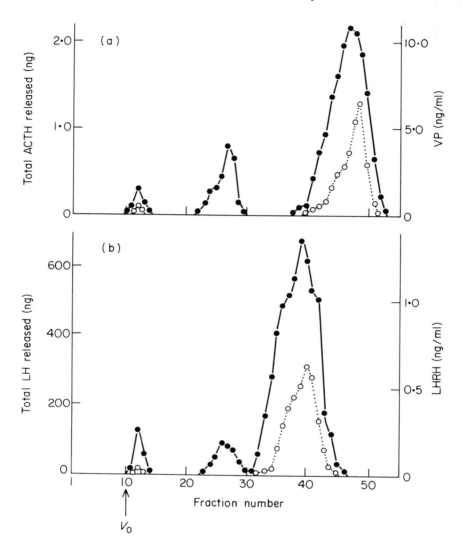

Fig. 2. Chromatography of rat SME on Bio-Gel P2 (200–400 mesh). Twenty rat stalk-median eminences (4mg wet weight per SME) were homogenized in 1.5ml of 10mM HCl. After addition of NaCl (9mg/ml) and centrifugation (3000g) the supernatant was applied to a column (1.5cm × 50cm) of Bio-Gel P2 (200–400 mesh) equilibrated with 10mM HCl containing NaCl (9mg/ml) and ascorbic acid (1mg/ml) at 4°C. The column was eluted with the same buffer and hourly fractions (2.5ml) were collected. Each fraction was neutralized with 25µl of 1.1M NaHCO₃ and was diluted 1:5 in the appropriate assay buffer. (a), CRF bioactivity, as measured by output of immunoactive ACTH from the cell column; O, AVP immunoactivity (ng of VP/ml in 1:5 dilution). (b), LHRH bioactivity as measured by output of immunoactive LH from the cell column; O, LHRH immunoactivity (ng/ml in 1:5 dilution). No significant amounts of ACTH nor LH were detected in any of the fractions. V_0, Void volume of column.

We were unable to investigate the CRF activity of a crude rat posterior lobe extract because the intermediate lobe peptides α-melanocyte-stimulating hormone (α-MSH; melanotropin) and corticotropin-like intermediate lobe peptide (CLIP), would seriously interfere in the ACTH immunoassay. However, human posterior lobe extract produced a dose–response curve typical for VP: flatter and significantly non-parallel to that for SME, and all CRF bioactivity of this extract could be accounted for by its immunoactive AVP content (Fig. 1).

We therefore concentrated on the stalk-median eminence region as our source of CRF.

CHROMATOGRAPHIC CHARACTERIZATION OF HYPOTHALAMIC CRF

In an attempt to characterize the CRF in normal rats, 20 or 50 normal rat SME's were chromatographed on Bio-Gel P2 in 10mm HCl containing 9mg of NaCl/ml and 1mg of ascorbic acid/ml[53]. All fractions were monitored for immunoactive LHRH, VP, luteinizing hormone (LH; lutropin) and ACTH, and the isolated pituitary cell column system was used to monitor the CRF and LHRH bioactivity in the column fractions. Fig. 2 shows that in all assays very small amounts of activity were found at the void volume, V_0. A minor CRF peak was eluted before a major CRF peak. The former appeared not to be specific for ACTH release as LH was also released by material from this region. This peak was not associated with immunoactive AVP or LHRH. The major peak of CRF bioactivity coincided with the peak of immunoactive AVP that eluted in the position expected for synthetic AVP. The main peak of LHRH bioactivity co-eluted with the peak of immunoactive LHRH and was well-separated from the main CRF/AVP peak. The recoveries were 35% for CRF bioactivity, 75% for AVP immunoactivity, 55% for LHRH bioactivity and 90% for LHRH immunoactivity. In the isolated pituitary cell column CRF bioassay the major CRF peak had the typical shallow log dose–response curve of synthetic VP and its CRF bioactivity may be fully accounted for by its immunoactive AVP content. Thus the major CRF peak behaves like synthetic AVP immunologically, chromatographically on Bio-Gel P2, and biologically in our CRF bioassay.

POTENTIATION OF CRF ACTIVITY OF VASOPRESSIN

The apparent loss of full agonistic properties of the major CRF peak may possibly be explained by the separation of a VP-CRF from a synergistic factor or factors during purification procedures.

This hypothesis was tested by recombining certain regions of the chromatogram. Fig. 3 shows that recombination of the so-called void region V_0, which possesses negligible CRF bioactivity, with the so-called major CRF peak, called the "AVP" peak because of its immunoactivity, produced a marked, highly significant, threefold potentiation of CRF activity. This system is analogous to that described by Pearlmutter, Rapino and Saffran[14]. However, they subdivided their chromatogram arbitrarily and the nature of the two regions that acted

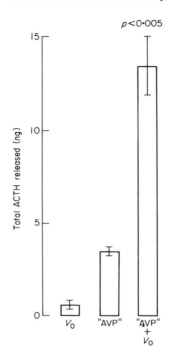

Fig. 3.   Potentiation of the CRF bioactivity of the AVP peak ("AVP") by material from the void region, V_0.

synergistically to produce CRF bioactivity were merely identified as a very-high-molecular-weight peptide, susceptible to hydrolysis, and a small non-peptide molecule or ion that acted with it in a manner similar to an enzyme–co-enzyme system. In a recent review, Saffran and Schally[54] reported that attempts to repeat these results of Pearlmutter and co-workers have been unsuccessful. We believe that our success may be due to the presence of ascorbic acid as an anti-oxidant in the chromatography system, as our earlier experiments without ascorbate showed no significant synergism. This observation suggests that some factor which is labile after chromatography contributes to the CRF bioactivity of crude stalk-median eminence extract.

The recombined V_0 and "AVP" peaks gave a log dose–response curve that was steeper than that for either peak alone and it was now parallel to the curve for crude SME extract[53]. A similar potentiation was also observed when synthetic AVP was used, which confirms the idea that the material in the major CRF peak was true vasopressin. Recombination of the V_0 peak with the so-called non-specific peak produced a variable potentiation of CRF bioactivity, which was greatly diminished after the fractions had been stored at $-20°C$ for 1 week.

PRELIMINARY INVESTIGATIONS ON THE NATURE OF THE SYNERGISTIC FACTOR

Crude SME and synthetic AVP were passed down a small (1 × 2cm) column of either thiol-activated Sepharose 4B, or Sepharose 4B eluted with 0.9% NaCl containing 10mM $NaHCO_3$. Table I shows that only in the case of SME passing through the thiol-activated column was the ratio of emerging CRF bioactivity to AVP immunoactivity significantly less than 1. In the light of the above experiments, this would suggest that VP in SME is modulated by factor(s) that require a free -SH group(s).

Table I. Percentage AVP immunoactivity and CRF bioactivity emerging from thiol-activated Sepharose 4B (SH) and Sepharose 4B (4B) columns.

Sample	% AVP immunoactivity	% CRF bioactivity	% CRF bioactivity *vs* % AVP immunoactivity
SME eluting from SH	47.6	15.1	0.32
SME eluting from 4B	74.2	49	0.66
AVP eluting from SH	65.6	47	0.72
AVP eluting from 4B	65.6	74	1.13

From these results it was concluded that the CRF activity of a crude stalk-median eminance extract is a multi-component complex consisting of VP whose potency is modulated by synergistic factors that have weak unstable inherent CRF bioactivity[53]. Thus it is no surprise that a pure peptide with potent CRF activity, distinct froms vasopressin, has not been found.

BRATTLEBORO RATS

Studies with the Brattleboro strain of rats that have diabetes insipidus have supported previous results[55]. Homozygous rats (DI homo) have no detectable immunoactive vasopressin either in their SME or their posterior lobes, and the heterozygotes (DI het) have significantly reduced amounts of vasopressin in both[34,55,56]. DI homo SME has only 20% and DI het only 60% of the CRF bioactivity of normal SME whether tested on normal, DI homo or DI het pituitary cell columns. Vasopressin gave the typical shallow log dose–response curve when tested on each type of cell column[55]. Similar results have been reported by Krieger *et al.*[34] DI homo SME was unstable after storage at $-20°C$ for a few weeks, whereas normal SME retained 75–95% of its activity after storage for 1 yr[55]. LHRH bio- and immuno-activity of Brattleboro SME was not significantly different from normal. It therefore appears that Brattleboro rats have a specific defect in the CRF activity of their SME which parallels a defect in the VP immunoactivity. Thus the genetic lesion responsible for the lack of antidiuretic hormone may also be responsible for the abnormal CRF.

Finally, chromatography of DI homo SME resulted in a chromatogram of CRF bioactivity identical to that for normal SME, except that the major AVP/CRF peak was missing[55]. The absolute sizes of the so-called V_0 and N_s peaks were not significantly greater than those for normal SME. The elution of LHRH bio-and immuno-activity was identical to that for normal SME. Once again, this shows that LHRH activity is normal in these rats and the CRF defect is associated with a lack of vasopressin. It is noteworthy that the CRF bio-activity of the recombined V_0 and N_s peaks of normal SME behaves in a similar way to the CRF activity in intact Brattleboro SME: namely that it is less potent and more labile than crude extracts of normal SME.

Thus we come to the conclusion once again that CRF is a multi-component system consisting of vasopressin plus synergistic factor or factors (as yet unidentified) which modulate the CRF bioactivity of median eminence vasopressin. In the absence of vasopressin, these factors account for the low activity labile CRF in Brattleboro SME. The fact that Brattleboro rats can respond at all to stress is used as evidence that VP cannot play an important role in that response. However, Yates *et al.*[32] have emphasized the importance of using submaximal stresses before a defect in the ACTH response of homozygous and heterozygous Brattleboro rats can be seen. Supramaximal stimuli may result in supramaximal release of the synergistic factors, or subsidiary CRF's, so that their low potency and instability would not be observable *in vivo*.

SUMMARY

A theory for the control of ACTH release, based on the biosynthesis of VP and NP described by Sachs *et al.* in 1969[57], is summarized in Fig. 4. VP and a CRF related to vasopressin ("VP-CRF") are probably identical, as suggested by the immunological, chromatographic and biological characteristics of the AVP/CRF peak[53]. We propose that VP and "VP-CRF" are synthesized at the ribosomes, probably in the supraoptic nucleus or paraventricular nucleus, as a large precursor molecule VP^1, which splits to give either the precursor for antidiuretic hormone (VP) or for CRF ("VP-CRF"). Brattleboro rats may have a genetic defect for synthesis of this molecule. These precursors become packaged into neurosecretory granules of diameter 130–180nM and 80–100nM respectively. This is in accordance with Zimmerman's[27] observation on the size of granules containing immunoactive vasopressin: the larger granules being found in the zona interna and the smaller granules being found in the zona externa of the median eminence. The true antidiuretic and CRF bioactivities are unmasked as the granules pass in their respective tracts to the posterior lobe of the pituitary and to the primary capillary beds of the hypothalamo-hypophyseal portal vessels. In the latter case the ACTH-releasing properties of vasopressin may be modulated by the synergistic factors, which could be concomitantly secreted into the vascular channels at the time of stress. It must be assumed that zona interna and zona externa vasopressin is normally under separate control from higher centres, to allow for independent control of

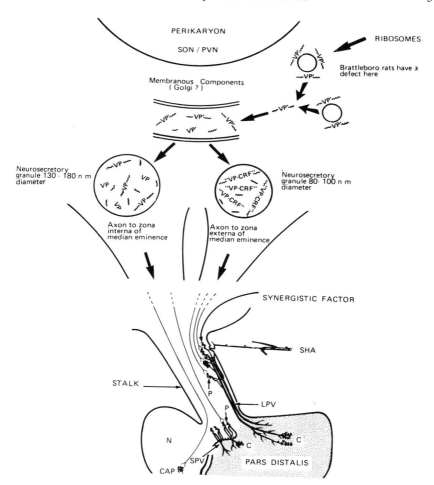

Fig. 4. ⌇VP'⌇, precursor molecule for vasopressin, neurophysin and CRF; ⌇VP⌇, precursor for posterior lobe vasopressin; VP, posterior lobe vasopressin; ⌇"VP-CRF"⌇, Pro-CRF; "VP-CRF", a CRF which may be identical in structure to posterior lobe vasopressin. P, primary capillary beds; LPV, SPV, long and short portal vessels; c, cells of the anterior lobe; cap., capillary bed; N, posterior lobe; SHA, superior hypophysial arteries.

antidiuresis and ACTH release. This multi-factor hypothesis, although relatively complicated, allows for a very precise and independent control of various stress situations (physiological, pathogenic, psychological) in addition to circadian rhythm. Such a fail-safe mechanism might well be expected for the control of ACTH release, which is the hormone most important to survival, and accounts for the elusive nature of CRF.

REFERENCES

1. Harris, G. W. (1948). *Physiol Rev.* **28**, 139.
2. Saffran, M. *et al.* (1955). *Endocrinology* **57**, 439.
3. Guillemin R. and Rosenberg, B. (1955). *Endocrinology* **57**, 599.
4. Schally, A. V. *et al.* (1973). *Science* **179**, 341.
5. Blackwell, R. E. and Guillemin, R. (1973). *Ann. Rev. Physiol.* **35**, 357.
6. Burgus, R. P. *et al.* (1973). *In* 'Advances in Human Growth Hormone Research, A Symposium', (Raiti, S. ed.), Baltimore Md, DHEW Publication No. (NIH) 74-612, pp. 144-158.
7. Porter, J. C. and Rumsfeld, H. W. (1959). *Endocrinology* **64**, 948.
8. Royce, P. C. and Sayers, G. (1960). *Proc. Soc. Exp. Biol. Med.* **103**, 447.
9. Schally, A. V. and Guillemin, R. (1963). *Proc. Soc. Exp. Biol. Med.* **112**, 1014.
10. Burgus, R. and Guillemin R. (1970). *Ann. Rev. Biochem.* **39**, 499.
11. Schally, A. V. *et al.* (1958). *Biochem. J.* **70**, 97.
12. Schally, A. V. *et al.* (1960). *Nature* **188**, 1192.
13. Chan, L. T. *et al.* (1969). *Endocrinology* **85**, 644.
14. Pearlmutter, A. F. *et al.* (1975). *Endocrinology* **97**, 1336.
15. Schally, A. V. *et al.* (1968). *Recent Prog. Horm. Res.* **24**, 497.
16. McCann, S. M. and Brobeck, J. R. (1954). *Proc. Soc. Exp. Biol. Med.* **87**, 318.
17. McDonald, R. K. and Weise, V. K. (1956). *Proc. Soc. Exp. Biol. Med.* **92**, 481.
18. Chan, L. T. *et al.* (1969). *Endocrinology* **84**, 967.
19. Portanova, R. and Sayers, G. (1973). *Proc. Soc. Exp. Biol. Med.* **143**, 661.
20. Buckingham, J. C. and Hodges, J. R. (1977). *J. Endocrinol.* **72**, 187.
21. de Wied, D. (1961). *Acta Endocrinol.* **37**, 288.
22. Hedge, G. A. *et al.* (1966). *Endocrinology* **79**, 328.
23. Rivier, C. *et al.* (1973). *Proc. Soc. Exp. Biol. Med.* **142**, 842.
24. Nichols, B. R. Jr. (1961). *Yale J. Biol. Med.* **33**, 415.
25. Martini, L. (1966). *In* "The Pituitary Gland", (Harris, G. W. and Donovan, B. T. eds.), Vol. 3, London Butterworths, pp. 535-577.
26. Goldman, H. M. and Lindner, L. (1962). *Separation Experientia* **18**, 279.
27. Zimmerman, E. A. (1976). *In* "Frontiers in Neuroendocrinology", (Martini, L. and Ganong, W. F. eds.), Vol. 4, New York, Raven Press, pp. 24-62.
28. Porter, J. C. *et al.* (1973). *Rec. Prog. Horm. Res.* **29**, 161.
29. Miller, R. E. *et al.* (1974). *Neuroendocrinol.* **14**, 233.
30. McCann, S. M. *et al.* (1966). *Endocrinology* **79**, 1058.
31. Arimura, A. *et al.* (1967). *Endocrinology* **81**, 235.
32. Yates, F. E. *et al.* (1971). *Endocrinology* **88**, 3.
33. Wiley, M. K. *et al.* (1974). *Neuroendocrinol.* **14**, 257.
34. Krieger, D. T. *et al.* (1977). *Endocrinology* **100**, 227.
35. Rumsfeld, H. W. and Porter, J. C. (1959). *Arch. Biochem. Biophys.* **82**, 473.
36. Dhariwal, A. P. S. *et al.* (1966). *Proc. Soc. Exp. Biol. Med.* **121**, 8.
37. Gillham, B. *et al.* (1975). *J. Endocrinol.* **65**, 12P.
38. Gillham, B. *et al.* (1976). *J. Endocrinol.* **71**, 60P.
39. Vale, W. and Rivier, C. (1977). *Abst. Amer. Endo. Soc. 59th Annual Meeting*, No. 321.
40. Synetos, D. *et al.* (1978). *J. Endocrinol.* **77**, 53P.

41. Schally, A. V. *et al.* (1977). *Abst. of Amer. Endo. Soc. 59th Annual Meeting*, No. 77.
42. Guillemin, R. *et al.* (1962). *Endocrinology* **70**, 471.
43. Lowry, P. J. (1974). *J. Endocrinol.* **62**, 163.
44. Gillies, G. and Lowry, P. J. (1978). *Endocrinology* **103**, 521.
45. Fehm, H. L. *et al.* (1975). *Acta Endocrinol. (Suppl.) (Kbh).* **193**, 129.
46. Gillies, G. *et al.* (1978). *Endocrinology* **103**, 528.
47. Zimmerman, E. A. *et al.* (1977). *Ann. N.Y. Acad. Sci.* **297**, 405.
48. Schally, A. V. and Bowers, C. Y. (1964). *Metabolism* **13**, 1190.
49. Guillemin, R. (1964). *Rec. Prog. Horm. Res.* **20**, 89.
50. McCann, S. M. (1957). *Endocrinology* **60**, 664.
51. Hiroshige, T. *et al.* (1968). *Jpn. J. Physiol.* **18**, 609.
52. Yasuda, N. and Greer, M. A. (1976). *Endocrinology* **99**, 944.
53. Gillies, G. and Lowry, P. J. (1979). *Nature* **278**, 463.
54. Saffran, M. and Schally, A. V. (1977). *Neuroendocrinol.* **24**, 359.
55. Gillies, G. and Lowry, P. J. (1979). *J. Endocrinol.* (in press).
56. Valtin, H. (1967). *Amer. J. Med.* **42**, 814.
57. Sachs, H. *et al.* (1969). *Rec. Prog. Horm. Res.* **25**, 447.
58. Watkins, W. B. *et al.* (1974). *Cell Tiss. Res.* **152**, 411.
59. Scharrer, E. and Scharrer, B. (1954). *Rec. Prog. Horm. Res.* **10**, 183.

7

CORTICOTROPIN-RELEASING FACTOR (CRF) AND VASOPRESSIN IN THE REGULATION OF CORTICOTROPIN (ACTH) SECRETION

†C. Mialhe, B. Lutz-Bucher, B. Briaud, R. Schleiffer and B. Koch

Laboratoire de Physiologie Général, Université Louis Pasteur, Strasbourg, France.

INTRODUCTION

Since Harris proposed his neurohumoral theory[1] the hypothalamus has been seen as the integrating centre of the brain that plays a key role in the modulation of the secretion of the anterior pituitary hormones. The existence of córticotro-pin-releasing activity in crude hypothalamic and posterior pituitary extracts was first described in 1955 by Saffran *et al.*[2] and by Guillemin and Rosenberg[3]. The corticotropin (ACTH)-releasing hormone (CRF; corticoliberin) remains one of those hypothalamic hormones yet to be characterized chemically. However, a hormone of known structure i.e. vasopressin (VP) has CRF-like activity[4]. The experiments described in this chapter focus on the importance relative to CRF of VP and include results of studies on their possible interaction in the release of ACTH from the anterior pituitary *in vitro*. In addition, we will report the results of experiments *in vivo* on the effect of 'neurogenic' stress in Brattleboro rats (animals that are unable to synthesize VP).

COMPARATIVE STUDIES ON THE CRF ACTIVITIES OF VP-FREE MEDIO-BASAL HYPOTHALAMIC (MBH) EXTRACTS AND VP

In all experiments anterior pituitaries from Wistar or Brattleboro rats were used in an incubation system described by Saffran and Schally[5]. Crude MBH extract (50μl, 0.1 M HCl/MBH) was added at different times to the incubation

64　　　　　　　　　　　　　　　　*C. Mialhe et al.*

medium, with or without specific arginine vasopressin antiserum (AVP-AS).
ACTH in the medium was measured by the isolated rat adrenal cell assay of
Sayers *et al.*[6]. VP contained in the anterior pituitary was extracted by the
method of Heller and Lederis[7] and was measured by radioimmunoassay (RIA)
as described previously[8].

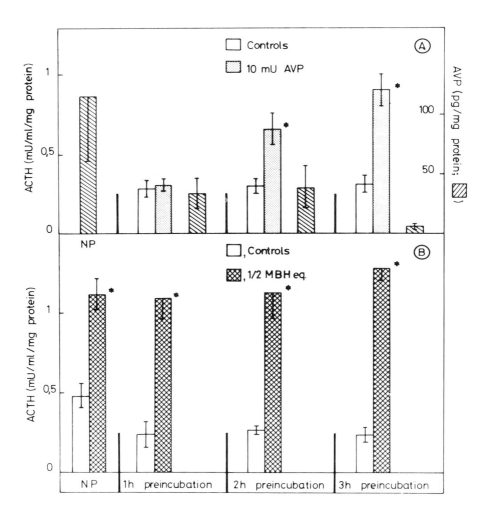

Fig. 1.　Relationship between ACTH release produced by incubated pituitaries (four
quarters/beaker) with VP (A) or VP-free MBH extract (B) in respect to time of preincubation and of VP pituitary content (striped columns) at the beginning of incubation.
NP, Not preincubated. Each column represents mean ± S.E.M. of eight assays (from two
independent experiments) * *p* < 0.01 *vs.* controls.

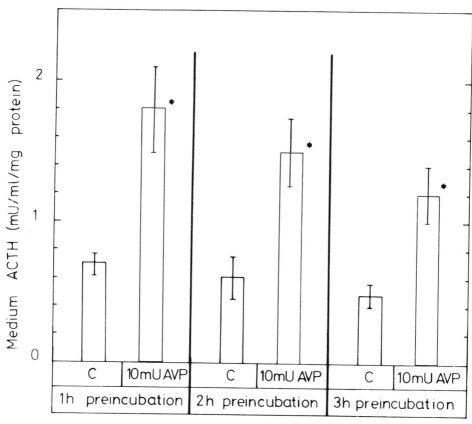

Fig. 2. VP-induced ACTH release from Brattleboro rat pituitary fragments after different times of preincubation. C, Controls. Each column represents mean ± S.E.M. of five assays. * *p* < 0.01 *vs.* controls.

CRF-like effect of VP and of VP-free MBH
extract *in vitro*

In an earlier experiment[8] we determined the amount of VP present in MBH extracts (about 12mU/MBH) and showed that the addition of an excess of AVP-AS did not significantly reduce the CRF activity in the extract. Next we demonstrated that AVP causes an increased ACTH release only when anterior pituitaries are preincubated for at least 2 h (Fig. 1). Such a preincubation is not necessary to evoke a response with MBH or VP-free MBH extracts (Fig. 1). Since VP has been reported to be present in the rat anterior pituitary[8-10], a possible explanation for these differences might be that saturation of VP receptor sites by the endogenous hormone occurs. That this view is a correct one is strengthened by our observation that the anterior pituitary VP content decreases as a function of the incubation time, concomitant with an increase in ACTH output in response

C. *Mialhe et al.*

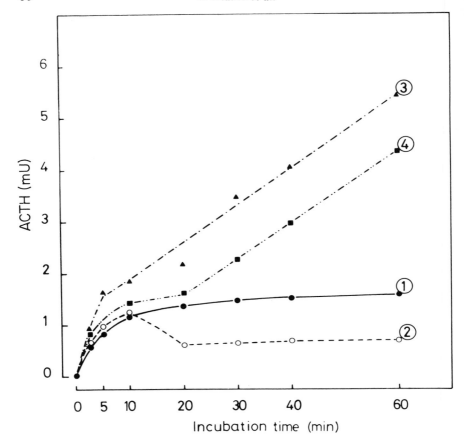

Fig. 3. Relationship between time of incubation and ACTH production by pituitary fragments incubated with MBH extract or VP in the presence of normal serum (curves 1 and 3) or of VP-antiserum (curves 2 and 4). Each point is the mean for duplicate assays. (Two other experiments gave the same type of results.) Preincubation time 3 h. •, AVP (20mU) + 10μl NS; ○, AVP (20mU) + 10μl AS; ▲, Extr. 2 MBH + 10μl NS; ■, Extr. 2 MBH + 10μl AS.

to exogenous VP. An additional argument in support of this hypothesis is given by an experiment using anterior pituitaries from Brattleboro rats, thus Fig. 2 shows that anterior pituitaries from these animals released significant amounts of ACTH in response to VP without preincubation. It has also been reported[11] that dispersed pituitary cells from these rats appear to be more responsive to VP than do those of normal animals. Thus occupancy of putative VP-receptor sites by the endogenous hormone seems to prevent the response of the tissue to exogenous hormone. Moreover, in two other experiments both a time- and a dose-dependent difference in the corticotropin-releasing activities was revealed when VP and VP-free MBH extracts were compared. First, VP-induced ACTH release reached a plateau in about 20 min, whereas VP-free MBH extract pro-

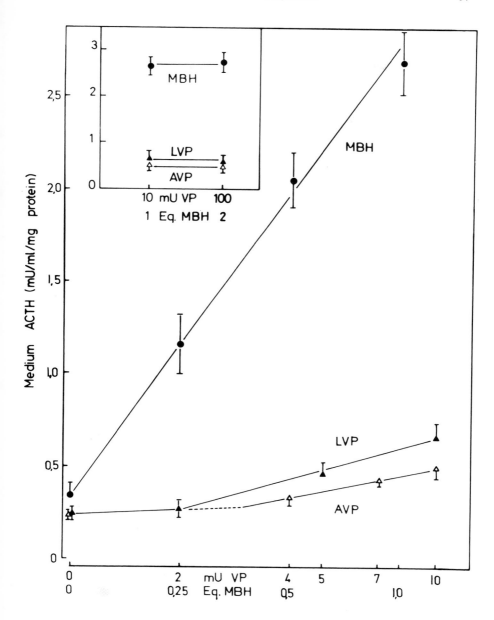

Fig. 4.   Semi-logarithmic dose–response curves for ACTH production by pituitary fragments incubated with an increasing amount of MBH extract or VP. Each point represents mean ± S.E.M. of four assays; the correlation coefficients are 0.996, 0.994 and 0.999 for MBH extract, lysine-vasopressin (LVP) and arginine-vasopressin (AVP) respectively. The insert shows that the secretion reached a plateau with 10mU of LVP or AVP, or with 1 MBH eq.

moted a continuous release throughout the whole period of incubation
(Fig. 3, curves 1 and 3). Secondly, when compared to the effect evoked by
increasing concentrations of VP-free MBH extracts, those of LVP or AVP were
characterized by a smaller maximal response and the dose–response curve was
shallower (Fig. 4). Similar results have been reported by Portanova and
Sayers[12].

Studies comparing the CRF activities of MBH extracts with and without VP

As shown in Fig. 5, anterior pituitaries respond in a similar fashion to MBH
extracts, whether VP is neutralized or not, when the experiment is performed
after 30 min preincubation of the tissue. After 3 h preincubation, however, the

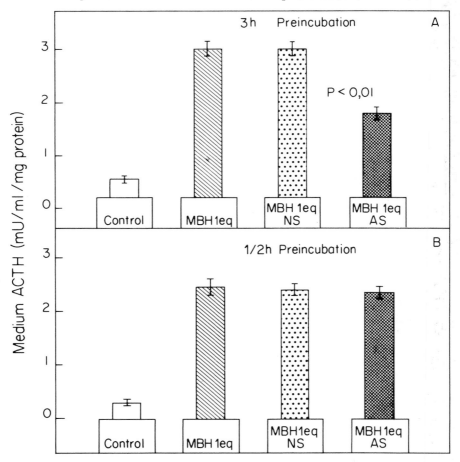

Fig. 5. ACTH released by pituitary fragments incubated with MBH extract alone, or with
MBH extract in the presence of normal serum (NS) or VP-antiserum (AS), after a preincubation of 3 h (A) or 30 min (B). Each column represents mean ± S.E.M. of eight assays (from
two independent experiments).

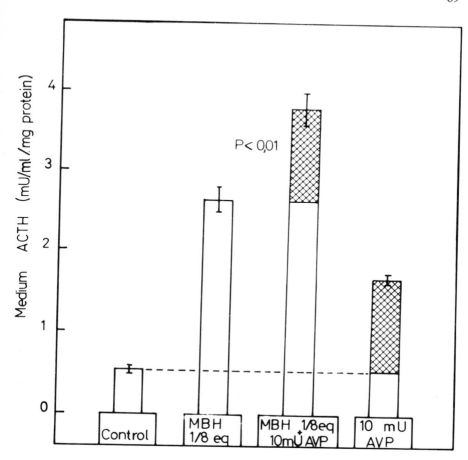

Fig. 6.   ACTH released by 3 h preincubated pituitaries, incubated with MBH extract, VP or MBH extract + VP. It can be seen that the effect of MBH extract + VP is the sum of the effects of MBH and VP when used separately. (VP present in 1/8 MBH eq. is negligible.) Each column represents mean ± S.E.M. of eight assays (from two independent experiments).

response to the 'neutralized' MBH extract is significantly less than to the untreated control. In another experiment (Fig. 6), where MBH extract and VP were added simultaneously to anterior pituitaries preincubated for 3 h, the response was equivalent to the sum of the effects of separate stimulations. Moreover, the concomitant addition of AVP-AS and MBH extracts or VP to anterior pituitaries caused a suppression of the CRF-like effect of VP which had decreased at 10 min and was abolished at 20 min (Fig. 3, curves 1 and 2). The parallelism of curves 3 and 4 and a comparison of the distances between those curves on the one hand and curves 1 and 2 on the other, clearly demonstrate that the effect of MBH extract is jointly due to VP and CRF. That is, the effect is additive not potentiating. This result is at variance with the observations *in vivo* of Yates *et al.*[13].

PUTATIVE CRF AND VP RECEPTOR SITES IN THE PITUITARY

To learn more about the differences in the modes of action of CRF and VP, anterior pituitaries were subjected to the influence of two successive stimulations, i.e. VP, VP; CRF, CRF; VP, CRF or CRF, VP. It can be seen in Fig. 7 that only on the first stimulations with VP did we get a good response to that hormone. The effect of VP was abolished or reduced considerably on a second stimulation. The magnitude of this inhibition depended on the amount of hormone used for the previous stimulation, presumably because this influenced the degree of uptake of VP by the tissue. For example, we found 38 ± 11.9 and 71 ± 16.2 pg of VP/mg of protein in the glands when the first incubation was with 10 or 100 mU VP respectively. The decreased ability of the tissue to respond to VP does not extend to CRF since successive responses were of about the same intensity when the regime was CRF, CRF. Similar results also come from the VP, CRF schedule. These various observations suggest the presence of putative receptors and/or binding sites for VP in the anterior pituitary, and that these are probably different from those mediating the CRF effect.

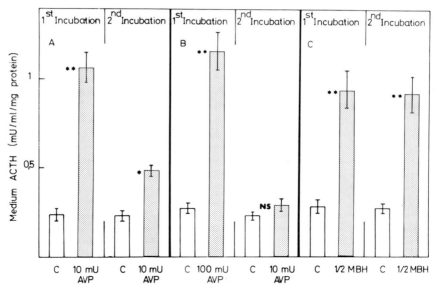

Fig. 7.   Effect of two successive stimulations produced by 10mU of AVP (A), 100mU of AVP (B) or MBH extract (C), on ACTH released from 3 h preincubated pituitary fragments. Each column represented mean ± S.E.M. of 16 assays. ** $p < 0.01$; * $p < 0.05$; NS, not significant.

SUBCELLULAR LOCATION OF CRF AND VP

Synaptosomes were obtained by subcellular fractionation of MBH extracts by differential and then discontinuous sucrose-gradient centrifugation[14]. CRF activity in the different fractions was evaluated, after suitable extraction, by

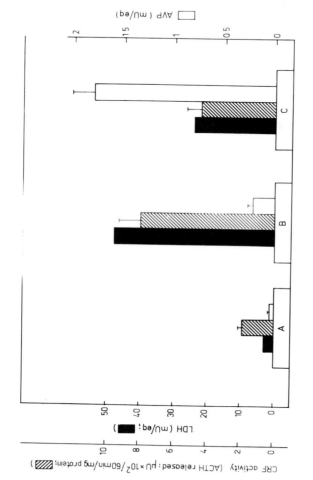

Fig. 8. Distribution of LDH, CRF and VP activities after subcellular fractionation of MBH extract: A (myeline), B (synaptosomes), C (mitochondria + synaptosomes) fractions. Each column represents the mean ± S.E.M. of five assays of one experiment.

C. Mialhe et al.

bioassay, and VP was determined by RIA. (Lactate dehydrogenase was the enzyme chosen as a synaptosomal marker[15].) As may be seen in Fig. 8, CRF and VP are present in synaptosomes, thus confirming the findings of Mulder *et al.*[16]. Our data demonstrate moreover that CRF and VP are concentrated mainly in nerve-terminals and probably in distinct populations for the two hormones.

STUDIES OF THE CRF-LIKE EFFECT OF VP *IN VIVO*

The CRF-like effect of VP suggests that this neurohormone, which is released rapidly after systemic or 'neurogenic' stimulation[17,18], may have a physiological role in the response to stress. Though the amount of VP utilized *in vitro* may appear supraphysiological it must be borne in mind that the amount of VP present in the hypophyseal portal vessels is about 300–1000 times greater than that in peripheral blood[19]. In this context our experiment may be physiologically reasonable, at least in conditions of severe stress. Against this is the fact that the CRF-like activity of VP is expressed only after a long preincubation *in vitro* and this seems incompatible with the situation *in vivo*. Nevertheless, an effect of VP *in vivo* has recently been demonstrated in hypophysectomized rats bearing pituitaries transplanted under the kidney capsule. In this case VP acts directly on the anterior pituitary, with a corticosteroid response similar to that observed during stress[20].

It has also been proposed that VP *in vivo* has an indirect effect on ACTH secretion, either through the hypothalamic CRF pathway or by potentiation of the CRF effect at the level of the anterior pituitary[21,22].

In order to extend our knowledge of the role of VP in the corticosteroid response to stress, we studied the effect of ether inhalation or histamine injection (classified as systemic stimuli) and sound (neurogenic stimuli) in Brattleboro rats. It is reported elsewhere[23,24] that these rats have a somewhat diminished corticosteroid response to stress. This was, indeed, observed by us in experiments involving systemic stress. However, we did not detect a significant corticotropic response to a neurogenic stimulus. Our results, using both intact and 7-day adrenalectomized (adx) Long Evans and Brattleboro rats, are outlined in Fig. 9. Each group included controls and rats subjected to neurogenic stimulus (sound). It can be seen that only in Brattleboro rats was the blood corticosterone level not significantly elevated either 10 or 20 min after stimulation. Moreover, blood ACTH levels, measured either 5 min (for Adx.) or 10 min (for intact) after onset of the stress, showed no increase. (Preliminary experiments had shown these times to be appropriate for maximal ACTH elevations in control animals.) These data show that the lack of corticosteroid response is associated with absence of increased ACTH secretion, and that this is particularly pronounced in Adx. rats.

An obvious question is whether the absence of VP is responsible for the lack of hypothalamo-hypophyseal activation as was suggested many years ago by de Wied[25]. The probable answer is 'yes'. Our data, however, do not exclude a role for intermediate lobe ACTH[26] as well, since Castel *et al.*[27] have recently produced immunocytological evidence for VP receptor sites in the pars intermedia.

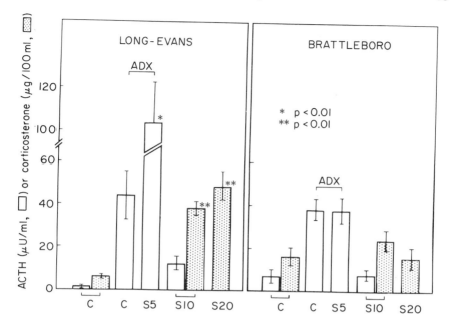

Fig. 9.   Corticosterone (μg/100ml) and ACTH (μU/ml) plasma level in intact Long Evans and Brattleboro rats submitted to a neurogenic stimulus for 10 or 20 min. ACTH plasma level in adrenalectomized (Adx.) Long Evans or Brattleboro rats killed 5 min after the beginning of a neurogenic stimulus. Sound: intensity 100Db, frequency 600c/s. Each column represents the mean ± S.E.M. for six to ten rats. ** $p < 0.001$, * $p < 0.05$; NS, not significant.

CONCLUSION

It may be concluded that CRF and VP are distinct entities, both having an effect on the stimulation of ACTH release *in vitro*. Their modes of action and their putative receptor and/or binding sites differ. It seems possible that VP, probably released by different nerve endings, is in some way involved, but its presence is not necessary for an increase in ACTH secretion *in vivo*, except perhaps in response to a neurogenic stimulus. Whether this effect on ACTH release is on the pars intermedia or the pars distalis remains to be determined.

ACKNOWLEDGEMENTS

The authors wish to thank Mrs. E. Fraquet, F. Herzog and A. Hoeft for their excellent technical assistance and Miss M. Porcherot who typed the manuscript. This work was supported by the Centre National de la Recherche Scientifique (CNRS, ERA178) and by the Institut National de la Sante et de la Recherche Medicale (INSERM contracts 5.74.25 and 87.1.227.4).

REFERENCES

1. Harris, G. W. (1948). *Physiol. Rev.* **28**, 139.
2. Saffran, M. *et al.* (1955). *Endocrinology* **57**, 439.
3. Guillemin, R. and Rosenberg, B. (1955). *Endocrinology* **57**, 599.
4. Saffran, M. and Schally, A. V. (1977). *Neuroendocrinol.* **24**, 359.
5. Saffran, M. and Schally, A. V. (1955). *Endocrinology* **56**, 523.
6. Sayers, G. *et al.* (1971). *Endocrinology* **88**, 1063.
7. Heller, H. and Lederis, K. (1959). *J. Physiol. (Lond.)* **147**, 299.
8. Lutz-Bucher, B. *et al.* (1977). *Neuroendocrinol.* **23**, 181.
9. Chateau, M. *et al.* (1973). *J. Physiol. (Paris)* **67**, 182.
10. Renlund, S. (1978). *Dissertations from the Faculty of Sciences,* Uppsala, Sweden.
11. Krieger, D. T. and Liotta, A. (1977). *Life Sci.* **20**, 237.
12. Portanova, R. and Sayers, G. (1973). *Proc. Soc. Exp. Biol.* **143**, 661.
13. Yates, F. E. and Maran, J. W. (1974). *In* 'Handbook of Physiology', (Greep, R. O. and Ashwood, eds.), Vol. 4 part 2, p. 367, American Physiological Society, Washington.
14. Whittaker, V. P. (1969). *In* 'Handbook of Neurochemistry', (Lajtha, A. ed.), Vol. 2, p. 327, Plenum, New York.
15. Johnson, M. K. and Whittaker, V. P. (1963). *Biochem. J.* **88**, 404.
16. Mulder, A. H. *et al.* (1970). *Endocrinology* **87**, 61.
17. Mirsky, I. A. *et al.* (1974). *Endocrinology* **94**, 1259.
18. Lutz, B. *et al.* (1969). *Horm. Metab. Res.* **1**, 213.
19. Zimmerman, E. A. *et al.* (1977). *Ann. N.Y. Acad. Sci.* **297**, 405.
20. Yasuda, N. *et al.* (1978). *Endocrinology* **103**, 328.
21. Hedge, G. A. *et al.* (1966). *Endocrinology* **79**, 328.
22. Hedge, G. A. and Smelik, P. G. (1969). *Neuroendocrinol.* **4**, 242.
23. Willy, K. *et al.* (1974). *Neuroendocrinol.* **14**, 257.
24. Yates, F. E. *et al.* (1971). *Endocrinology.* **88**, 3.
25. de Wied, D. (1960). *First. Int. Cong. Endoc. Copenhagen.* p. 119.
26. Mialhe, C. and Briaud, B. (1976). *J. Physiol. (Paris)* **72**, 261.
27. Castel, M. and Hochman, J. (1976). *Sixth Eur. Cong. on Electron Microscopy,* Jerusalem, p. 606.

8

NEURAL PATHWAYS CONTROLLING RELEASE OF CORTICOTROPIN (ACTH)

Donald S. Gann*, David G. Ward, and Drew E. Carlson*

*The Johns Hopkins University School of Medicine,
Baltimore, Md. 21205, U.S.A.*

INTRODUCTION

The response of corticotropin (ACTH) release to diverse peripheral stimuli such as changes in blood volume, pain and injury imply the presence of ascending neural pathways in the brainstem governing the control of release of ACTH. However, the details of these neural pathways have eluded description. Recently it has proven possible to define these pathways by bringing together neurophysiological and neuronanatomical techniques and the direct measurement of ACTH in plasma [1,2]. We have focused particularly on the identification of central neurons responsive to hemodynamic changes because it had been shown previously that the response to these changes was dependent on changes in right atrial and arterial receptor activity [3,4] and because the location and termination of the primary afferents from these receptors were known [5]. We have tested the responsiveness of ACTH to electrical stimulation of areas containing neurons responsive to hemodynamic changes and their surrounds. Our working hypothesis was that pathways mediating the response of ACTH to hemodynamic stimuli could be identified by demonstrating the presence of neurons responsive to hemodynamic stimuli in a given area in which electrical stimulation led to changes in ACTH. Further, we hoped to demonstrate physiological and anatomical connectivity of a given area implicating the control of ACTH to other areas also related to the control of release of that hormone. As indicated below, we have been able to meet these criteria for some areas in the brainstem and to postulate a set of pathways mediating the release of ACTH in response to hemodynamic stimuli.

*Present address: Section of Surgery, Brown University, Rhode Island Hospital, Providence, R.I. 02902, USA.

In addition, we have identified other brainstem areas active in the control of
ACTH but not containing neurons responsive to hemodynamic changes. These
areas are probably implicated in the control of ACTH in response to other
sensory stimuli.

METHODS

To examine the role of central neural areas in the control of ACTH, we have
stimulated electrically those areas and surrounding areas in cats anesthetized with
chloralose/urethane. Small bipolar coaxial electrodes were placed stereotaxically.
Stimulations (20 sec, $100-200\mu A$, 0.2m sec, 100 Hz) were carried out at several
points along an electrode track that was marked with electrolytic lesions at its
upper and lower bounds for histological localization. Before stimulation and at
several times after stimulation of each site, plasma samples were collected for
measurement of ACTH by radioimmunoassay (RIA). Arterial pressure was
measured at intervals during and after stimulation. Sites of stimulation were
plotted on representative sagittal and coronal planes of the brainstem and
hypothalamus of the cat. Contiguous areas were defined that contained sites that
consistently either increased or decreased ACTH. In some cases areas were defined
that increased or decreased arterial pressure. The values and changes of ACTH for
each of these areas were then analyzed by analysis of variance corrected for
repeated measures over time in the same subjects[6]. In other studies of neural
control in response to hemodynamic changes that change ACTH, single neurons
were recorded from microelectrodes placed stereotaxically in ACTH active areas
and in other areas of the brainstem. Changes in venous return induced by constriction of the vena cava and changes in right atrial stretch induced by volume
pulsation have been used to identify neurons that are responsive and to characterize the response of these neurons to these stimuli. In some cases, efferent and
afferent connections of these neurons were defined by examining the responses
of neurons to stimulation of other sites in the nervous system. It was possible to
distinguish efferent projections from a neuron by acquiring evidence for anti-
dromic activation from a distant site. Sites of neurons and of stimulations were
plotted on identical sagittal and coronal planes of the brainstem and hypothalamus.

RESULTS

Earlier anatomical and physiological studies have indicated that signals from
cardiovascular receptors first reach the solitary region of the dorsal medulla[5,7,8].
Accordingly, to determine if these structures might be part of a central neural
pathway mediating changes in ACTH in response to hemodynamic change, the
dorsal medulla was stimulated electrically and the response of ACTH was
observed[9] as shown in Fig. 1. There is a lateral area coincident with the region
of the lateral solitary nucleus where electrical stimulation led to inhibition of
ACTH. There is also a medial inhibitory area coincident with the posteromedial
portion of nucleus intercalatus. Between these two inhibitory areas there is an
area coincident with the anterolateral nucleus intercalatus, the dorsal motor

nucleus of the vagus and the underlying reticular formation, where electrical stimulation led to facilitation of ACTH release.

If areas of the central nervous system that mediate the release of ACTH are part of pathways mediating the release of ACTH in response to hemodynamic change, they must contain neurons responsive to hemodynamic change. Further, these neurons should be connected to *other* ACTH active areas of the central nervous system. Accordingly, experiments were designed to specify changes in activity of neurons in ACTH active areas of the dorsal medulla in response to hemodynamic change and to establish connectivity to other areas of the brainstem. Our earlier studies described neurons whose activity changed in response to stretch of the right atrium[10]. Of 70 neurons tested, the activity of 16 increased and the activity of 11 decreased in response to stretch of the right atrium. Of those neurons tested, all responded to hemorrhage with a change in firing rate in the opposite direction. One-half of the responsive neurons projected directly to the dorsal rostral pons. However, recent studies[11] suggest that another population of neurons may exist whose activity changes in response to constriction of the vena cava (a stimulus analogous to hemorrhage) but not in response to stretch of the right atrium (unless the vena cava is constricted). As shown in Fig. 1, neurons stimulated by atrial stretch and projecting rostrally are located in the two ACTH inhibitory areas of the medulla, whereas neurons inhibited by atrial stretch and projecting rostrally are located in the intermediate ACTH facilitatory area. Since atrial stretch inhibits ACTH, the directions of the changes in neural activity are consistent with the directions of change in ACTH in response to electrical stimulation.

The neurons in the ACTH active areas of the medulla appear to project into or through a hypothetical cylinder with a diameter of 0.5mm which passes through the principal locus coeruleus, through a portion of the locus subcoeruleus and through an area ventral to the periaqueductal gray[10]. Accordingly, to determine if these structures might be part of a central neural pathway mediating the release of ACTH, the dorsal rostral pons was stimulated electrically and the response of ACTH was observed. Three major responsive areas were defined[12]. As shown in Fig. 1, there is a lateral area where electrical stimulation led to inhibition of ACTH. This area includes a parvicellular region in part lateral to and in part anterior to the principal locus coeruleus. The anterolateral locus coeruleus and part of the locus subcoeruleus lie within this area. This region is adjacent to the brachium conjunctivum and to the mesencephalic nucleus of the trigeminal nerve. There is also a medial inhibitory area that includes the dorsal raphe nucleus, the superior central nucleus of the raphe and a portion of the dorsal tegmental nucleus. This region appears continuous anteriorly with the lateral inhibitory area. Finally, there is a lateral facilitatory area. This area is a magnocellular region that includes the principal locus coeruleus, the medial nucleus of the brachium conjunctivum and the rostral extent of the gigantocellular tegmental field.

If these areas are part of a pathway mediating the release of ACTH in response to hemodynamic change, they must contain neurons responsive to hemodynamic change. Experiments were designed to specify the responses of neurons in ACTH active areas of the dorsal pons. Of 76 neurons tested in the lateral pons, the activity of 26 increased and the activity of two decreased in

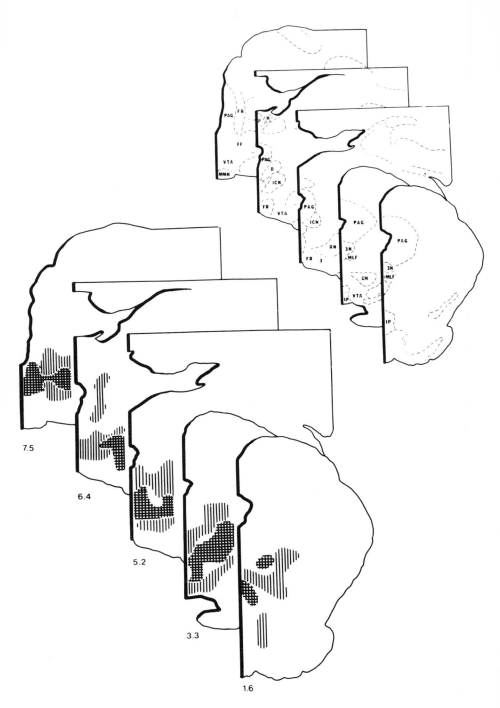

Fig. 1. (for legend see p. 81).

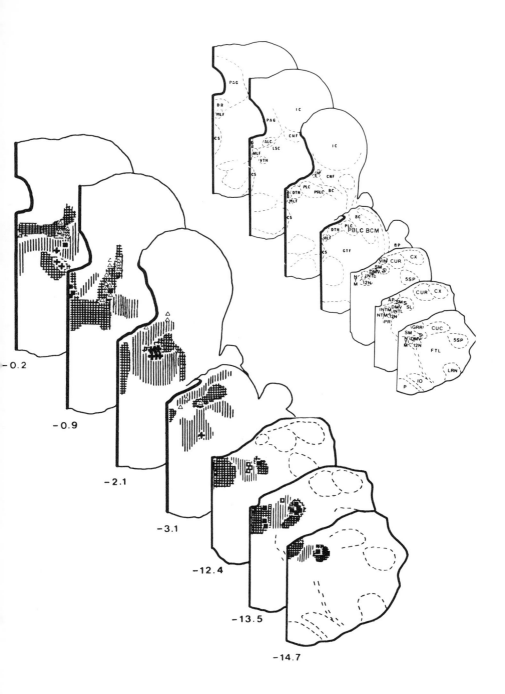

-0.2

-0.9

-2.1

-3.1

-12.4

-13.5

-14.7

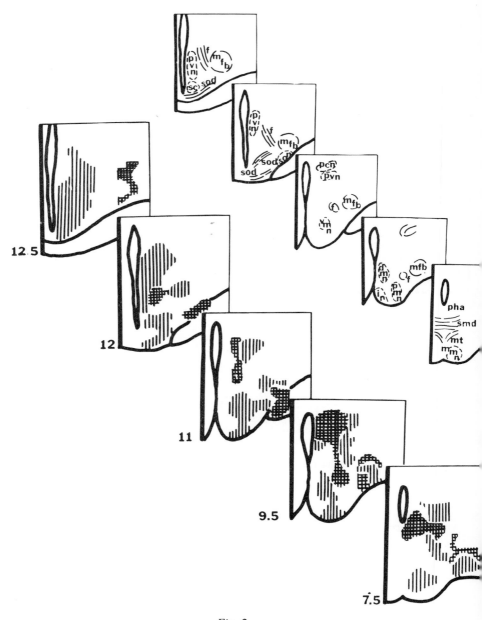

Fig. 2.

Fig. 1. ACTH-active areas of the brainstem projected on coronal planes (from the atlas of Berman[38]) of the medulla at 14.7, 13.5 and 12.4mm posterior to stereotaxic zero; of the pons at 3.1, 2.1, 0.9 and 0.2mm posterior to stereotaxic zero; and of the midbrain at 1.6, 3.3, 5.2, 6.4 and 7.5mm anterior to stereotaxic zero. Areas inhibiting the release of ACTH are shown with cross hatching. Areas facilitating the release of ACTH are shown with vertical shading.

The locations of medullary neurons responsive to right atrial pulsation that were activated antidromically from sites in the dorsal rostral pons are shown superimposed on the ACTH-active areas of the medulla. Neurons whose firing rates increased in response to right atrial pulsation are indicated by solid squares. Neurons whose firing rates decreased in response to right atrial pulsation are shown by open squares.

The locations of pontine neurons responsive to caval constriction or to right atrial pulsation are shown superimposed on the ACTH-active areas of the pons. Neurons whose firing rates increased in response to caval constriction are indicated by solid pluses. Neurons whose firing rate increased in response to right atrial pulsation and/or decreased in response to caval constriction are indicated by solid squares.

Neural features shown on the coronal drawings of the medulla on the right side are: 12N, hypoglossal nucleus; DMV, dorsal motor nucleus of the vagus; SM, medial solitary nucleus; S, solitary tract; GRR, nucleus gracilis; CUC, nucleus cuneatus; AP, area postrema; SL, lateral solitary nucleus; NTM, nucleus intermedius; INTM, medial extent of nucleus intercalatus; INTL, lateral extent of nucleus intercalatus; VIN, vestibular nucleus; FTL, tegmental reticular field; SSP, spinal tract, trigeminal-nerve; LRN, lateral reticular nucleus; IO, inferior olive; P, pyramidal tract; PR, paramedian reticular nucleus; CX, nucleus cuneatus, external division; CUR, nucleus cuneatus, rostral division. Neural features shown on the coronal drawings of the pons on the right side are: DR, dorsal nucleus of the raphe; DTN, dorsal tegmental nucleus of Gudden; VTN, ventral tegmental nucleus of Gudden; MLF, medial longitudinal fasciculus; PAG, periaqueductal gray; P, pyramids; CS, central nucleus of the raphe; TRN, tegmental reticular nucleus; BP, brachium pontis; GTF, gigantocellular tegmental field; TRF, tegmental reticular field; PLC, principal locus coeruleus; ALC, anterior locus coeruleus; SLC, locus subcoeruleus; 5M, mesencephalic nucleus of the trigeminal nerve; IC, inferior colliculus; CNS, cuneiform nucleus; BC, brachium conjunctivum; BCM, medial parabrachial nucleus; PBLC, parabrachial extent of anterior locus coeruleus.

Neural features shown on the coronal drawings of midbrain on the right side are: VTA, ventral tegmental area of Tsai; FF, fields of Forel; RN, red nucleus; 3, oculomotor nerve; SN, substantia nigra; PG, pontine gray; TRN, tegmental reticular nucleus; TRF, tegmental reticular field; SLC, locus subcoeruleus; ALC, anterolateral locus coeruleus; 5M, mesencephalic nucleus of the trigeminal nerve; 5MT, mesencephalic tract of the trigeminal nerve; IC, inferior colliculus; MM, mammillary bodies; MT, mammillothalamic tract; FR, fasciculus retroflexus; ICA, interstitial nucleus of Cajal; VTL, lateral extent of the ventral tegmental nucleus of Gudden; MLC, medial extent of the principal locus; PHA, posterior hypothalamic area; IP, interpeduncular nucleus; BCX, decussation of the brachium conjunctivum; VTM, medial extent of the ventral tegmental nucleus of Gudden; DTN, dorsal tegmental nucleus of Gudden; DR, dorsal raphe nucleus; 4N, nucleus of the trochlear nerve; MLF, medial longitudinal fasciculus; PAG, periaqueductal gray.

Fig. 2. ACTH-active areas of the hypothalamus projected on five representative coronal planes (from the atlas of Snider and Niemer[39]) from 7.5mm to 12.5mm anterior to stereotaxic zero. Areas inhibiting or facilitating ACTH are indicated as in Fig. 1. Neural features shown on the coronal drawings of the hypothalamus on the right side are: mmn, medial mammillary nucleus; mfb, medial forebrain bundle; mt, mammillothalamic tract; smd, supramammillary decussation; pha, posterior hypothalamic area; ff, fields of Forel; in, infundibular nucleus; pmn, premammillary nucleus; f, fornix; dmn, dorsomedial nucleus; vmn, ventromedial nucleus; pvn, paraventricular nucleus; pcn, parvocellular nucleus; sod, supraoptic decussations; son, supraoptic nucleus; sc, suprachiasmatic nucleus.

response to constriction of the vena cava[13]. None of the neurons stimulated by constriction of the vena cava responded to stretch of the right atrium. In contrast, neurons inhibited by caval constriction were facilitated by atrial pulsation alone. Six of nine responsive neurons tested responded to constriction of the vena cava during partial servocontrol of arterial pressure. A quantitative analysis suggested that these neurons respond to changes in venous return as well as to changes in arterial pressure. As shown in Fig. 1, most neurons responsive to constriction of the vena cava are located within the hypothetical cylinder. Neurons responsive to caval constriction are located at or near the junction of the ACTH stimulatory and ACTH inhibitory areas of the pons.

Signals from the pons that reach the hypothalamus for control of ACTH must pass through midbrain structures. In order to determine areas of the midbrain that may contain pathways mediating the release of ACTH, the medial regions of the midbrain were stimulated electrically and the responses of ACTH were observed[14]. Three major responsive areas were identified. As shown in Fig. 1, there is a dorsal area where electrical stimulation led to facilitation of ACTH. This region is coincident, in large part, with the lateral division of the dorsal longitudinal fasciculus and appears to be continuous with the ACTH facilitatory area of the pons. Ventrally, there is a second ACTH facilitatory area that is coincident with the ventral tegmental area of Tsai. The caudal portion of this area appears to be a continuation of the facilitatory area of the pons. There is also an intermediate ACTH inhibitory area that is coincident with portions of the central tegmental tract and of the mammillary peduncle. It appears continuous with both lateral and medial inhibitory areas of the pons.

So far, we have stimulated electrically over 850 sites throughout the hypothalamus. Many hypothalamic areas appear to be ACTH-active. Fig. 2 consists of five representative coronal planes which show the anatomical locations and organization of these areas. Areas not shaded in this figure were inert with respect to release of ACTH in response to electrical stimulation.

In the most caudal plane, similarity with the most rostral plane of Fig. 1 is apparent. The dorsal facilitatory region, coincident with the fields of Forel, has ascended from the lateral division of the dorsal longitudinal fasciculus. The inhibitory region of the mammillary peduncle and central tegmental tract is coursing into the posterior hypothalamic area. Laterally and ventrally, the medial forebrain bundle appears to have both facilitatory and inhibitory components. The medial mammillary nucleus also appears to be facilitatory, and it may be continuous with the medial forebrain bundle laterally.

The dorsal areas course rostrally, and at 9.5mm anteriorly, the dorsal inhibitory area projects ventrally to a facilitatory area coincident with the lateral aspect of the dorsomedial nucleus. This projection extends anteriorly to impinge on the laterodorsal aspect of the ventromedial nucleus as well (not shown). The multicomponent medial forebrain bundle is again evident. However, our findings to date suggest no continuity of the medial forebrain bundle with the medial ventral facilitatory areas that include the premammillary and infundibular nuclei.

In the three rostral planes, convergence of the facilitatory areas on the median eminence is evident. The dorsal areas, which include the parvocellular and paraventricular nuclei, appear to descend to the median eminence. The medial forebrain bundle feeds into the supraoptic decussations to reach the suprachiasmatic and thence to the median eminence. There appears to be posterior projections of this pathway to the ventromedial, dorsomedial infundibular and periventricular nuclei. The dorsal inhibitory areas pass through the dorsal hypothalamic area and project ventrally to the posterior aspects of the anterior paraventricular and suprachiasmatic nuclei. The inhibitory component of the medial forebrain bundle appears to surround the caudal and lateral aspects of the supraoptic nucleus. This same area is facilitatory for vasopressin[15]. In the most rostral plane, an inhibitory area is seen on the lateral aspect of the medial forebrain bundle.

The mediodorsal region, which extends from the posterior hypothalamic area to the dorsal paraventricular nucleus, contains cells that respond to stretch of the right atrium. Significantly, the majority of these cells are only responsive during periods of carotid occlusion, suggesting convergence of atrial and arterial baroreceptors[16]. Further, we have located many cells throughout the medial hypothalamus which are driven orthodromically by stimulation with single shocks in the ACTH-active region of the dorsal pons. The most prominent connection appears to be excitatory, so that stimulation in ACTH-facilitatory areas in the pons excites cells in ACTH-facilitatory areas in the hypothalamus. Similar projections are observed between inhibitory areas, and some inhibitory projections connect regions of opposite polarity with respect to release of ACTH[17].

DISCUSSION

These experiments have demonstrated the presence of a number of apparently connected areas implicated in the control of ACTH in regions of the brainstem extending from the medulla to the hypothalamus. In selected regions of most areas examined, neurons have been identified that are responsive to hemodynamic changes. It is important to note, however, that the demonstration of neurons responsive to such changes in areas mediating release of ACTH does not implicate those neurons in the control of ACTH. Other neurons in the same area with different afferent connections might be involved. Since it is impossible to measure a change in ACTH in response to stimulation of a single neuron, it is not at present technologically possible to implicate a neuron in the control of ACTH. Nevertheless, the consistent finding of neurons driven by hemodynamic signals within ACTH active areas makes it reasonable to hypothesize that the changes in the release of ACTH in response to hemodynamic changes are mediated by changes in activity of these neurons.

The present studies suggest several general features of the organization of central neural pathways controlling the release of ACTH. Throughout the brainstem and hypothalamus there are multiple anatomically segregated parallel pathways that converge on the median eminence. There are pathways that facilitate ACTH and pathways that inhibit ACTH. Thus the release of ACTH may be adjusted by the integration of facilitatory and inhibitory signals.

The ascending pathways which convey hemodynamic signals appear to be characterized by convergence and divergence. At the level of the medulla, primary afferents from cardiovascular receptors terminate in the lateral solitary nucleus. Secondary projections terminate in medial and intermediate regions of the solitary complex. From these regions paths appear to converge on a highly localized region in the locus coeruleus and locus subcoeruleus. Anatomical studies indicate that neurons in the solitary complex also project laterally to the parabrachial region of the pons[18]. Thus signals from the dorsal medulla may ascend also in parallel paths to the pons. However, anatomical studies say nothing about the signals carried in these pathways. From the pontine areas, signals may diverge again to project to medial and lateral regions of the rostral pons and then to ascend to the hypothalamus in multiple paths. Other anatomical studies indicate that neurons in the solitary complex project directly to the hypothalamus[19] and to the median eminence[20]. Thus signals for the control of ACTH may reach the hypothalamus in at least two modes. First, the signals ascend to the pons and interact with other sensory modalities before ascending to the hypothalamus. Second, the signals may ascend to the hypothalamus from the medulla unaltered by other signals. This pattern of organization provides an anatomical substrate for differential processing of information.

As indicated above, neurons in some areas appear primarily responsive to large hemodynamic signals, whereas others appear more responsive to small signals and to changes in the rate of stimulation. Earlier work in this laboratory suggested the presence of parallel paths ascending in the brainstem with different thresholds to hemodynamic stimulation[21]. The present findings provide anatomical and physiological evidence for such pathways and for their differential sensitivity.

All neurons that have been found to be responsive to hemodynamic manipulation have been located in areas implicated in the control of ACTH. The release of other hormones of the pituitary, including vasopressin[22], growth hormone[23] and prolactin[24] are also responsive to hemodynamic changes. Similarly, the sympathetic nervous system, and through it the release of hormones including the catecholamines, glucagon and insulin, also is modulated by changes in baroreceptor activity. The failure to demonstrate ascending hemodynamic pathways in areas not implicated in the control of ACTH suggest that the hemodynamic control of this entire set of functions may be shared by common ascending pathways. This would provide an anatomical and physiological substrate for a coordinated neuroendocrine response to hemodynamic changes.

On the other hand, neurons sensitive to cardiovascular changes have been found in highly discrete areas within larger ACTH-active areas. These findings suggest strongly that other sensory modalities may ascend through pathways parallel to but different from those conveying hemodynamic information. Although there may be some convergence of these pathways at various levels of the brainstem, such convergence cannot be complete in regions caudal to the hypothalamus.

The dorsal and ventral facilitatory areas of the hypothalamus converge in the region of the supraoptic decussations before projecting to the median eminence. Accordingly, Makara and colleagues have blocked the release of ACTH mediated by pain with anterolateral cuts that sever the supraoptic decussation[25]. However, Stark and colleagues have shown that stresses of sufficient intensity are effective even after an anterolateral cut[26]. Moreover, our findings indicate that the inhibitory extensions that project ventrally from the posterior and dorsal hypothalamic areas would escape destruction after such a cut. We have suggested previously that the dorsal pathways may represent a high threshold route by which potent stimuli such as large hemorrhage induce release of ACTH even in the presence of steroid suppression[21].

All of the hypothalamic nuclei that we have found to be facilitatory are said to contain significant corticotropin-releasing activity[27,28], except for the medial mammillary nucleus. Further, some cells in these nuclei may project to the median eminence by way of the supraoptic decussation[29]. Projections from the medial mammillary nucleus may join projections from the subthalamic area and from the ventral tegmental area of Tsai in the medial forebrain bundle, as suggested by the findings of Brodal and Rossi[30].

The inhibitory areas of the dorsal hypothalamus are juxtaposed to four nuclei that may contain corticotropin-releasing factors (CRH; corticoliberin), the dorsomedial, ventromedial, paraventricular and suprachiasmatic. Thus the proposed inhibitory pathway may act to inhibit CRH neurons in these nuclei. Further, some inhibitory projections may be entirely intrahypothalamic. Short projections from the posterior hypothalamic area to the dorsal paraventricular nucleus have been documented[31]. Alternatively, there may be direct inhibition of the release of CRH in the ventrobasal hypothalamus. The ventral extensions shown in Fig. 2 suggest such a mechanism. As with all the ACTH-active areas that we have found, stimulation in the medial forebrain bundle may act through descending projections to ACTH active regions in the brainstem[32]. The lateral area seen most rostrally in Fig. 2 may represent an inhibitory projection from forebrain and limbic structures. Finally, any of the inhibitory areas could mediate release of a corticotropin-inhibiting factor.

Stimulation surrounding the caudal pole of the supraoptic nucleus inhibits ACTH but leads to moderate increases in the peripheral concentration of vasopressin[15]. In contrast, stimulation in the area of the paraventricular nucleus facilitates both hormones. It has been proposed that the retrograde flow of blood from the neurohypophysis to the median eminence and thence to the portal circulation might provide a pathway whereby vasopressin influences the release of ACTH[33]. Because stimulation of the paraventricular or of the supraoptic nucleus is equally effective in releasing vasopressin but is differentially effective in releasing ACTH, it is unlikely that retrograde flow from the posterior pituitary plays a significant role in the short-term control of ACTH during moderate changes in vasopressin release.

ACTH release may be mediated in part by a direct projection from vaso-pressinergic neurons in the paraventricular nucleus to the external zone of the median eminence. Zimmerman and colleagues have documented this projection in several species, and have shown further that no similar pathway originates from the supraoptic nucleus[34]. They have also found that significant amounts of vasopressin are released into the portal vessels in the monkey[35]. In preliminary studies, Dornhorst and co-workers have found that infusion of vasopressin anti-serum into the third ventricle blocks the release of ACTH in the response to electrical stimulation of the paraventricular nucleus. Together, these results suggest strongly that the paraventricular–median eminence pathway can mediate release of ACTH. Vasopressin may act by potentiating the action of CRH[36] or it may act by increasing the release of CRH from the median eminence[37].

The work on which this paper is based was supported in part by NIH grant AM14952.

REFERENCES

1. Gann, D. S. *et al.* (1977). *Ann. N.Y. Acad. Sci.* **297**, 477.
2. Gann, D. S. *et al.* (1978). *Rec. Progr. Horm. Res.* **34**, *(in press).*
3. Cryer, G. L. and Gann, D. S. (1974). *Am. J. Physiol.* **227**, 325.
4. Baertschi, A. J. *et al.* (1976). *Am. J. Physiol.* **231**, 692.
5. Baertschi, A. J. *et al.* (1975). *Brain Res.* **93**, 189.
6. Winer, B. J. (1972). Statistical Principles in Experimental Design, McGraw-Hill, New York.
7. Crill, W. E. and Reis, D. J. (1968). *Am. J. Physiol.* **214**, 269.
8. Cottle, M. A. (1964). *J. Comp. Neurol.* **121**, 329.
9. Ward, D. G. and Gann, D. S. (1976). *Endocrinology* **99**, 1213.
10. Ward, D. G. *et al.* (1977). *Am. J. Physiol.* **232**, R.116.
11. Lefcourt, A. M. *et al.* (1979). *Fed. Proc.* **38**, 1201.
12. Ward, D. G. *et al.* (1976). *Endocrinology* **99**, 1220.
13. Ward, D. G. *et al.* (1978). *Fed. Proc.* **37**, 743.
14. Ward, D. G. *et al.* (1978). *Endocrinology* **102**, 1147.
15. Dornhorst, A. *et al.* (1978). *Neurosci. Abstr.* **4**, 344.
16. Grizzle, W. E. *et al.* (1975). *Am. J. Physiol.* **228**, 1039.
17. Carlson, D. E. *et al.* (1976). *Neuroscience Abstr.* **2**, 647.
18. Loewy, A. D. and Burton, H. *J. Comp. Neurol.* **181**, 421.
19. Ricardo, J. A. and Koh, E. T. (1978). *Brain Res.* **153**, 1.
20. Palkovits, M. (1977). *Ann. N.Y. Acad. Sci.* **297**, 455.
21. Gann, D. S. and Cryer, G. L. (1972). *Adv. Biomed. Engr.* **2**, 1.
22. Claybaugh, J. R. and Share, L. (1973). *Am. J. Physiol.* **224**, 519.
23. Meyer, V. and Knobil, E. (1967). *Endocrinology* **80**, 163.
24. MacLeod, R. M. (1976). *In* 'Frontiers in Neuroendocrinology', Vol. 4, (L. Martini and W. F. Ganong, eds.), pp. 169–194, Raven, New York.
25. Makara, G. B. *et al.* (1969). *J. Endocrinol.* **44**, 187.
26. Stark, E. *et al.* (1970). *Acta. Physiol. Acad. Sci. Hung.* **38**, 43.
27. Lang, R. E. (1976). *Neurosci. Letters* **2**, 19.
28. Krieger, D. T. and Zimmerman, E. A. (1979). *In* 'Clinical Neuroendocrinology', (Besser, M. and Martini, L. eds.), Academic Press, New York, *(in press),*
29. Makara, G. B. and Hodacs, L. (1975). *Brain Res.* **84**, 23.
30. Brodal, A. and Rossi, G. (1955). *Arch. Neurol. Psychiat.* **74**, 68.
31. Woods, W. H. *et al.* (1969). *Brain Res.* **12**, 26.
32. Crosby, E. C. and Woodburne, R. T. (1951). *J. Comp. Neurol.* **94**, 1.
33. Oliver, C. *et al.* (1977). *Endocrinology* **101**, 598.
34. Zimmerman, E. A. and Antunes, A. L. (1976). *J. Histochem. Cytochem.* **24**, 807.
35. Zimmerman, E. A. *et al.* (1973). *Science* **182**, 925.
36. Yates, F. E. *et al.* (1971). *Endocrinology* **88**, 3.
37. Hedge, G. A. *et al.* (1966). *Endocrinology* **79**, 328.
38. Berman, A. L. (1968). *The Brain Stem of the Cat,* U. Wisconsin Press, Madison.
39. Snider, R. S. and Niemer, W. G. (1961). *A Stereotaxic Atlas of the Cat Brain,* V. Chicago Press, Chicago.

9

CHANGES IN BRAIN AMINES DURING STRESS

M. Palkovits

*1st Department of Anatomy, Semmelweis University Medical School,
Budapest, Hungary*

INTRODUCTION

In recent years the role played by biogenic amines in neuroendocrine mechanisms, including the stress response, has been studied intensively. This paper attempts to summarize what is known about the response of biogenic amines in the central nervous system to stressful stimuli.

It is generally accepted that various forms of stress affect brain biogenic amines and activate the sympatho-adrenal system in the periphery. The stress-induced increase in activity of the adrenal medullary catecholamine-synthesizing enzymes is associated with increased plasma concentration of catecholamines. Levels of norepinephrine and epinephrine in rat plasma have been shown to be increased severalfold after acute stress[1].

A great variety of stresses result in immediate and definitive changes in the concentrations of biogenic amines in the central nervous system. A number of authors have reported significant alterations in the biosynthesis of norepinephrine, dopamine[2-5], epinephrine[6] and serotonin (5-HT; hydroxytryptamine)[7-9] in the central nervous system following acute or repeated stressful procedures. The possible sites, mechanisms and course of the central actions of stressful stimuli are detailed in the subsequent pages.

SITE OF THE ACTION OF STRESS ON BRAIN BIOGENIC AMINES

Two major questions are to be answered. (1) Whether stress-induced changes in the level and synthesis of biogenic amines are general or focal in the central nervous system, and (2) whether the stressor affects aminergic cell bodies or their terminals.

GENERAL AND FOCAL CHANGES

The effects of various stressors on brain amine content and metabolism have usually been studied only in whole brain or in large segments such as the forebrain or brainstem. Measurements of the amine content or the activity of their synthesizing enzymes in whole brain may fail to detect alterations in distinct areas of the brain. Most authors have reported a fall in norepinephrine concentrations and increased turnover in the whole brain. In the case of dopamine, the concentration has been found to be unchanged, whereas turnover has been described as increased, decreased or unchanged. Contradictory data have also been reported for brain 5-HT concentrations after stressful stimuli.

When amine levels or enzyme activities were measured in individual brain regions or nuclei, the following observations were made.

(a) After acute stress, the concentration of norepinephrine was reduced selectively in the hypothalamus, especially in the arcuate and ventromedial nuclei[3-5].

(b) Under the influence of acute stress, dopamine concentration was significantly reduced in the arcuate nucleus[3,4] and areas that contain dopaminergic cell bodies, e.g. substantia nigra and A8-catecholaminergic cell group in the midbrain[5].

(c) Acute stress (4 h immobilization) induced a decrease in epinephrine levels in certain hypothalamic nuclei, e.g. periventricular, anterior hypothalamic, ventromedial and arcuate nuclei[6].

(d) 5-HT concentration rapidly decreased in the hypothalamus after certain stress stimuli. However, unlike the decrease in catecholamine concentrations, this fall was found not only in the hypothalamus, but also in many other brain regions[8,9].

(e) Under the condition of repeated stress there was an increase in tyrosine hydroxylase activity in the arcuate nucleus[3], in the brain stem (including the locus coeruleus)[10,11], and increased norepinephrine levels particularly in hypothalamic nuclei[6].

(f) Repeated stress tended to elevate tryptophan hydroxylase activity in the dorsal raphe nucleus[12]. Accelerated 5-HT metabolism in various brain areas has also been reported following different stressors[9,13-16].

Changes in norepinephrine, dopamine and epinephrine concentrations in some hypothalamic nuclei under the influence of stress indicate that catecholamines, particularly in the medial-basal hypothalamus (arcuate and ventromedial nuclei), may be involved in the regulation of neuroendocrine processes activated by stress. The fact that after stress 5-HT content diminished not only in the medial-basal hypothalamus but in many other brain regions suggests that stress affects brain 5-HT more diffusely than brain catecholamines.

EFFECTS ON CELL BODIES AND AXONS

Norepinephrine

The acute-stress induced reduction of epinephrine and norepinephrine levels in the hypothalamic nuclei must reflect diminished amine concentration in nerve terminals since epinephrine and norepinephrine-containing cell bodies are outside the hypothalamus. This reduction indicates an enhanced release from the nerve terminals. Previous authors have usually reported a fall in norepinephrine concentrations with intense activation of norepinephrine neurons and increased turnover in the whole brain[2,17-19]. It has been hypothesized that stress causes both increased release and synthesis of norepinephrine. If stress is sufficiently severe, brain norepinephrine synthesis is unable to keep pace with release and catabolism. Consequently, reduced norepinephrine concentrations in nerve terminals suggests that after acute stress, release exceeds synthesis.

A slight decrease in the norepinephrine concentration has been observed in the locus coeruleus after acute immobilization. Repeated stress produced an increase in both the norepinephrine level and tyrosine hydroxylase activity in this cell group. To determine the contribution of this nucleus to the changes in norepinephrine turnover observed after stress in the nerve terminals, various experimental studies were performed in the rat. Stimulations of the locus coeruleus resulted in a rapid drop in the levels of norepinephrine in the cerebral cortex and hippocampus[20]. Surgical transections of dorsal and ventral noradrenergic bundles prevented the acute stress-induced fall of the norepinephrine concentrations in the hypothalamic nuclei (Palkovits *et al.*, in preparation). These results indicate that the locus coeruleus plays a major role in controlling the changes in hypothalamic norepinephrine.

Dopamine

Dopamine concentration, under the influence of acute immobilization, was significantly reduced in areas that contain dopaminergic cell bodies (arcuate nucleus, A8-cell groups, substantia nigra) but was unaltered in the hypothalamic regions that contain the dopamine in nerve terminals[3,4,5]. Bliss *et al.*[13] demonstrated that the stress of foot-shock accelerates the metabolism of dopamine and 5-HT to the same degree as norepinephrine. However, although dopamine and 5-HT were rapidly resynthetized, norepinephrine was regenerated at a slower rate.

5-HT

Various acute stressful stimuli are followed by a temporary reduction of 5-HT concentrations in both 5-HT nerve terminals and cell bodies. However, following repeated stress, slight increase of 5-HT concentration or tryptophan hydroxylase activity has been observed only in the midbrain, where 5-HT-containing cell bodies are concentrated.

ACTION OF STRESSORS ON AMINERGIC NEURONS

It is generally accepted that stress induces a rapid release of biogenic amines from the nerve terminals together with a subsequent increase in their turnover during recovery.

Immobilization for 5 min results in a marked decrease of catecholamine concentrations in the hypothalamus which are further reduced over extended time intervals. This decrease in catecholamine concentration was inversely correlated with the elevated plasma corticotropin (ACTH) and corticosterone levels[4]. Immobilization for 20 min or injection with formalin 30 min before resulted in depletions of norepinephrine and dopamine concentrations in certain hypothalamic and midbrain nuclei[3,5].

These data suggest a rapid depletion of endogenous catecholamine levels in the nerve terminals and this is followed by an accelerated synthesis. Norepinephrine levels were unchanged in the ventromedial nucleus after 180 min of immobilization, whereas a 20 min stress produced significant amine reduction in this nucleus[4,5]. The stores of norepinephrine depleted by stress were replenished chiefly by newly synthetized norepinephrine.

The accelerated turnover of norepinephrine persisted for several hours after acute stress, resulting in a restoration of the amine content in the nerve terminals. Such an increased synthesis most probably represents a response to release of

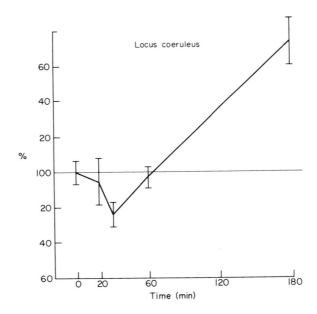

Fig. 1. Time course of norepinephrine concentrations in the locus coeruleus during immobilization stress. Animals were killed immediately after indicated intervals of stress. Data are expressed as mean value of six animals as a percentage of values in related intact controls (100%).

catecholamines in acute stress. Repeated stress resulted in increased dopamine β-hydroxylase activity in the whole brain[21] and in the hypothalamus[4] as well as in elevated norepinephrine concentrations in various hypothalamic nuclei[4,5]. The increased synthesis and turnover occured mainly in the catecholamine-containing cell bodies in the brain stem (Fig. 1). The newly synthetized nore-pinephrine appeared to be utilized preferentially in this brain region[22]. After stress, tyrosine hydroxylase activity was reported as being increased in a pontine tissue blocks containing the locus coeruleus[11] in the medulla oblongata[23] and in the arcuate nucleus[3]. These findings could be interpreted as enhanced synthesis in adrenergic cell bodies, but not in the nerve terminals. The increase of tyrosine hydroxylase in the arcuate nucleus after repeated immobilization is con-sistent with increased aminergic synthesis in this hypothalamic cell group which contain dopamine cell bodies beside norepinephrine- and probably dopamine-containing nerve terminals (Fig. 2).

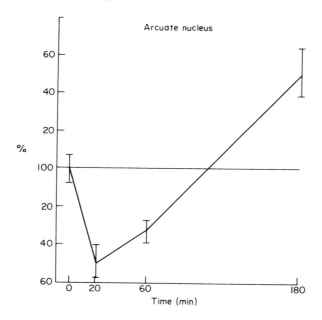

Fig. 2.   Time course of dopamine concentrations in the arcuate nucleus during immobili-zation stress[3,4,5]. Data are expressed as a percentage of values in related intact controls (100%).

Acute stress (10–30 min) induced a decrease in endogenous serotonin levels of various brain regions. The rapid depletion is followed by a rapid restoration as a result of a stress-induced increase of 5-HT synthesis (Fig. 3). At 30–120 min after stress, 5-HT concentrations returned to normal or were slightly elevated [7,20,19]. Repeated stress increased the synthesis of 5-HT in the brain stem-mesencephalon[18], especially in the dorsal raphe nucleus[9,12].

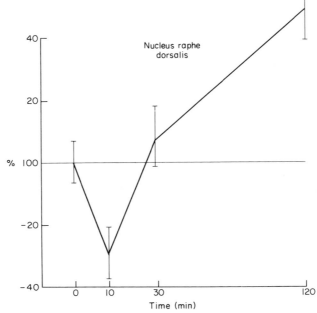

Fig. 3. Time course of 5-HT concentrations in the dorsal raphe nucleus during immobili-zation stress[9,12]. Data are expressed as a percentage of values in related intact controls (100%).

POSSIBLE MECHANISM OF STRESS-INDUCED CHANGES IN BRAIN AMINES

The exact mechanism of the stress-induced changes in the brain aminergic neurons is still unknown. Data on the possible inputs to aminergic neurons may be placed in two categories, namely neural or humoral inputs.

Neural Inputs

The neuronal pathways certainly constitute important components of mechanisms involved in stress-induced changes of brain amines. Stressors with peripheral sites of action enter the spinal cord *via* the peripheral nerves or the brain stem *via* the cranial nerves. The course of these fibres, as well as their neuronal connections within the brainstem, is not known. A high proportion of the presently known aminergic cell groups are located in the lower brain stem. Axons or axon collaterals of peripheral or cranial fibres with sensor functions might terminate in these cells. The mechanism of this probable input, as well as the neurotransmitters involved, have still to be elucidated.

Humoral Inputs

The effects of ACTH and adrenal corticoids on the biosynthesis of adrenal and brain catecholamines have recently been summarized by Axelrod[24] and Van

Loon *et al.*[25]. Present data, however, do not enable us to say whether the changes in the adrenal axis and brain amines have a cause–effect relationship or are simply parallel responses to stressful stimuli.

ACTH can affect catecholamine levels in the median eminence, ventromedial nucleus and locus coeruleus as rapidly as 10–20 min after a single injection of ACTH (3U/rat)[26]. At 3 h after ACTH injection, an elevated norepinephrine content in the locus coeruleus and decreased level of this amine could be observed in the arcuate and ventromedial nuclei. Dopamine levels were not changed in any brain areas examined[26,28].

ACTH and adrenocortical hormones do not have similar effects on brain amines. Thus the effect of ACTH on the norepinephrine cell bodies (increased norepinephrine turnover in the locus coeruleus) is independent of the adrenocortical secretion[28,29]. The acute effects of ACTH on brain amine levels could not be mimicked by acute glucocorticoid treatment[26,28].

In contrast to the ACTH-corticoid effects on brain catecholamines, a single dose of corticosterone increased the hypothalamic 5-HT content[7], whereas a single dose of ACTH had no effect.

POSSIBLE ROLE OF BIOGENIC AMINES IN STRESS RESPONSE

In recent years there have been many reports on the possibility that catecholamines participate in the regulation of ACTH secretion. They are very extensive studies from which it had been concluded that norepinephrine and 5-HT have inhibitory effects on ACTH secretion, whereas dopamine exerts no appreciable effect[25,30–38]. Parallel to the stress-induced changes in the ACTH–corticosteroid system, amine concentrations and their synthesizing enzyme activities in certain brain regions will also change. However, as mentioned earlier, this correlation does not prove a casual relationship and it is possible that these two phenomena are parallel but independent results of the stress.

Neither the mechanism nor the sites of action of biogenic amines on ACTH-corticosterone system is known. It seems clear that norepinephrine or epinephrine does not act directly on the pituitary. Systematically administered catecholamines have no direct effect on ACTH cells, nor do they alter the ACTH release from the pars intermedia cells[39,40] or from the pars distalis[41]. Microinjection of biogenic amines directly into the rat pars distalis is without effect on ACTH release, except for epinephrine at unphysiological infusion doses of $10–100\mu g$[42]. Although observations indicate that brain catecholamines do not play an essential role in stress-induced activation of the pituitary–adrenal system[43], there is considerable evidence that the catecholamines, particularly norepinephrine, inhibit the ACTH–corticosteroid system[3,31,30,43,44]. It seems likely that norepinephrine rather than dopamine is the mediator in stress and that central α-adrenergic receptors are involved.

A number of observations support Ganong's hypothesis[30,31,35,43,44] that central norepinephrine regulates ACTH secretion at the hypothalamic level, probably by inhibiting corticotropin-releasing factor (CRF; corticoliberin) release. It has been suggested that the noradrenergic neurons end on the cell bodies and dendrites of the putative CRF-secreting neurons and act on them to inhibit their secretion. In studies *in vitro*, this inhibitory effect of norepinephrine was demonstrated directly on the hypothalamus[45,46]. Some observations argue for an intrahypothalamic localization of CRF-producing cell bodies[47,48]. Others, in contrast, claim that CRF cells are situated outside the medial-basal hypothalamus (in other hypothalamic areas or even outside it, see Makara, this volume) and that the high CRF activity found there[48,51] is due to the CRF stored in nerve terminals[49,50]. There has been considerable speculation[50,31] that norepinephrine modifies CRF release *via* axo-axonal synapses in the median eminence. However, stress failed to produce any changes either in norepinephrine or in dopamine concentrations in the median eminence[3,5]. In contrast, stress affected catecholamines in the arcuate nucleus: both norepinephrine and dopamine levels decreased acutely[3,5] and their synthesis rates increased in this nucleus but not in the median eminence.

It has been assumed that dopamine, in contrast to norepinephrine, exerts no appreciable effect on ACTH regulation[30,35]. However, the dopamine content in certain medial-basal hypothalamic cell groups, especially in the arcuate nucleus, decreases on stress stimuli, whereas it does not change in the other brain region studied[1,3,4]. Ether stress increases the dopamine synthesis rate in the arcuate nucleus but not in the residual hypothalamus[52]. Dopamine appears to stimulate other hypothalamic neuronal peptides (PIH (prolactostatin), LH-RH (luliberin)). Since stress affects both dopamine concentrations in the hypothalamus and a number of hypothalamic peptide activities[50], it is supposed that dopamine might participate in mediating stress-induced neurohormonal secretion other than that of CRF.

5-HT has been implicated in the control of ACTH secretion for a long time, but there are divergent views as to the character of its effect. Several investigators have proposed that 5-HT normally inhibits ACTH secretion[7,53,54], but others have been led to the opposite conclusion[46,55,56]. The overall response of 5-HT secretion to stressful stimuli in the central nervous system[8,9,12] suggests that 5-HT does participate in many aspects of the functioning of the neuroendocrine system including CRF–ACTH regulation.

CONCLUSION

Recent information indicates that stressful stimuli induce acute and chronic changes in the release and synthesis of biogenic amines in the central nervous system and suggest that biogenic amine-containing neurons may participate in the control of the CRF–ACTH secretory mechanism. The general importance of these mechanisms remains to be determined.

REFERENCES

1. Kvetňanský, R. *et al.* (1977). *The Pharmacologist* **19**, 241.
2. Stone, E. A. (1973). *J. Neurochem.* **21**, 589.
3. Palkovits, M. *et al.* (1975). *Neuroendocrinology* **18**, 144.
4. Kvetňanský, R. *et al.* (1976). *In* 'Catecholamines and Stress', (Usdin, E. *et al.* eds.), pp. 39–50 Pergamon, Oxford.

5. Kvetňanský, R. *et al.* (1977). *Neuroendocrinology* **23**, 257.
6. Kvetňanský, R. *et al.* (1978). *Brain Res.* **155**, 387.
7. Vermes, I. *et al.* (1974). *Acta. Physiol. Acad. Sci. Hung.* **43**, 33.
8. Telegdy, G. and Vermes, I. (1976). *In* 'Catecholamines and Stress', (Usdin, E. *et al.* eds.), pp. 145–156 Pergamon, Oxford.
9. Palkovits, M. *et al.* (1976). *Neuroendocrinology* **22**, 298.
10. Musacchio, J. M. *et al.* (1969). *Proc. Nat. Acad. Sci. USA.* **63**, 1117.
11. Zigmond, R. E. *et al.* (1974). *Brain Res.* **70**, 547.
12. Palkovits, M. *et al.* (1976). *In* "Catecholamines and Stress". (Usdin, E. *et al.* eds.), pp. 51–58, Pergamon, Oxford.
13. Bliss, E. L. *et al.* (1968). *J. Pharmacol. exp. Ther.* **164**, 122.
14. Thierry, A. M. *et al.* (1968). *Eur. J. Pharmacol.* **4**, 384.
15. Weiss, B. L. and Aghajanian, G. K. (1971). *Brain Res.* **26**, 27.
16. Bourgoin, S. *et al.* (1973). *Eur. J. Pharmacol.* **22**, 209.
17. Korf, J. *et al.* (1973). *Neurpharmacol.* **12**, 933.
18. Thierry, A. M. *et al.* (1968). *J. Pharmacol. Exp. Ther.* **163**, 163.
19. Stoner, H. B. and Elson, P. M. (1971). *J. Neurochem.* **18**, 1837.
20. Korf, J. *et al.* (1973). *Eur. J. Pharmacol.* **23**, 276.
21. Van Loon, G. R. (1976). *In* "Catecholamines and Stress", (Usdin, E. *et al.* eds.), pp. 77–78, Pergamon, Oxford.
22. Thierry, A. M. *et al.* (1970). *Eur. J. Pharmacol.* **10**, 129.
23. Thoenen, H. (1970). *Nature (London).* **228**, 861.
24. Axelrod, J. (1977). *Ann. N.Y. Acad. Sci.* **297**, 275.
25. Van Loon, G. R. *et al.* (1977). *Ann. N.Y. Acad. Sci.* **297**, 284.
26. Herman, J. P. *et al.* (1977). *Pol. J. Pharmacol.* **29**, 323.
27. Fekete, M. *et al.* (1976). *In* "Catecholamines and Stress", (Usdin, E. *et al.* eds.), pp. 69–75, Pergamon, Oxford.
28. Fekete, M. I. *et al.* (1978). *Neurosci. Lett.* **10**, 153.
29. Versteeg, D. H. G. and Wurtman, R. J. (1975). *Brain Res.* **93**, 552.
30. Ganong, W. F. (1972). *In* "Brain-Endocrine Interaction", (Knigge, K. M. *et al.* eds.), pp. 254–266, Karger, Basel.
31. Ganong, W. F. (1974). *In* "The Neurosciences: Third Study Program", (Schmidt, F. E. and Worden, F. G. eds.), pp. 549–563, Cambridge, Mass.
32. Vermes, I. and Telegdy, G. (1972). *Acta. Physiol. Acad. Sci. Hung.* **42**, 49.
33. Van Loon, G. R. (1973). *In* "Frontiers in Neuroendocrinology", (Ganong, W. F. and Martini, L. eds.), pp. 209–247, Oxford, New York.
34. Van Loon, G. R. (1974). *In* "Recent Studies of Hypothalamic Function", (Lederis, K. and Cooper, K. E., eds.), pp. 100–113, Karger, Basel.
35. Ganong, W. F. (1977). *Ann. N. Y. Acad. Sci.* **297**, 509.
36. Krieger, D. T. (1977). *Ann. N.Y. Acad. Sci.* **297**, 527.
37. Palkovits, M. (1977). *Ann. N.Y. Acad. Sci.* **297**, 455.
38. Van Loon, G. R. and Kragt, C. L. (1970). *Proc. Soc. Exp. Biol. Med.* **133**, 1137.
39. Vernikos-Danellis, J. *et al.* (1977). *Ann. N.Y. Acad. Sci.* **297**, 518.
40. Kraicer, J. and Morris, A. R. (1976). *Neuroendocrinol.* **21**, 175.
41. Saffran, M. and Schally, A. V. (1955). *Can. J. Biochem. Physiol.* **33**, 408.
42. Hiroshige, T. and Itoh, S. (1968). *Hokkaido Univ. Med. Library Series* **1**, 21.
43. Van Loon, G. R. *et al.* (1971). *Endocrinology* **89**, 1464.
44. Scapagnini, U. *et al.* (1972). *Neuroendocrinology* **10**, 155.
45. Jones, M. T. and Hillhouse, E. W. (1977). *Ann. N.Y. Acad. Sci.* **297**, 536.
46. Jones, M. T. *et al.* (1972). *Neuroendocrinology* **10**, 155.
47. Yasuda, N. and Greer, M. A. (1976). *Neuroendocrinology* **22**, 38.

10

THE SITE OF ORIGIN OF CORTICOLIBERIN (CRF)

G. B. Makara

Institute of Experimental Medicine, Hungarian Academy of Sciences
Budapest, Hungary

INTRODUCTION

Hypothalamic control of the pituitary–adrenal axis is currently thought to be mediated by an as-yet-unidentified corticotropin-releasing factor (corticoliberin, CRF), which is presumed to be produced by nerve cells located in the medial basal hypothalamus (MBH). With appropriate stimulation, CRF is released from axon terminals into the primary portal plexus of the median eminence (ME), and transported to the anterior pituitary lobe where it stimulates the release of corticotropin (ACTH) from the corticolipotrope cells. The consensus in this field is based on a body of evidence derived from various experiments which have used lesions, electrical stimulation and hypothalamic knife cuts and have tested both basal and stress-induced changes in ACTH and corticosteroid release as indices of CRF secretion.

The various other hypothalamo–pituitary–target organ systems were also thought to be organized along similar lines, the release of pituitary hormones being, in some cases, controlled by the interplay of stimulatory and inhibitory hypothalamic mediators whose cell bodies were believed to lie in the MBH. With the availability of refined bioassays and immunoassays as well as immunocyto-chemical methods for the chemically identified hypothalamic mediators, the hypothalamic organization of luteinizing hormone-releasing hormone (LHRH, luliberin), thyrotropin-releasing hormone (TRH, thyroliberin) and somatostatin-producing nerve cells have been studied in detail. Recent results have revealed widespread distribution of LHRH, TRH and somatostatin cell bodies not only within but outside of the MBH[1-3].

In the light of the findings that LHRH, TRH and somatostatin cell bodies lie outside of the MBH, although processes of all funnel to the median eminence

region, we have re-examined the evidence that CRF cell bodies and projections
are contained within the MBH.

Table I summarizes the main lines of evidence used to support the concept
that CRF-producing cells with their axonal projections are contained within the
MBH. An alternative hypothesis is that CRF-containing fibers come from some
other hypothalamic or extrahypothalamic brain areas and the fibers only traverse
the MBH on their way towards the stalk- median eminence (SME) and the neural
lobe (NL). We will argue that some of the evidence is ill-suited for distinguishing
between the two alternatives, and that other evidence for the established view
are not corroborated by recent studies in this laboratory.

Table I.   Evidence for the dominant role of the medial basal hypothalamus
(MBH) in the control of ACTH release from the anterior pituitary gland.

a. CRF activity is concentrated in the MBH and the SME[8,9].
b. Lesions of the MBH decrease resting pituitary–adrenal function[4].
c. Widespread lesions in the MBH block ACTH-release in response to some stressful stimuli[5].
d. Electrical stimulation of the MBH results in ACTH release[10,11].
e. Pituitary–adrenal function is best maintained if pituitary transplants are placed
   in the MBH in hypophysectomized rats[6,7].
f. Surgical isolation of the MBH is compatible with increased basal release of
   ACTH[12].
g. Surgical isolation of the MBH does not abolish ether-induced ACTH release,
   whereas removal of the viable MBH tissue prevents ether-induced release of
   ACTH[13-16].
h. CRF activity of the MBH is unchanged or elevated in rats with surgical
   isolation of the MBH[9,17].

Until histological methods can be developed for tracing the CRF-containing
fibers we have to rely on indirect evidence derived from biochemical and
endocrinological studies using various experimental interventions.

In this respect, not all the evidence carries the same weight since, in theory,
some experimental manipulations do not discriminate between these alternatives
(Table I, a–e). Under both hypotheses we would expect that CRF activity ought
to be mostly concentrated in the regions where the fibers release it into the
circulation, since it is well known that a variety of neurohormones and transmitters are most concentrated in those parts of the neuron where they are
released, i.e. the terminal arborization. In contrast, much smaller amounts of
CRF would be expected in areas containing dendrites and cell bodies. Similarly,
lesions placed in the MBH may destroy parts or all of the CRF-containing
system equally well under both hypotheses. Electrical stimulation in the MBH
should also indiscriminately activate the fibers and terminals of the CRF neurons
irrespective of whether the cell bodies are inside or outside the MBH. Stimulation
of other hypothalamic or extrahypothalamic regions also fails to differentiate
between the possibilities of activating the CRF cells or some excitatory pathways
to these cells. Studies of distribution of CRF-like activity in various areas of the
hypothalamus[8,9] may give some lead, but finding significant CRF activity in
areas outside the MBH may be explained also by postulating collaterals to various

hypothalamic nuclei besides the main projection to the SME (and neural lobe), or that in various areas of the brain CRF-like substances may subserve functions not related to the control of ACTH secretion.

Similarly, the fact that pituitary fragments transplanted to the "hypophysio-trophic area" can maintain some degree of adrenocortical activity may simply indicate that either the special blood circulation of the median eminence, pituitary stalk, and the arcuate–periventricular region[18,19] is best suited to maintain some degree of "autonomous" pituitary function or, more likely, that CRF is most concentrated in that region of the hypothalamus and thus it reaches the ACTH cells of the graft in sufficient amounts only when the tissue is placed in the immediate vicinity of the median eminence.

Theoretically, in the absence of specific histological methods, the experiments on animals with neurally isolated parts of the hypothalamus can give us the best evidence for the location of the CRF-producing perikarya, which project to the SME (Table I, f–h).

BASAL PITUITARY–ADRENAL FUNCTION IN RATS WITH PARTIAL OR COMPLETE SURGICAL ISOLATION OF THE MBH

The first studies demonstrated a significant increase in the morning levels of plasma corticosterone[12] and a substantial elevation of anterior pituitary content of ACTH at various times after placing a complete cut (CC) around the MBH[20]. Since it is well known that large lesions of the MBH result in a decrease of basal pituitary adrenal function[16], these data can be used as strong support for the hypothesis that the surgically isolated MBH contains all elements necessary for the basal control of ACTH secretion, and that the input from other brain regions play a predominantly inhibitory role[12]. Only the unchanged adrenal weight of these animals did not seem to fit into this hypothesis, implying chronically increased ACTH output.

Subsequent studies generated a controversy, since some laboratories consis-tently found increased basal corticosterone levels, whereas others, including our own, failed to find any change (see ref. 21). Careful re-evaluation of basal pituitary–adrenal function after isolation of the MBH, with special attention focused on the completeness of the surgical isolation, demonstrated no significant increase in plasma corticosterone level or in ACTH content of the anterior pituitary[21]. In a recent study[22] we realized the importance of meticulous care in the histological control of hypothalamic cuts, especially in the basal part of the lateral retrochiasmatic area (RCAL) where a small gap (as little as 50–100 μ) along the circumference of the cut seems to be sufficient to allow a stress-induced rise of plasma corticosterone. The simplest explanation for the above-mentioned controversy would be that, with the histological methods used in the earlier studies, small slabs of intact tissue were overlooked and thus the cuts were supposed to be complete; however, the unnoticed gaps allowed some stimulatory influence to reach the MBH and consequently the ACTH-secreting cells.

DIRECT CHEMICAL OR ELECTRICAL STIMULATION OF
THE ISOLATED MBH

If CRF-containing perikarya exist mainly within the MBH with their axons projecting directly to the SME, one would expect that either after surgical isolation of the MBH *in vivo*, or by incubating or culturing the MBH *in vitro* some basal CRF release would be maintained. Additionally, electrical stimulation or application of excitatory neurotransmitters should result in increased release of CRF under these conditions. Conversely, if the MBH after acute isolation contains only amputated axons, electrical stimulation would release CRF but we would expect no, or very little, response to excitatory transmitters, because these normally act at postsynaptic sites on dendrites and cell bodies; chronic isolation of the MBH should decrease or prevent both basal and stimulated release of CRF.

The first studies on the chemical sensitivity of ACTH release in rats with chronic CC around the MBH showed that some ACTH release can be elicited by convulsants antagonizing GABA action[23]. Surprisingly, however, intraventricularly infused glutamic acid[24] or various cholinomimetics, including acetylcholine, failed to increase ACTH release[25]. In parallel studies, Hillhouse *et al.* [26] showed that the whole hypothalamus, including some preoptic nuclei, releases CRF *in vitro* and that release can be stimulated by both acetylcholine[26] and serotonin[27,28] in minute amounts. In contrast, CRF release from a smaller hypothalamic fragment (essentially the MBH + SME) was unchanged by these putative excitatory transmitters[27]. Thus results obtained with chemical stimulation argue against the existence of a substantial number of CRF-containing cells within the MBH; although one can devise alternative explanations, too[25].

In the first experiments deliberately designed to test the postulated location of the CRF cells, we used electrical stimulation in rats with various cuts around the MBH[29]. Rats with CC or anterolateral cut (ALC) around the MBH were implanted with electrodes 7 to 8 days after hypothalamic surgery and subjected to various stimulation protocols (see legends of Figs. 1 and 2) designed to activate most of the intrahypothalamic nerve fibers Blood was withdrawn from a vein before and 30 min after the stimulation and the difference in corticosterone level between the two samples was used as an index of ACTH secretion. In some experiments the rats were pretreated with dexamethasone, morphine and Nembutal[R][11] to maintain low basal levels when the prestimulus corticosterone level might have been elevated by the stressful manipulation involved in the placement of the electrode(s).

Electrical stimulation in controls, both with and without pharmacological pretreatment, produced significant and similar increments of plasma corticosterone (see controls in Figs. 1 and 2). Rats with CC had low prestimulus corticosterone levels even without pretreatment, which agrees with previous findings[22]. Only one of the 19 test rats showed an increment of plasma corticosterone above $0.3\mu mol/1$, whereas the mean increment in the controls was well above that. Since 9 of the 19 rats with CC were stimulated with an electrode array at six different points within the isolated MBH, we think that most of the isolated tissue was reached by the stimulation (Fig. 1).

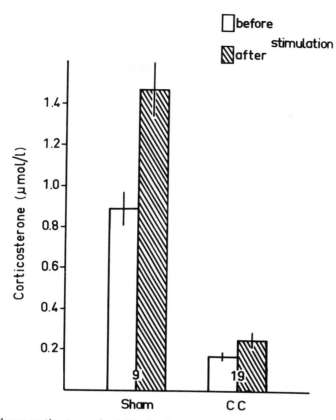

Fig. 1. Plasma corticosterone level 30 min after electrical stimulation in pentobarbitone-anesthetized rats. Sham, sham-operated controls; CC, rats with a complete cut around the MBH, 7–8 days postoperatively. About half of the rats in each group were stimulated with ± 200 μA, 60/sec, 10 sec on – 10 sec off, for 10 min. Other half received ± 100 μA trains for 1 min through each of three electrode pairs. In this and all subsequent Figures, columns denote the mean and bars, the S.E.M.

Similar results were obtained when the posterior and some posterolateral pathways to the MBH were left intact by the anterolateral cut (ALC). Animals in which the knife did not interrupt all fibers in the RCAL were grouped separately. Electrical stimulation of the MBH in rats with ALC was ineffective in raising plasma corticosterone whereas in those rats in which the RCAL was not transected on at least one side a significant rise was obtained (Fig. 2). The lack of response to electrical stimulation was maintained also at 3 weeks after the operation and also if after unilateral ALC the electrodes were placed in the ipsilateral half of the MBH. This latter finding suggests that no substantial crossing of fibers containing CRF occurs within the MBH. Parasagittal cuts leaving anterior fibers intact also blocked the response to stimulation (Fig. 2).

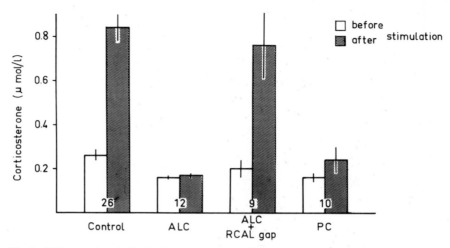

Fig. 2. Effect of electrical stimulation (200 μA; 60/sec; 10 sec on- 10 sec off for 10 min) on plasma corticosterone levels in pharmacologically blocked rats. ALC, anterolateral cut around the MBH; RCAL, lateral retrochiasmatic area; PC, parasagittal cuts through RCAL.

These results clearly show that the effectiveness of electrical stimulation to elicit ACTH release is dependent on intact connections coming from an antero-lateral direction and also that a significant portion of the necessary fibers enter the MBH through the RCAL. One possible way to reconcile these data with an intra-MBH location of the CRF cells is to postulate that the surgery produced a selective loss of excitatory elements (fibres and cells) in the MBH and left intact a dominant local inhibitory circuit which is so powerful that after electrical stimulation it is able to suppress even the electrically activated release of CRF. We tried to exclude this possibility by collecting corroborative evidence using different approaches.

CRF CONTENT IN THE STALK-MEDIAN EMINENCE (SME) OF THE ISOLATED MBH

If the bulk of the CRF-containing fibers in the SME originated from perikarya within the MBH then we would expect CRF to be present in substantial amounts even after surgical isolation of this region, irrespective of whether the balance of excitation and inhibition of the tissue is shifted towards inhibition. Thus measurements of CRF in the chronically isolated MBH may be a valuable aid in localizing the origin of the CRF fibers

We used manual micro-dissection of the SME from fresh unfrozen brain and analyzed the sections from paraffin-embedded hypothalamus to determine both the extent of the excisions and the configuration of the cut (Fig. 3). CRF was extracted by ice-cold 0.1 M HCL and the freeze-dried extracts were individually assayed by a miniaturized version of a bioassay using cultured anterior pituitary

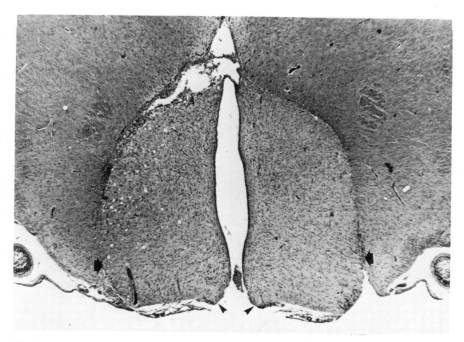

Fig. 3.   Coronal section through the anterior median eminence. Arrows point to the cut (ALC), arrowheads point to lateral border of excised SME.

cells[30,31]. ACTH released into the medium was measured by a radioimmuno-assay that was validated by parallel bioassay on dispersed adrenal cells.

In the first experiment, none of the extracts (0.4 SME equivalents (equ.)) from eight rats with CC contained detectable CRF activity, whereas all control extracts stimulated ACTH release at a dose of 0.1 SME equ. In a second experiment, extracts taken 7 or 8 days postoperatively from rats with ALC showed no detectable activity with 0.25 SME equ., whereas in the controls one-tenth of this dose (0.025 SME equ.) caused significant ACTH release (Fig. 4). CRF was also undetectable in 0.25 SME equ. derived from rats with ALC when the samples were taken at the end of, or 30 min after, a 2 min exposure to ether vapour[32]. In preliminary experiments even 1.25 SME equ. of a pool collected from rats with ALC failed to release significant amount of ACTH. These data suggest that at least 90% of the CRF activity disappears from the neurohemal regions of the SME within 8 days after transecting all nerve fibers entering the MBH from anterior and/or lateral directions, presumably due to disappearance of the degenerated nerve fibers. In the hypothalamus, fibre degeneration is known to proceed rapidly so that most of the fibers are eliminated between 2 and 3 days after transection. Similarly, the antidiuretic activity of the neural lobe decreases significantly between 1 and 3 days after transecting the hypothalamic-neurophysophyseal tract by stalk lesions[33]. The time course of the change in CRF activity of the SME after placing an ALC seems to be roughly parallel with

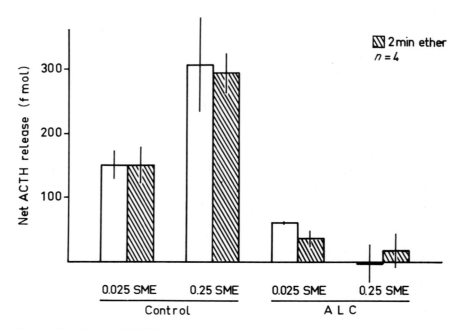

Fig. 4. Net release of ACTH in anterior pituitary cell cultures after addition of SME extract from rats with an anterolateral cut (ALC) around the MBH. Basal release in the presence of equivalent amount of cerebral cortical extract is subtracted.

these findings (Fig. 5). On the first postoperative day, there was no significant change, but a significant decrease had occurred after 3 days when the SME still contained detectable CRF activity, which disappeared by day 7.

These results agree well with those obtained by direct electrical and chemical stimulation of the isolated MBH but are in sharp contrast with two sets of reports, claiming: 1. that *CRF content of the MBH* is unchanged or even elevated[9,17] in rats with CC, and 2. that ether inhalation in CC rats stimulates ACTH release[13–16].

In our opinion, the discrepancy between the CRF results of others and our own can be explained by either one or both of two essential differences in design. First, in both studies a large piece of MBH was extracted together with unspecified amounts of median eminence and stalk tissue, whereas we used the anatomically specified median eminence and the stalk (SME). The MBH contains significantly less CRF per unit volume than the SME, and it might contain a substantial background of non-specific substances so that the relatively large non-specific influence of tissue extract may mask any specific change in the SME. Also, if CRF remains in the MBH but disappears from the SME, CRF-like material in the MBH may not fulfill a hormone-releasing role since according to the established neurohumoral theory of pituitary control, any mediator should first be transported to the periportal pools of the SME (and neurohypophysis) and then be released into the blood for transport to the pituitary.

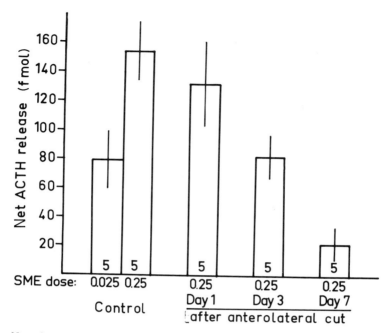

Fig. 5.   Net release of ACTH in anterior pituitary cell cultures in response to SME from rats with hypothalamic surgery.

The second difference between experiments of others and our own is that in one of the cited studies histological check of the hypothalamic cuts was omitted[17] and in the other it was performed on widely spaced (300μm) cryostat sections[9]. Cryostat sections are by necessity inferior in quality to good paraffin sections and, because of the spacing, even large contingents of uncut fibers entering the MBH (and SME) from outside might have remained undetected.

Although CRF content is probably not a good indicator of the ability of the MBH to release CRF (and consequently ACTH) it is nevertheless difficult to reconcile the large fall in CRF content of the SME in rats with CC with the compelling argument that pituitary-adrenal response to ether anesthesia is normal in rats with CC. This prompted us to re-investigate whether rats with histologically demonstrated CC or ALC do release ACTH in response to ether inhalation.

THE PITUITARY-ADRENAL RESPONSE TO ETHER AFTER ISOLATION OF THE MBH

As most of the earlier studies used plasma corticosterone as an index of ACTH secretion, we first repeated those studies using postoperative periods ranging from 1 to 28 days, groups of female as well as male rats and various sampling

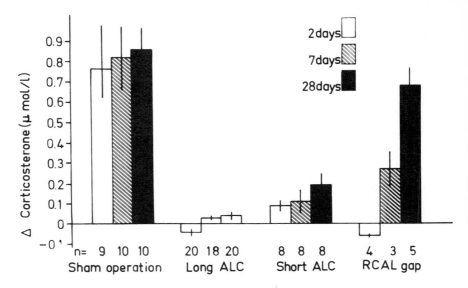

Fig. 6. Pituitary-adrenal response to ether–venesection stress in rats with short or long anterolateral cuts (ALC) around the MBH at various times after the operation. Δ, Increment over basal level.

protocols[34]. In five of the six experimental series ether was completely ineffective in raising plasma corticosterone levels in rats with either CC or ALC 1, 2, 7 or 28 days after the operation. In a single experiment, the response of female rats with ALC was strongly inhibited but not completely prevented. Results from a representative experiment are shown in Fig. 6. The configuration of the hypothalamic cut was studied on frequently taken coronal section of MBH and the rats were grouped as having a long ALC (extending behind the level of the middle median eminence), short ALC (ending at the level of the anterior ME) or RCAL gap with some uncut fibers entering the MBH in this region. Both the short and the long ALC prevented the ether-induced rise of plasma corticosterone although in the rats with short ALC a tendency to respond appeared by the 28th day. In contrast, the group with RCAL gap showed significant stress-induced increments by the 7th postoperative day and the response returned to almost normal by the 28th day.

A substantial ether-induced rise in immunoreactive plasma ACTH level was reported by Allen *et al.*[35] in adrenalectomized rats with either CC or ALC. We used rats in which adrenalectomy and hypothalamic cuts were performed in one session[36]. At 7 to 8 days later, some of the rats were anesthetized with ether for 3 min and plasma ACTH was measured by radioimmunoassay. Ether induced a rise in plasma ACTH *only* if some fibers in the RCAL remained uncut (Table II).

Possible reasons for disagreement between the present data and most previous studies are discussed elsewhere[34]; here we would only emphasize again the difference in the histological control. The frozen sections used by others[13,15] precluded evaluation of fine morphological details; thus the simplest explanation

Table II.   The effect of 3 min of ether inhalation on the plasma ACTH level of adrenalectomized (adrex) rats with antero-lateral cut (ALC) around the MBH.

Group	Immunoreactive ACTH (pg/ml of plasma)	
	Basal	After 3 min of ether
Adrex + hypothalamic sham operation	592 ± 84 (13)[a]	1590 ± 187 (12)[b]
Adrex + ALC with gap in the RCAL	193 ± 128 (3)	600 ± 96 (4)[c]
Adrex + ALC	94 ± 15 (10)[d]	109 ± 19 (9)

[a]   Mean ± S.E.M. (number of rats).
[b]   Significantly different from control in the same row ($p < 0.01$).
[c]   Significantly different from control in the same row ($p < 0.05$).
[d]   Significantly different from sham-operated basal level ($p < 0.01$).

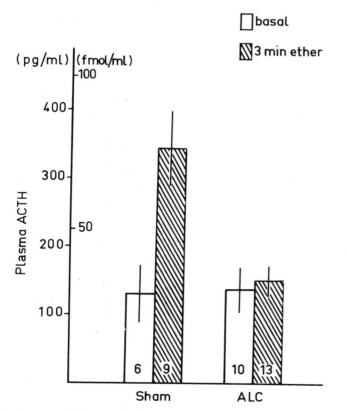

Fig. 7.   Plasma ACTH levels after 3 min of ether exposure in rats 2 h after cutting anterolateral fibre connections of the MBH.

for the discrepancy is that previously observed pituitary–adrenal responses in rats with CC or ALC were due to some unnoticed fibers entering the MBH island somewhere along the RCAL.

The question remains, however, whether the fibers coming from the direction of the RCAL carry CRF to the SME or some trophic influence to the cells of the MBH. If it is the loss of a trophic influence that in the rats with ALC prevents ACTH release from occurring normally after ether inhalation, then one would expect a normal response to ether a few hours after transection of the fibers, partly because CRF within the SME is known to be available within 24 h of placing an ALC. To choose between these alternatives, an experiment was performed 2 h after placing an ALC under ether anesthesia, with some rats reexposed to ether for 3 min before decapitation. The basal levels of plasma ACTH were similar in the sham-operated and the ALC groups, but ether anesthesia raised plasma ACTH only in the former group (Fig. 7). These results argue for the alternative that the cut amputated the CRF fibers from their perikarya since the site of ether action is probably not at the axon terminals but at the soma–dendritic level or at neural elements that give rise to synaptic input to the CRF cells.

In Table III we have summarized the arguments that support the idea that most of the CRF fibers in the SME originate from outside the MBH.

Table III.   Evidence for CRF-perikarya being outside the MBH.

a. No rise in basal ACTH release in rats with CC or ALC[21].
b. Serotonin and acetylcholine stimulate CRF release *in vitro* only when hypothalamic fragments are larger than the MBH[27].
c. Intraventricular acetylcholine or glutamate fails to release ACTH in rats with CC[24,25].
d. Electrical stimulation of MBH fails to release ACTH after cutting the anterolateral connections to the MBH[29].
e. Ether fails to release ACTH if *all* anterolateral connections to the MBH are cut, but does so in rats with RCAL gap[34,36].
f. CRF content of the SME *proper* falls in rats with CC or ALC[32].

THE STATUS OF NEUROHYPOPHYSIAL CRF

Although it has been known for a long time that a substantial amount of CRF activity is present in the neural lobe (NL) of the pituitary gland, very little is known about its origin and role in controlling the pituitary adrenal activity. Recent mapping studies[8,9] found significant amounts of CRF-like activity in the supraoptic, suprachiasmatic and paraventricular nuclei and since the magno-cellular nuclei have well-known projections to the NL, the question arises whether CRF in the neurohypophysis (NL-CRF) originates from the magnocellular neurones.

When considering this question, two points should be emphasized. First, it seems clear that vasopressin itself is not the physiological CRF[37]. Secondly, a number of workers have shown that neurosecretory material, neurophysin and vasopressin fibres that originate in the paraventricular nuclei, terminate in the external zone of the SME and that their staining intensity varies apparently in parallel with the activity of the pituitary–adrenal axis (for ref. see 38–40).

Recent measurements[31,41] of NL-CRF and SME-CRF agree that the amounts in the neural lobe are of the same order of magnitude as in the SME. In our hands, NL-CRF seems to comprise about a quarter of all CRF present in the whole neurohemal complex of the rat[31]. However, there are virtually no data on whether NL-CRF is ever released into the blood and can stimulate the corticotroph cells.

Electrical stimulation of the NL appears to be a method suitable for studying this problem. We used rats in which the response to the surgical stress associated with the placing of electrodes via the parapharyngeal approach was blocked by pretreatment with dexamethasone, morphine and Nembutal, and sampled venous blood both before and 20 min after 3 min of electrical stimulation[42]. The procedure itself had no ACTH-releasing effect in the pharmacologically blocked animals when the electrodes were simply pushed against the surface of the anterior lobe; however, stimulation in the NL sharply raised plasma corticosterone levels (Fig. 8), and this rise was completely prevented by cutting anterior and lateral afferents to the MBH. If such cuts completely transect the RCAL, they result in a virtually complete loss of neurosecretory material from the NL. A substantial concomitant atrophy of the NL develops, which is probably due to the peculiar anatomical arrangement of the fibers of the paraventricular magnocellular neurones. The tract of neurosecretory fibers leaves this nucleus near its upper lateral pole and first it is directed laterally then down toward the far lateral

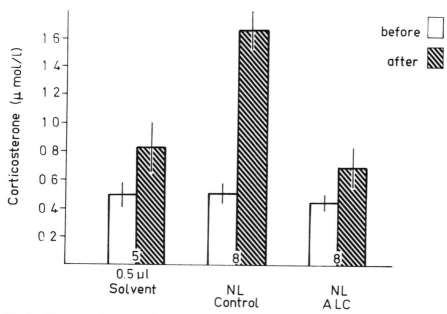

Fig. 8.   Plasma corticosterone level before and 20 min after electrical stimulation (200 μA; 60/sec; 3 min) or the anterior lobe (AL) or the neural lobe (NL) of the pituitary in pharmacologically blocked rats. ALC, anterolateral cut.

retrochiasmatic area where it joins the fibers coming from the supraoptic nuclei; thus sections of the RCAL can transect most, if not all, the fibers coming from the main magnocellular nuclei.

In parallel studies we placed large or small knife lesions in the region of the paraventricular nuclei. Large lesions destroyed an inverted cone of tissue of about 3.5 mm in diameter, whereas the small lesions destroyed all the paraventricular magnocellular cells and their immediate surroundings. When, 7 to 8 days later, the NL of the lesioned rats was stimulated under pharmacological blockade, a rise in plasma corticosterone occurred but it was significantly smaller than that observed in the control animals, irrespective of the lesion size (Fig. 9).

These studies provided the first experimental demonstration that neural lobe CRF can be released *in vivo* to stimulate ACTH secretion and that the nerve fibers that contain the NL-CRF originate from outside the MBH; moreover, a significant portion of these fibers probably come from or through the region of the paraventricular nuclei.

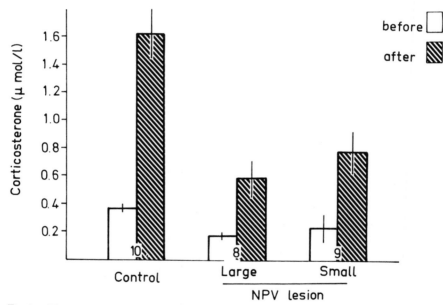

Fig. 9.   Plasma corticosterone level before and 20 min after electrical stimulation (± 200 μA; 60/sec; 3 min) of the neural lobe of rats 7–8 days after lesions of the paraventricular nucleus (NPV).

The conclusion about the origin of the NL-CRF is partly supported by bioassay of CRF in extracts from NL taken 7 to 8 days after transection of the anterior and lateral fiber connections of the MBH[43]. In such an experiment it is necessary to clean the NL from any adherent intermediate lobe tissue since the latter contains ACTH and related peptides that may interfere both in the bioassay and the subsequent radioimmunoassay of the secreted ACTH. Removal of the intermediate lobe tissue was performed by suction through a fine tube under high magnification of a dissecting microscope. Individual neural lobes were extracted with 0.1M HCl, freeze-dried and assayed on a tissue culture of anterior lobe cells[31]. At 7 days after anterolateral isolation of the MBH, neural lobe CRF content was undetectable and the comparison with the activity in the control extracts suggests that at least 90% of the CRF activity is lost (Fig. 10).

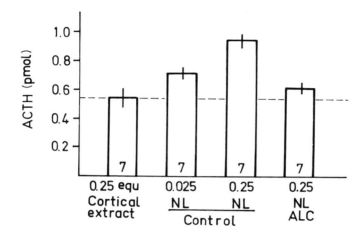

Fig. 10.   ACTH release by anterior pituitary cell cultures after addition of neural lobe (NL) extract from rats with anterolateral cut (ALC) around the MBH.

Although these studies seem to exclude an intra-MBH origin for the NL-CRF, they fail to prove that the origin is in the magnocellular neurones. It is equally possible that CRF is transported within axons that run along the hypothalamo-neurohypophysial tract but originate from the parvicellular neurons.

Also, we can only speculate about the possible routes whereby NL-CRF may reach the ACTH-producing cells. Theoretically, there are several possibilities. In the rat, substances from the neural lobe might reach nearby ACTH cells by diffusion, by the blood circulating through the short vessels bridging the layer of intermediate lobe that separates the neural and anterior lobes, or by the blood from the neural lobe, which may reach the plexus in the stalk and median eminence *via* the interconnected vascular system[44] where it may be mixed with the flow that irrigates the sinusoids of the anterior lobe. In addition, one should also consider the possibility that CRF-containing axons that reach the NL may give off several collaterals in the SME and such collaterals may release CRF when the action potential generated in the NL excite them antidromically. With such an anatomical arrangement, the CRF fibers of the NL should work in parallel with some CRF fibers in the SME, each releasing its mediator into the blood in different parts of the same interconnected vascular system.

In conclusion, recent studies with hypothalamic regions isolated *in vivo* or *in vitro* suggest that the fibers that release CRF in the SME and the NL originate predominantly from outside the MBH. Placing anterolateral or complete cuts around the MBH when the knife transects *all* nerve fibers along the intended cuts, results in no elevation in resting plasma corticosterone levels or ACTH content of the anterior pituitary and loss of CRF release after electrical, direct chemical or ether-induced stimulation.

At this point, however, it should be emphasized that the physiological neurohumoral mechanism that mediates the control of the hypothalamic-pituitary–adrenal system can also be bypassed by various routes and thus animals may respond with ACTH release to various stimuli even after transection or complete destruction of the CRF-containing elements of the hypothalamus. Some stimuli such as bacterial endotoxin[45,46] or severe surgery[47] are capable of inducing adrenocortical activation even after removal or destruction of the whole medial hypothalamus, although the physiological relevance of this phenomenon might be questioned. Similarly, rats with complete hypothalamic cuts around the MBH respond to drugs that interfere with neurotransmitter metabolism or action even when the RCAL is completely transected[23,48]. All these phenomena suggest that if the stimulation is really powerful and/or lasting either "tissue CRF"[49] or CRF of neural origin may reach the pituitary *via* the systemic circulation, possibly *via* diffusion or *via* newly formed vascular channels.

ACKNOWLEDGEMENTS

The data and ideas presented in this Chapter resulted from studies conducted in collaboration with Prof. E. Stark, Mrs. E. Fellinger, Drs. M. Karteszi, M. Palkovits and G. Rappay.

REFERENCES

1. Brownstein, M. J. *et al.* (1976). *Endocrinology* **98**, 662.
2. Brownstein, M. J. *et al.* (1975). *Proc. Nat. Acad. Sci. USA*, **72**, 4177.
3. Brownstein, M. J. *et al.* (1977). *Endocrinology* **100** 246.
4. Szentágothai, J. *et al.* (1978). *In* "Hypothalamic Control of the Anterior Pituitary", pp. 220–248, Akademiai Kiado, Budapest.
5. Brodish, A. (1963). *Endocrinology* **73**, 727.
6. Halász, B. *et al.* (1965). *Endocrinology* **77**, 343.
7. Csernus, V. *et al.* (1975). *Neuroendocrinol.* **17**, 18.
8. Lang, R. E. *et al.* (1976). *Neurosci. Lett.* **2**, 19.
9. Krieger, D. T. *et al.* (1977). *Endocrinology* **100**, 227.
10. Redgate, E. S. and Fahringer, E. E. (1973). *Neuroendocrinol.* **12**, 334.
11. Dunn, J. and Critchlow, V. (1973). *Endocrinology* **93**, 835.
12. Halász, B. *et al.* (1967). *Neuroendocrinol.* **2**, 43.
13. Feldman, S. *et al.* (1970). *Acta Endocrinol.* **63**, 405.
14. Greer, M. A. and Rockie, C. (1968). *Endocrinology* **83**, 1247.
15. Palka, Y. *et al.* (1969). *Neuroendocrinol.* **5**, 333.
16. Dunn, J. and Critchlow, V. (1973). *Proc. Soc. Exp. Biol. Med.* **142**, 749.

17. Yasuda, N. and Greer, M. A. (1976). *Neuroendocrinol.* **22**, 48.
18. Ambach, G. *et al.* (1976). *Acta Morph. Acad. Sci. Hung.* **24**, 93.
19. Sétalo, G. *et al.* (1976). *Acta Morph. Acad. Sci. Hung.* **24**, 79.
20. Halász, B. *et al.* (1967). *Endocrinology* **81**, 921.
21. Stark, E., Makara, G. B., Palkovits, M., Kórteszi, M. and Mihaly, K. (1978). *Endoc. Exp.* **12**, 209.
22. Palkovits, M. *et al.* (1976). *Neuroendocrinol.* **21**, 280.
23. Makara, G. B. and Stark, E. (1974). *Neuroendocrinol.* **16**, 178.
24. Makara, G. B. and Stark, E. (1975). *Neuroendocrinol.* **18**, 213.
25. Makara, G. B. and Stark, E. (1976). *Neuroendocrinol.* **21**, 31.
26. Hillhouse, E. W. *et al.* (1975). *Neuroendocrinol.* **17**, 1.
27. Jones, M. T. and Hillhouse, E. W. (1977). *Ann. N.Y. Acad. Sci.* **297**, 536.
28. Jones, M. T. *et al.* (1976). *In* "Frontiers of Neuroendocrinology", Vol. 4. (Martini, L. and Ganong, W. F. eds.), Raven Press, New York.
29. Makara, G. B., Stark, E. and Palkovits, M. (1978). *Neuroendocrinol.* **27**, 109.
30. Takebe, K. *et al.* (1975). *Endocrinology* **97**, 1248.
31. Kórteszi, M., Stark, E., Makara, G. B., Fazekas, I. and Rappay, G. (1979). *Endocrinol. Exp.* **12**, 204.
32. Makara, G. B., Stark, E., Rappay, G., Karteszi, M. and Palkovits, M. (1979). *Endocrinology* **12**, 204.
33. Laszlo, F. A. and De Wied, D. (1966). *J. Endocrinol.* **36**, 125.
34. Makara, G. B., Stark, E. and Palkovits, M. (1979). *Neuroendocrinol. (in press)*
35. Allen, C. F. *et al.* (1974). *Proc. Soc. Exp. Biol. Med.* **146**, 840.
36. Kórteszi, M., Makara, G. B. and Stark, E. (1979). *Acta Endocrinol.* Submitted.
37. Saffran, M. and Schally, A. V. (1977). *Ann. N.Y. Acad. Sci.* **297**, 95.
38. Bock, R. and Jurna, I. (1977). *Cell Tiss. Res.* **185**, 215.
39. Zimmerman, E. A. *et al.* (1977). *Ann. N.Y. Acad. Sci.* **297**, 405.
40. Vandesande, F. *et al.* (1977). *Cell Tiss. Res.* **180**, 443.
41. Yasuda, N. *et al.* (1977). *J. Endocrinol.* **75**, 293.
42. Fellinger, E., Stark, E. and Makara, G. B. *In preparation.*
43. Kórteszi, M., Stark, E., Rappay, G., Szabo, D., Fellinger, R. and Makara, G. B. *In preparation.*
44. Page, R. B. and Bergland, R. M. (1977). *Am. J. Anat.* **148**, 345.
45. Makara, G. B. *et al.* (1971). *Endocrinology* **88**, 412.
46. Stark, E. *et al.* (1973/4). *Neuroendocrinol.* **13**, 224.
47. Lymangrover, J. R. and Brodish, A. (1973). *Neuroendocrinol.* **12**, 225.
48. Makara, G. B. and Stark, E. (1978). Role of GABA in the hypothalamic control of the pituitary gland. *In* "Interactions Between Putative Neurotransmitters in the Brain". (Garattini, S., *et al.* eds.), pp. 263–281, Raven Press, New York.
49. Brodish, A. (1977). *Ann. N.Y. Acad. Sci.* **297**, 420.

11

THE SECRETION OF CORTICOTROPIN-RELEASING HORMONE IN VITRO: EFFECTS OF NEUROTRANSMITTER SUBSTANCES, DRUGS AND CORTICOSTEROIDS

Julia C. Buckingham and J. R. Hodges

Neuroendocrine Unit,
Royal Free Hospital, Clinical Sciences Building,
London NW3 2QG, UK.

INTRODUCTION

The secretion of corticotropin (ACTH) is dependent on the functional integrity of the hypothalamus and is controlled by a corticotropin-releasing hormone or factor (CRH or CRF, corticoliberin) which is secreted by neurons in the median basal hypothalamus and conveyed to the adenohypophysis by the hypothalamo–hypophyseal portal vessels. The activity of the CRH-producing neurons is under the control of various excitatory and inhibitory nervous pathways from higher centres in the brain and many parts of the central nervous system are now known to affect profoundly the secretion of ACTH. Although many experimental methods (e.g. placing lesions in or stimulation of discrete areas of the brain) have been used, our knowledge still does not enable us to define clearly the importance of the various regions of the brain in the regulation of hypothalamo-pituitary–adrenocortical activity.

EFFECTS OF NEUROTRANSMITTERS AND DRUGS ON THE RELEASE OF CRH

A new approach to the study of hypothalamic pathways and the receptors which they innervate was made by Bradbury, Burden, Hillhouse and Jones[1] and Jones, Hillhouse and Burden[2] which showed that the rat hypothalamus is

capable of producing releasing hormones *in vitro* and responds to various neurotransmitter substances with changes in the degree of its functional activity. We
have extended their work and improved the method by using a more sensitive
and precise assay for CRH. Hypothalami were removed from rats immediately
after decapitation, incubated in an artificial medium and challenged with
neurotransmitter substances and drugs as described by Buckingham and Hodges[3].
The CRH concentrations in the hypothalami and the medium in which they had
been incubated were determined immediately by a method which depends on the
ability of the releasing hormone to stimulate anterior pituitary tissue to synthesize
and release ACTH[4].

Acetylcholine (1 pM – 1 nM), other cholinomimetic drugs and 5-hydroxy-
tryptamine (1 nM – 1 μM; 5-HT) increase both the content of CRH in the
hypothalami and the amount of hormone released into the medium; their effects
are dose-related. Of the many polypeptides and other neurotransmitter substances
tested, only angiotensin II and its 5-isoleucine analogue resemble cholinomimetic
substances and 5-HT in their ability to increase significantly both the CRH release
and content of the hypothalamus. On the other hand, noradrenaline significantly
reduces the spontaneous release of CRH into the medium. It also reduces the
rises in hypothalamic CRH release and content induced by acetylcholine or 5-HT.
These data suggest the presence in the hypothalamus of cholinoceptors, 5-HT
receptors and adrenoceptors all of which are concerned with the control of the
synthesis and release of CRH.

Although it is well established that the release of CRH is under the stimulatory
influence of cholinergic fibres, the role of 5-HT is still controversial. Our work
agrees with the bulk of the evidence that 5-HT, like acetylcholine, stimulates
CRH release. The results with noradrenaline support the hypothesis[5] that the
amine plays an inhibitory role in the control of hypothalamo–pituitary–adrenocortical activity.

The cholinoceptors exist as a mixed population of muscarinic and nicotinic
receptors since, although nicotine and bethanechol cause dose-related increases
in CRH secretion, their maximal effects are considerably less than those of
acetylcholine. Further, the actions of bethanechol and nicotine are completely
inhibited by their competitive antagonists atropine and pempidine respectively,
whereas those of acetylcholine are reduced by either antagonist but completely
inhibited only when the two are given together (Fig. 1). These results are not
in complete agreement with those of Hillhouse, Burden and Jones[6] who claimed
that the cholinoceptors are predominantly nicotinic since bethanechol did not
stimulate CRH secretion in their preparation. 5-HT evokes CRH secretion by
stimulating specific receptors since its effects are competitively antagonized by
methysergide and by cyproheptadine. The suggestion has been made[2] that the
actions of 5-HT are effected by intermediary cholinergic neurons because they
are inhibited by hexamethonium. Our data do not agree with the existence of
such an intermediary nervous pathway since the effects of 5-HT are not affected
by pempidine or hexamethonium in concentrations that maximally antagonize
the actions of acetylcholine.

It is generally agreed that noradrenergic nervous pathways exert an inhibitory
influence on the secretion of CRH, but it is not yet established whether the effect
is mediated via α- or β-adrenoceptors. Our results, like those of Jones *et al.*[6],
showed that only α-adrenoceptors are important in this respect since the actions

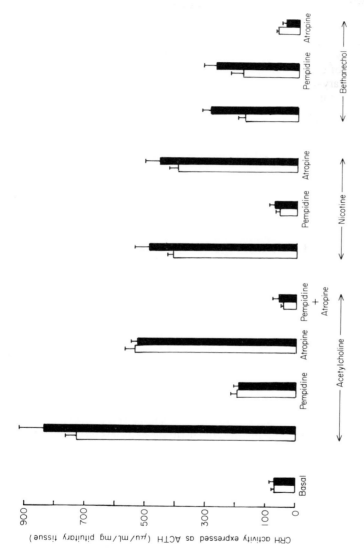

Fig. 1. The effects of pempidine (10 nM) and atropine (20 nM) on hypothalamic CRH production induced by acetylcholine (0.1 nM), nicotine (1 μM) or bethanechol (5 μM). □, CRH release; ■, CRH content. Each column is the mean of five determinations and is shown with its standard error.

of noradrenaline are mimicked by adrenaline and the specific α-adrenoceptor agonists phenylephrine and methoxamine, but not by the β-adrenoceptor agonist isoprenaline. Further, they are antagonized by the α-adrenoceptor antagonist phentolamine, but not by the β-adrenoceptor antagonist atenolol.

EFFECT OF CORTICOSTEROIDS ON THE RELEASE OF CRH

The importance of corticosteroids in controlling the functional activity of the hypothalamo–pituitary–adrenocortical system is well recognized but their site and mode of action is not clear. In one of our studies[7] we found that adrenalectomy caused a rise, corticosterone treatment a fall and stress a fall followed by a rise in hypothalamic CRH content in the rat. Also, stress-induced changes in hypothalamic CRH content, like those in pituitary and plasma ACTH, were exaggerated in adrenalectomized rats but normal in adrenalectomized rats maintained on corticosterone. Further, the ability to synthesize and release CRH *in vitro* was enhanced in hypothalami removed from adrenalectomized rats but was reduced in those removed from corticosterone-treated animals. The data suggest that the corticosteroids act on the hypothalamus or on higher centres in the brain to modulate the stress-induced release of corticotropin.

Experiments in which corticosterone was added to the incubation medium containing the rat hypothalami showed that the steroid does not influence the basal activity of the hypothalamus, but like noradrenaline it reduces the amount of CRH released into the medium when the hypothalami are challenged with acetylcholine or 5-HT. However, in contrast to noradrenaline, corticosterone potentiates the rise in hypothalamic CRH content induced by acetylcholine or 5-HT. Thus the steroid inhibits the release but not the synthesis of CRH. Many other workers have suggested the presence of corticosteroid receptors in the hypothalamus but there is a considerable amount of evidence to suggest that they also exist elsewhere in the central nervous system.

Although data from experiments *in vitro* cannot always be translated to the situation *in vivo*, the use of the isolated hypothalamus as a physiological model for studying the mechanisms controlling its functional activity has obvious advantages over more conventional methods (e.g. lesioning and implantation techniques) because these usually involve the disturbance of less-discrete, ill-defined areas of the brain.

The production of CRH by the isolated hypothalamus in response to neurotransmitter substances is very consistent, and the use of a sensitive and precise bioassay method for its determination has yielded data with remarkable precision. Studies on the effects of steroids, neurotransmitter substances and drugs, which mimic or antagonize their effects, on the production of releasing hormones will inevitably lead to a better understanding of the physiology of the hypothalamus.

REFERENCES

1. Bradbury, M. W. B. *et al.* (1974). *J. Physiol.* **239**, 269.
2. Jones, M. T. *et al.* (1976). *J. Endocrinol.* **69**, 1.
3. Buckingham, J. C. and Hodges, J. R. (1977). *J. Physiol.* **272**, 469.

4. Buckingham, J. C. and Hodges, J. R. (1977). *J. Endocrinol.* **72**, 187.
5. Ganong, W. F. (1975). *In* "Hypothalamic Hormones" (Motta, M. *et al.* eds.), Academic Press, New York.
6. Hillhouse, E. W. *et al.* (1975). *Neuroendocrinol.* **17**, 1.
7. Buckingham, J. C. (1979). *J. Physiol.* **286**, 331.

12

THE ROLE OF γ-AMINOBUTYRIC ACID (GABA) IN CONTROLLING CORTICOLIBERIN (CRF) SECRETION

G. B. Makara

*Institute of Experimental Medicine, Hungarian Academy of Sciences
Budapest, Hungary*

INTRODUCTION

The likely candidacy of γ-aminobutyric acid (GABA), as an inhibitory transmitter involved in the regulation of CRF and consequently corticotropin (ACTH) secretion has been reviewed recently[1,2], so here I will only summarize briefly the more recent advances.

To date, most experiments have produced only indirect evidence consistent with the proposal that GABA may take part in one way or another in the neural chains controlling the pituitary–adrenal axis. That manipulation of the GABA-sensitive and/or GABA-ergic neurons produce changes in the CRF secretion is not at all surprising if two well-known features of the brain are taken into account. First, both GABA and its synthetizing enzyme glutamic acid decarboxylase (GAD) are widely and yet unevenly distributed in the forebrain, including the hypothalmus[2], and GABA is able to inhibit most if not all neurons in the forebrain including the neurosecretory cells of the supraoptic nucleus. Secondly, CRF is very labile and is stimulated by a large variety of neuronal influences, probably involving several neuronal circuits in which GABA-ergic neurons seem likely to be interposed. Therefore, when speaking about experimental evidence for the role of GABA one should always ask the question where in the brain is the site of the postulated action?

EXOGENOUS GABA

The effect of exogenous GABA on CRF release has been studied both *in vitro* and *in vivo*. Incubated whole hypothalami release CRF at an enhanced rate when stimulated with acetylcholine or serotonin and the stimulatory effects of both substances can be prevented by the addition of nanomolar concentrations of GABA, a finding indicating that some hypothalamic cells involved are sensitive to GABA-ergic inhibition[1]. *In vivo*, when GABA is infused into the third ventricle the stress-induced rise of plasma corticosterone in rats is inhibited[2], and this effect is not duplicated by the administration of glycine. These findings only show that exogenous GABA can inhibit some cells in the hypothalamus that are involved in the control of CRF release but do not allow further conclusions about the role of endogenous GABA.

DRUGS THAT MODIFY THE METABOLISM OR EFFECTS OF GABA

Pharmacological manipulation of ACTH release with drugs modifying the effects or the metabolism of GABA also provide supporting evidence. The antagonists of GABA action, picrotoxin and bicuculline, are also powerful stimulants of CRF secretion *in vivo* even when given as intracerebroventricular (i.c.v.) infusions to rats with a complete cut (CC) around the medial basal hypothalamus (MBH)[2,3]. At the time these experiments were published, the data were interpreted as suggesting the involvement of GABA-ergic neurons located within the MBH. Since then, we have discovered the large fall in the CRF content of the SME caused by the transection of fibers entering the MBH, and in the light of these data the previous interpretation ought to be modified.*

There are several possible ways of accounting for the findings and here two of the more likely will be considered. If a small portion of CRF cell bodies lie within the MBH then these may not be sufficient to maintain CRF stores in the SME but may be able to stimulate ACTH release as a consequence of the application of powerful direct neural excitants. Alternatively, the drugs that remain effective even in rats with CC that have been checked carefully may act to stimulate CRF cells outside the MBH and the released mediator may reach the anterior pituitary either *via* the systemic circulation or through vascular channels that are newly formed in response to the surgery and bridge the scar surrounding the isolated tissue[4,5]; the blood enriched in CRF could thus enter the island and be mixed with the blood perfusing the arcuate-periventricular region of the MBH; this region, in turn, has connections to the portal system, which has been described recently[6]. Although these considerations preclude the localization of the primary site of action of drugs in such experiments, nevertheless the data from manipulation of the GABA-ergic system *in vivo* may support the role of this transmitter somewhere in the neuronal ensemble contributing to the control of ACTH secretion.

In rats with CC, i.c.v. infusion of picrotoxin and bicuculline, as well as intraperitoneal (i.p.) injection of the GAD blocker 3-mercaptopropionic acid (3-MP), lead to the stimulated release of ACTH; moreover, their effects could be inhibited

---

*See also chapter 10, this volume.

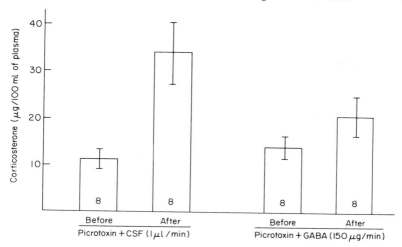

Fig. 1.   Assessment of the release of ACTH in rats with complete cuts around the medial basal hypothalamus. Left hand side of the figure shows plasma corticosterone levels before and after infusions i.c.v. of picrotoxin. Right hand side shows a similar experiment but with added GABA in the infusion medium.

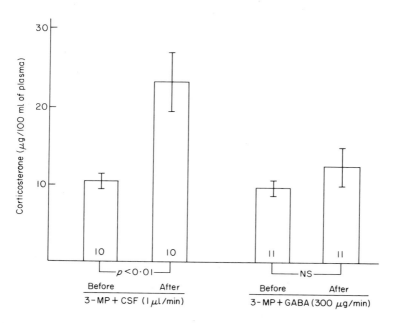

Fig. 2.   Assessment of the release of ACTH in rats with complete cuts around the medial basal hypothalamus. Left hand side of the figure shows plasma corticosterone levels before and after i.p.-injection of 3-mercaptopropionate (3-MP). Right hand side shows a similar experiment but with added GABA in the infusion medium.

strongly by a simultaneous i.c.v. infusion of GABA (Figs. 1 and 2). Jones and Hillhouse[1] have shown that in rats with intact hypothalami picrotoxin and bicuculline potentiate ACTH release induced by the stress of unilateral adrenalectomy, whereas intracarotid injection of GABA or the i.p. injection of aminooxyacetic acid (known to raise brain GABA stores) reduced stress-induced ACTH release.

However, there are also two dissenting reports. In the conscious cat, implantation of cristalline GABA[7] or the infusion of GABA into the lateral ventricle[8] resulted in *elevation* rather than decrease of plasma cortisol levels. These authors implicated GABA in excitatory mechanisms of CRF secretion. The difference between the rat and cat experiments may reflect either a true species difference in the organization of neural control of ACTH secretion, or, alternatively, that in those experiments GABA did not reach the CRF-secreting cells but disrupted normal CNS function near its site of administration and this led indirectly to an activation of the CRF cells. It is worth mentioning that GABA penetrates the ventricular wall only poorly and due to avid uptake, autoradiographs show a steep gradient in the hypothalamus within 500 μm of the ventricle. Thus i.c.v. GABA might not reach CRF cells in large animals as it does in the rat. With localized cristalline implants it may happen that the sites where presently unknown CRF cells are located were not among the restricted number of implantation sites[7].

ENDOGENOUS GABA

At present there are only two findings that implicate endogenous GABA in the control of CRF release. *In vitro*, nipecotic acid, an inhibitor of GABA uptake, was shown to inhibit the serotonin-induced release of CRF[1], and this fact suggests that hypothalamic cells may release GABA in amounts sufficient to inhibit CRF secretion. Based on evidence *in vivo*, GABA has also been implicated in the mediation of the feed-back effects of corticosteroids. Acs and Stark[9] postulated that corticosteroids may induce the formation of the enzyme GAD and thus enhance the synthesis of GABA. If this is the case, then an inhibitor of GAD, such as 3-MP should interfere with the dexamethasone-induced inhibition of the stress-induced rise of plasma corticosterone. When injected into rats 3 h after dexamethasone, 3-MP raised basal levels and partially restored the corticosterone response to sham adrenalectomy or an injection of formaldehyde. Since the effects of 3-MP were not duplicated by a non-specific stressful stimulus (i.p. injection of histamine), these data are consistent with the proposal that GAD inhibition prevented the effects of corticosteroids on GABA synthesis. Unfortunately, these data do not permit anatomical localization of the site where the relevant interaction between glucocorticoids and GABA synthesis might occur.

CONCLUSION

In summary, the evidence presently available for the participation of GABA in the control of ACTH secretion is predominantly indirect. It is clear that the neurons involved are sensitive to GABA-ergic inhibition and that GABA-ergic neurons are either involved in the control processes or are closely coupled with the neuronal circuits involved. However, in the future more specific hypotheses with anatomically specified proposals should be elaborated and experimentally tested if real progress is to be made.

REFERENCES

1. Jones, M. T. and Hillhouse, E. W. (1977). *Ann. N.Y. Acad. Sci.* **927**, 536.
2. Makara, G. B. and Stark, E. (1978). *In* "Interactions Between Putative Neurotransmitters in the Brain" (Garattini, S. *et al.* eds.), pp. 263–281,
3. Makara, G. B. and Stark, E. (1974). *Neuroendocrinology* **18**, 213.
4. Makara, G. B. *et al.* (1970). *J. Endocrinol.* **47**, 411.
5. Lengavári, I. and Halász, B. (1974). *Acta. Morph. Acad. Sci. Hung.* **22**, 1.
6. Ambach, G. *et al.* (1976). *Acta. Morph. Acad. Sci. Hung.* **24**, 93.
7. Krieger, H. P. and Krieger, D. T. (1970). *Amer. J. Physiol.* **218**, 1632–1641.
8. Garcy, A. M. and Morotta, S. F. (1978). *Neuroendocrinology* **25**, 343.
9. Acs, Z. and Stark, E. (1978). *J. Endocrinol.* **77**, 137.

13

MODIFICATIONS OF THE SENSITIVITY OF RECEPTORS INVOLVED IN THE REGULATION OF THE HYPOTHALAMO-PITUITARY-ADRENAL AXIS

U. Scapagnini, L. Angelucci, I. Gerendai, P. Valeri, P. L. Canonico, M. Palmery, F. Patacchioli, and B. Tita

Department of Pharmacology, Faculty of Medicine, University of Catania and Department of Pharmacology, Faculty of Pharmacy, University of Rome Italy

INTRODUCTION

There is a considerable evidence in the literature that suggests that norepinephrine (NE) is responsible for the inhibition of corticotropin (ACTH) secretion and that the NE is acting *via* an α-adrenergic receptor mechanism[1,2]. Some evidence suggests that norepinephrine has an excitatory role, but these results are mainly drawn from experiments in which catecholamines (CAs), which barely cross the blood–brain barrier, were administered systemically and might therefore exert their effects by the peripheral stimulation of α-adrenergic receptors. Experiments where CAs have been administered into the third ventricle have consistently shown inhibition of ACTH secretion[1]. However, when brain CAs have been depleted by pharmacological manipulations, the results have often been contradictory. Indeed, where long-lasting depletion of brain CA has been induced, little evidence has been found consistent with the hypothesis that NE exerts an inhibitory influence on ACTH secretion.

Collectively, the results when dealing with acute manipulations of brain CA levels and/or turnover with relatively short-term evaluation of adrenocortical activity favour the hypothesis of a central norepinephrinergic (NE) mechanism tonically inhibiting the corticoliberin (CRF)–ACTH secretion[1,2]. In contrast, the hypothesis of a tonic NE inhibition appears less tenable in conditions of long-lasting depletion of brain CA. In fact, after a single dose of reserpine a long-lasting depletion of brain CA was induced but there was only a short-term activation of the hypothalamo–pituitary–adrenal axis (HHAA)[3,4]. The same discrepancy was present after repeated injections of reserpine. In rats, daily intraperitoneal (i.p.) administration of low doses of reserpine (0.5mg/kg for 9 days) markedly depleted hypothalamic NE content, whereas plasma corticosterone (B) levels after an initial rise progressively decreased to reach control values after 5 days of treatment[5,6,7].

The dissociation between the immediate and prolonged effects of depletion in brain CA can best be explained in terms of various compensatory changes within the CA system. Such changes might be characteristic of all monaminergic systems and so we have investigated such changes in both CA and serotoninergic systems.

COMPENSATION CHANGES WITHIN THE MONOAMINERGIC SYSTEM

Catecholamines

There are several possible compensatory changes within the CA system under conditions of prolonged depletion. First, there may be re-appearance of a small functional NE pool produced as a consequence of increased tyrosine hydroxylase (TH) activity due to feed-back stimulation. It has been shown, in fact, that long-term treatment with low doses of reserpine progressively increased TH activity in the brain stem and this was reflected by the rate of HHAA function. In rats pretreated for 9 days with reserpine, the injection of α-methyl-p-tyrosine (α-MpT), at a dose of 100mg/kg, restored the elevated levels of plasma B. Under these conditions α-MpT suppressed the small NE pool still functioning after the depleting effects of reserpine[6]. It should be mentioned that this dose of α-MpT has no effect on the HHAA in control rats.

The same type of reasoning can be applied to explain the lack of activation of the CRF–ACTH system found after central injection of 6-hydroxydopamine (6-OHDA)[8,9,10,11]. Evaluation of the effects of centrally injected 6-OHDA in rats, shortly after drug administration (24 h), revealed a marked depletion of hypothalamic NE content which was accompanied by adrenocortical activation[8,12,13] and an enhanced response to stress[14]. In contrast, 3, 15 and 30 days later, in spite of the sustained depletion of hypothalamic NE, corticosterone levels were not modified[5,12]. However, as in the reserpine-pretreated rats, in these animals injection of a low dose of α-MpT induced activation of HHAA. Therefore, even after selective degeneration of CA nerve terminals, a pool of NE responsible for the functional inhibition of the HHAA can still be present. The maintenance of a functionally active pool could be attributed to the hyperactivity of NE-containing neurons surviving the degenerative effects of 6-OHDA.

Another possible reason in the interpretation of this phenomenon could be the appearance of receptor supersensitivity following specific degeneration of the NE neurons. In fact, in experiments *in vitro*, the appearance of this supersensitivity has been demonstrated (Jones, *personal communication*). Rats treated intraventricularly with 6-OHDA were killed 14 days later and the hypothalami were dissected for subsequent studies *in vitro* according to Jones' technique (see in

this volume). These hypothalami showed a higher sensitivity to the inhibitory
action of NE on CRF release when compared with controls.

In a recent experiment, we have investigated the nature and the specific
anatomical location of the NE pathways responsible for the effects seen after
6-OHDA intraventricular administration. Histochemical fluorescence studies
have revealed that the midbrain gives rise to anatomically complex ascending
monoaminergic pathways of which the ventral NE tract (VNAT) represents one
of the major ascending NE systems with cell bodies situated in the medulla
oblongata and the pons. The VNAT innervates the whole hypothalamus, the
internal layer of the median eminence, the retrochiasmatic and preoptic areas[16].
The neurotoxic agent 6-OHDA (10 μg in 2 μl) was injected into the VNAT at
the level of the medial lemniscus and its effect on the plasma B levels and on NE
hypothalamic content was observed 1, 3 and 15 days later. As shown in Fig. 1,

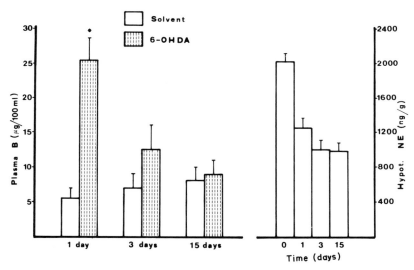

Fig. 1.   Effect of injection of 6-OHDA into the VNAT on plasma B (left part of the Fig.)
and on hypothalamic NE (right part of the Fig.) * $p < 0.01$ if compared with the corresponding controls.

the injection of 6-OHDA into the VNAT produced on the HHAA and on the
hypothalamic NE content an effect similar to the one elicited by the injection
of 6-OHDA into the third ventricle. These results stress the specificity of the
former experiment with 6-OHDA and focus attention on the importance of
the VNAT as a determinant component in the mechanism (NE in nature) tonically
inhibiting the HHAA activity. The fact that the adrenocortical activation is
observed only after 24 h but not after 3 and 15 days, can be explained in a
similar way to the effect of the intraventricular injection of the neurotoxic agent;
with the appearance of postdenervation receptor supersensitivity.

Serotonin

Unlike CA[5], serotoninergic (5-HT) neurotransmission does not seem to be involved predominantly in acute response to stress but in the control of circadian periodicity of adrenocortical secretion. A diurnal fluctuation of 5-HT has been demonstrated in the whole brain as well as in specific brain areas of several mammalian species[2]. A positive correlation between 5-HT content in the limbic system and plasma corticosterone (B) rhythm (characterized by a peak at 20.00 h) was found in the rat, suggesting that 5-HT may play a role in the regulation of diurnal fluctuation of ACTH secretion[17,18]. However, the existence of a simple correlation between brain monoamines (MA) and plasma hormone levels does not demonstrate a causal relationship.

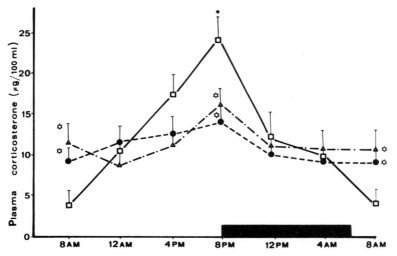

Fig. 2. Effect of PCPA (●; 300 mg/kg i.p. 48 h before death) and PCPA-methyl ester (▲; 200 mg/kg i.p. 24 h before death) on plasma B levels. ☆ $p < 0.01$ if compared with the corresponding controls (□).

Experiments in which central 5-HT activity was modified by surgical or pharmacological means provided more direct information on the role of 5-HT in the ACTH diurnal rhythm. p-Chlorophenylalanine (PCPA), a blocker of 5-HT synthesis, eliminated the diurnal fluctuation of plasma corticosteroids in birds, rats and cats[2]. It was demonstrated that the insoluble form of PCPA (300 mg/kg) given 48 h before, or PCPA methyl-ester (200 mg/kg) given less than 24 h before, resulted in constant plasma B levels throughout the day with elevated morning and normal evening levels (Fig. 2). Interestingly, 48–72 h after PCPA injection, in spite of the continual depletion of brain 5-HT levels, a normal diurnal rhythmicity of plasma B was restored[19].

These data can be explained by the reappearance of a small functional pool produced as a consequence of the induction of tryptophan hydroxylase activity

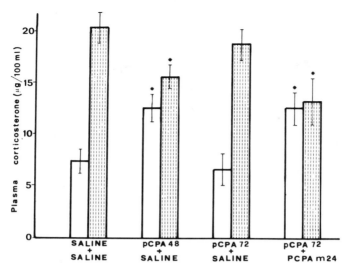

Fig. 3. Effect of PCPA (300 mg/kg i.p. 48 and 72 h before death) and of PCPA (300 mg/kg 72 h before death) + PCPA-methyl ester (50 mg/kg 24 h before death) on the plasma B levels at 08.00 h (□) and 20.00 h (▦). * $p < 0.01$ compared with the corresponding controls.

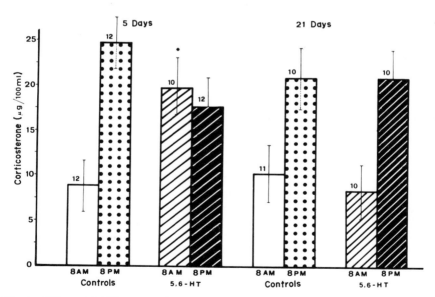

Fig. 4. Effect of 5,6-DHT (50 μg/animal into the third ventricle) on plasma B levels at 08.00 h (8 a.m.) and 20.00 h (8 p.m.) 5 and 21 days after the injection. * $p < 0.01$ compared with the corresponding controls.

due to feed-back stimulation after PCPA administration[2]. In fact, in rats pre-treated 72 h before with insoluble PCPA (300 mg/kg), an injection of PCPA methyl ester, at a dose (50 mg/kg), that is unable to modify the HHAA activity in control rats, abolished the diurnal rhythmicity of plasma B (Fig. 3). Intra-ventricular injection of the neurotoxic tryptamine derivative 5,6-dihydroxytryp-tamine (5,6-DHT) produced a blunting of the circadian rhythm detectable 5 but not 21 days after the treatment (Fig. 4). In recent experiments the use of 5-HT agonist quipazine allowed us to suggest that the 5-HT receptors develop super-sensitivity 3 weeks after 5,6-DHT treatment. In normal animals quipazine is able to increase the morning levels of plasma B, the lowest active dose being 5 mg/kg.

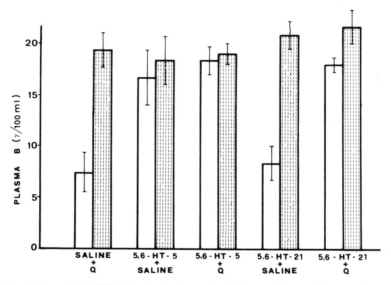

Fig. 5. Effect of 5,6-DHT (50 μg/animal into the third ventricle 5 and 21 days before death) and of 5,6-DHT (50 μg/animal 5 and 21 days before death) + quipazine (Q, 1 mg/kg) on plasma B levels at 08.00 h (□) and 20.00 h (▤).

When a *per se* inactive dose of quipazine (1 mg/kg) was given to animals pretreated 21 days before with 5,6-DHT, the morning values of plasma B were greatly increased (Fig. 5) probably due to the appearance of receptor supersensitivity.

Also, in experiments in which the impairment of the 5-HT pathways was performed by neurosurgery, it was possible to observe the restoration of the altered endocrine functions. In fact the transection of the fornix[20,21] or septal lesion[22] resulted in disappearance of the usual circadian rhythm with intermediate (fornix) or high (septum) B levels. However, 3 weeks after fornix transection the diurnal B variation reappeared[21] in spite of the fact that at this time the hippocampal 5-HT content was as low as after 1 week. This phenomenon can be justified by the appearance of receptor supersensitivity 3 weeks after fornical transection. Our

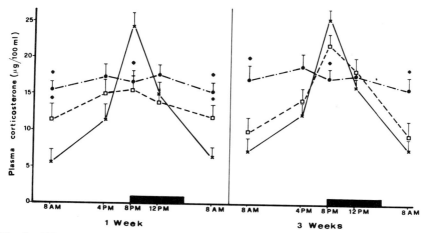

Fig. 6. Effect of the fornix cut (□) and of the fornix cut + roof cut (●) on the diurnal variation on plasma B. * $p < 0.01$ compared with the corresponding controls (X).

recent results showed that in animals submitted to so-called roof-cuts (disconnections of all afferents to the hypothalamus from dorsal brain areas), fornix cuts abolished the circadian rhythm of plasma B and this also lasted for 3 weeks (Fig. 6), indicating that an accessory pathway can take over the function when the main regulatory pathway is lesioned.

In conclusion, from the above-mentioned results it appears likely that in conditions of severe central MA depletion the postsynaptic receptors responsible for the hypothalamic control of CRF-ACTH release can develop supersensitivity in order to keep the homoeostasis of the system.

Interactions Between 5-HT and Corticosterone Uptake in Hippocampus and Septum

Different levels of the hypophyseal–adrenocortical activity in mice and rats are accompanied by variations in the specific corticosterone uptake (SBU) in the hippocampus and septum[23]. A direct correlation exists between plasma B levels and uptake *in vivo* (SBU) or binding of the hormone *in vitro* in the hippocampus and septum[24]. The SBU in the hippocampus is not affected by dexamethasone and fluctuates throughout 24 h[25]. In 4–10 h adrenalectomized (ADREX) animals the trough phase was found at about 08.00 h and a peak between 12.00 and 16.00 h, namely at the time preceding the surge of plasma B in normal animals. At this range of survival time the SBU rhythm in the hippocampus was independent of the post-ADREX interval but dependent on the day time of measurement. This phenomenon would appear to be an intrinsic property of the hippocampus.

We have studied the relationship between the changes in the circadian B rhythm and those of hippocampal SBU after serotoninergic impairment. In this experi-

Table I. Brain MAs and metabolites in the brain 5 and 21 days after 5, 7-DHT treatment. Morning (M) and evening (E) mean values ± S.E.M. in ng/mg tissue. In each pair the upper value is the control value. $^a p < 0.05$, $^b p < 0.01$ and $^c p < 0.001$.

		HIPPOCAMPUS		HYPOTHALAMUS (1)		AMYGDALA		MESENCEPHALON(2)	
		day 5	day 21	day 5	day 21	day 5	day 21	day 5	day 21
NA	M	409 ± 15 408 ± 14	437 ± 15 396 ± 19	2128 ± 55 1970 ± 55	2177 ± 51 2170 ± 46	820 ± 31 851 ± 22	790 ± 30 695 ± 36	1155 ± 36 1228 ± 24	1164 ± 53 1091 ± 42
	E	431 ± 14 392 ± 10	415 ± 17 417 ± 11	2102 ± 49 1993 ± 46	2154 ± 49 2112 ± 45	824 ± 31 900 ± 42	794 ± 30 698 ± 41	1140 ± 56 1241 ± 67	1179 ± 30 1067 ± 34
DA	M	2269 ± 58 2401 ± 185	2294 ± 112 2586 ± 90^a	3694 ± 84 4016 ± 70	3746 ± 47 3846 ± 57	2242 ± 121 2444 ± 158	2158 ± 101 2384 ± 114	786 ± 21 847 ± 23	764 ± 36 730 ± 29
	E	2254 ± 107 2491 ± 110	2293 ± 54 2775 ± 140^a	3646 ± 72 3992 ± 97	3795 ± 53 3936 ± 79	2169 ± 122 2318 ± 127	2231 ± 102 2505 ± 76	805 ± 21 847 ± 10	746 ± 33 771 ± 29
5-HT	M	751 ± 19 581 ± 11^c	677 ± 28 562 ± 13^b	910 ± 16 792 ± 14^a	916 ± 17 806 ± 25^a	1114 ± 17 1098 ± 23	1100 ± 11 1070 ± 18	817 ± 9 718 ± 8^c	790 ± 3 710 ± 15^b
	E	732 ± 19 620 ± 18^b	695 ± 28 479 ± 23^b	916 ± 19 793 ± 24^b	909 ± 15 798 ± 26^a	1147 ± 25 1119 ± 24	1178 ± 20 1102 ± 17	816 ± 7 731 ± 5^c	793 ± 4 712 ± 3^b
HVA	M	163 ± 3 177 ± 5	159 ± 11 186 ± 5						
	E	173 ± 7 186 ± 2	156 ± 10 183 ± 6						
DOPAC	M	237 ± 16 266 ± 10	274 ± 7 292 ± 4						
	E	235 ± 12 262 ± 14	279 ± 5 297 ± 6						
5-HIAA	M	371 ± 11 235 ± 18^c	359 ± 15 234 ± 14^b	568 ± 10 473 ± 12^b	576 ± 13 471 ± 14^b	400 ± 13 397 ± 5	397 ± 8 395 ± 4	387 ± 8 298 ± 3^c	388 ± 6 292 ± 2^c
	E	361 ± 14 301 ± 10^a	368 ± 13 284 ± 19^b	573 ± 12 488 ± 11^b	571 ± 12 504 ± 14^a	402 ± 7 403 ± 8	410 ± 8 401 ± 8	350 ± 11 307 ± 3^c	345 ± 4 303 ± 2^c

ment the 5-HT depletion was obtained by the administration of 5,7-dihydroxy-tryptamine (5,7-DHT) after protection of the NE endings by nortryptiline. The injection of 5,7-DHT produced a decrease of 5-HT and 5-hydroxyindolacetic acid (5-HIAA) concentrations in the hippocampus, hypothalamus and mesen-cephalon but not in the amygdala. The decrease in 5-HT and 5-HIAA obtained 5 days after the lesion was still present at 21 days. The biochemical lesion appeared quite selective since NE and dopamine (DA) as well as DOPAC and HVA concentrations in various brain areas were unaffected by 5,7-DHT. Curiously enough, DA concentration in the hippocampus increased 21 days after treatment (Table I).

As in the experiment with 5,6-DHT, the plasma B levels at 5 days showed little circadian fluctuation due to an increase in the morning values. The rhythm returned to normal 21 days later in spite of the still pronounced depletion of 5-HT.

At 5 days after 5,7-DHT treatment, the evening level of SBU in the hippo-campus was much higher than in the controls, so that circadian fluctuations were abolished at high levels. Conversely 21 days after the treatment the morning levels of SBU were depressed so that the rhythm was abolished at low levels (Fig.7).

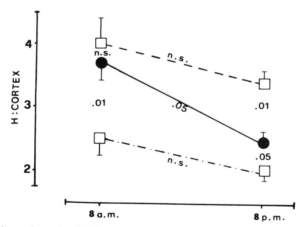

Fig. 7.   Morning and evening SBU in the hippocampus (d.p.m./mg; ratio to brain cortex) 5 (– – –) and 21 (–·–·–) days after 5,7-DHT treatment compared with controls (•).

This study seems to suggest that there is a correlation between the central serotoninergic tone and the circadian SBU activity in the hippocampus since a disruption of the 5-HT endings results in a modification of the SBU daily fluctuation.

Finally, if the intensity of SBU reflects the degree of sensitivity of the corti-costerone receptors, these receptors display hyper- or hypo-sensitivity 5 and 21 days after selective degeneration of 5-HT neurons.

CONCLUSION

It appears that depletion of monoamines in the brain results in compensatory changes in both the pre- and post-synaptic elements. The presynaptic adjustments include the increased synthesis of the neurotransmitter in the remaining neuronal pool. At the postsynaptic level the receptors develop supersensitivity to the released neurotransmitter. There is some indication that removal of the adrenal glands may result in corticosteroid receptor supersensitivity in the hippocampus and septum.

REFERENCES

1. Preziosi, P. and Scapagnini, U. (1978). *In* "The Endocrine Function of the Human Adrenal Cortex" (V. H. T. James, *et al.* eds.), p. 91, Academic Press, London.
2. Müller, E. *et al.* (1977). *In* "Neurotransmitters and Anterior Pituitary Function", Academic Press, New York.
3. Carr, L. A. and Moore, K. E. (1968). *Neuroendocrinol.* 3, 285.
4. Montanari, R. and Stockham, M. P. (1962). *Brit. J. Pharmacol.* 18, 337.
5. Scapagnini, U. (1974). *In* "The Neurosciences: Third Study Program". (F. O. Schmidt and F. G. Worden, eds.), p. 565, MIT Press, Cambridge, Massachussetts.
6. Scapagnini, U. *et al.* (1976). *Neuroendocrinol.* 20, 243.
7. Hodges, J. R. and Vellucci, S. V. (1975). *Brit. J. Pharmacol.* 53, 555.
8. Scapagnini, U. and Preziosi, P. (1973). *Prog. Brain Res.* 39, 171.
9. Kaplanski, J. and Smelik, P. G. (1973). *Res. Commun. Chem. Pathol. Pharmacol.* 5, 263.
10. Kaplanski, J. *et al.* (1974). *Neuroendocrinol.* 13, 123.
11. Kumeda, H. *et al.* (1974). *J. Endocrinol.* 62, 161–170.
12. Cuello, A. C. *et al.* (1974). *Brain Res.* 78, 57.
13. Ganong, W. F. (1974). *In* "The Neurosciences: Third Study Program" (F. O. Schmidt and F. G. Worden, eds.), p. 549, MIT Press, Cambridge, Massachussetts.
14. Fuxe, K. *et al.* (1973). *In* "Brain–Pituitary–Adrenal Interrelationships" (A. Brodish and E. S. Redgate, eds.), p. 239, S. Karger, Basel.
15. Uretsky, N. J. *et al.* (1971). *J. Pharmacol. exp. Ther.* 176, 489.
16. Ungerstedt, U. (1971). *Acta. Physiol. Scand. Suppl.* 367, 1.
17. Scapagnini, U. *et al.* (1971). *Neuroendocrinol.* 7, 90.
18. Simon, M. L. and George, R. (1975). *Neuroendocrinol.* 17, 125.
19. Vernikos-Danellis, J. *et al.* (1973). *Prog. Brain Res.* 39, 301.
20. Moberg, G. P. *et al.* (1971). *Neuroendocrinol.* 7, 11.
21. Lengvari, I. and Halasz, B. (1973). *Neuroendocrinol.* 11, 191.
22. Harrington, R. J. *et al.* (1973). *J. Anim. Sci.* 37, 313.
23. Valeri, P. *et al.* (1978). *Neurosci. Lett.* 9, 249.
24. Angelucci, L. and Valeri, P. (1978). *Ann. 1st Sup. Sanita* XIV, 40.
25. Angelucci, L. *et al.* (1978). Second European Neuroscience Meeting, Florence, Italy, September 4–9, Abst. in *Neurosci. Lett.* Suppl. 1, S198.

14

GLUCOCORTICOSTEROID AND MINERALOCORTICOSTEROID HORMONE TARGET SITES IN THE BRAIN: AUTORADIOGRAPHIC STUDIES WITH CORTICOSTERONE, ALDOSTERONE AND DEXAMETHASONE

Walter E. Stumpf and Madhabananda Sar

Department of Anatomy, University of North Carolina,
Chapel Hill, North Carolina, U.S.A.

INTRODUCTION

The thaw-mount and dry-mount autoradiographic techniques, introduced by Stumpf and Roth[1,2] and Stumpf and Sar[3], were used to study the localization of genomic target cells for steroid hormones and to establish the patterns of brain distribution for estrogen, androgen, progestagen and adrenal hormones. Reviews on the autoradiographic localization of sex steroids in peripheral tissues and nervous tissues have been published[4,5,6]. This brief report compares the topography of target cells in the rat brain for corticosterone and aldosterone. Data on dexamethasone uptake and distribution are included.

DISTRIBUTION AND UPTAKE

Male Sprague-Dawley rats, weighing 150–200 g and adrenalectomized 48 h before were injected *via* the jugular vein under ether anesthesia. The steroids given were (0.5 to 1.0 μg/100 g body wt.): [^{3}H] corticosterone (specific radioactivity 55–80 Ci/mmol), [^{3}H] aldosterone (specific radioactivity 80–120 Ci/mmol) or [^{3}H] dexamethasone (specific radioactivity 27 Ci/mmol). Animals were decapitated 30 min or 1 h after [^{3}H] corticosterone or [^{3}H] aldosterone

137

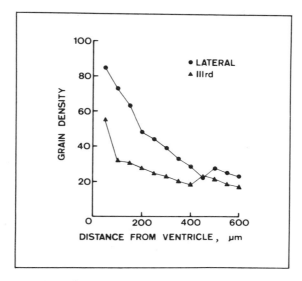

Fig. 1. Diffusion gradient [³H] dexamethasone from ventricle to brain at 30 min after the intravenous injection of 3 μg/100 g body weight. The silver grain density was measured at different distances medially from the lateral ventricle at the septal region and laterally from the third ventricle at the level of the central hypothalamus. At 3 h after the injection no such gradient is observed. Reproduced from Rees *et al.*[7].

and 30 min or 3 h after [³H] dexamethasone. Brains were removed, dissected and freeze-mounted on tissue holders, sectioned and thaw-mounted on emulsion-coated slides as described in detail by Stumpf and Sar[3]. After 6 to 12 months exposure, the autoradiograms were photographically processed, stained and examined under the microscope.

After [³H] corticosterone or [³H] aldosterone injection, a clear topographic pattern of target neuron distribution can be recognized. In contrast, after [³H]-dexamethasone no such distinct pattern is obtained. Unlike the natural adrenal steroid hormones the synthetic glucocorticoid dexamethasone does not penetrate readily through capillaries into the brain, apparently because of a blood–brain barrier for this compound. In the case of [³H] dexamethasone entry into the brain seems to occur mainly *via* the capillaries of the choroid plexus and the cerebrospinal fluid[7]. At 30 min a steep gradient of radioactivity can be seen in the brain neuropil in periventricular regions parallel to the ependyma or the surface of the brain (Fig. 1). At this time glial cells and neurons in this periventricular zone show some nuclear concentration of radioactivity. At 3 h, the level of radioactivity appears almost uniform throughout the brain, with weak but widespread nuclear labelling of glial cells and neurons in apparently non-select regions. In comparison, after [³H] corticosterone (Fig. 2) or [³H] aldosterone (Fig. 3) a neuronal nuclear labelling with graded topographical distinction is found. The distribution of the labelled neurons after injection of [³H] corticosterone or [³H] aldosterone is depicted on opposite pages for comparison: for the forebrain Figs. 4–6 and Figs. 7–9 respectively, and for the midbrain, hindbrain and spinal cord Figs. 10–12, 16–17 and 13–15, 18–19, respectively.

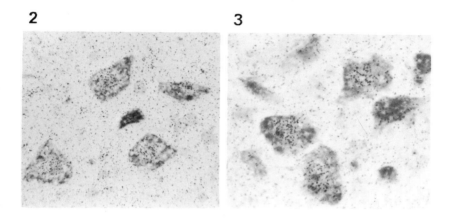

Figs. 2 and 3.   Autoradiograms after injection of [³H] corticosterone (Fig. 2) or [³H]-aldosterone (Fig. 3), showing concentration of radioactivity in nuclei or neurons of the fifth and the twelfth motor nerve respectively. Stained with methyl green pyronin. Exposure times 365 days (Fig. 2, specific radioactivity 54.5 Ci/mM, 0.9 μg/100 g body wt.), 176 days (Fig. 3, specific radioactivity 120 Ci/mM, 0.85 μg/100 g body wt.).

The wide distribution in the central nervous system of neurons that retain and concentrate radioactivity after labelled glucocorticoid or mineralcorticoid administration is noteworthy. The nuclear radioactivity probably represents mainly [³H] corticosterone after [³H] corticosterone and mainly [³H] aldosterone after [³H] aldosterone injection rather than the respective metabolites. This can be inferred from chemical characterization of radioactivity extracted from nuclear fractions of brain tissue[8] as well as from competition experiments conducted in our laboratory with an excess of unlabelled corticosterone, aldosterone or dihydrotestosterone.

In the forebrain, for both [³H] corticosterone and [³H] aldosterone the highest nuclear uptake is seen in neurons in the pre-, supra- and post-commissural hippocampus, followed by the dorsal septum, certain nuclei of the amygdala and widespread regions of the pallium. The caudate-putamen contain target neurons for both hormones.

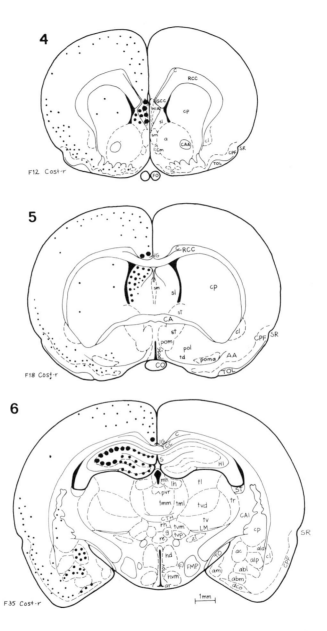

Figs. 4–19. Topographical distribution of target neurons after injection of [³H] corticosterone (Figs. 4–6, 10–12, 16–17) or [³H] aldosterone (Figs. 7–9, 13–15, 18–19). Schematic drawings of rat brain cross sections—including forebrain, midbrain, hindbrain and cervical spinal cord—prepared from thaw-mount autoradiograms. For comparison the results obtained after [³H] corticosterone and [³H] aldosterone are depicted on opposite pages. For explanation of abbreviations see reference [6].

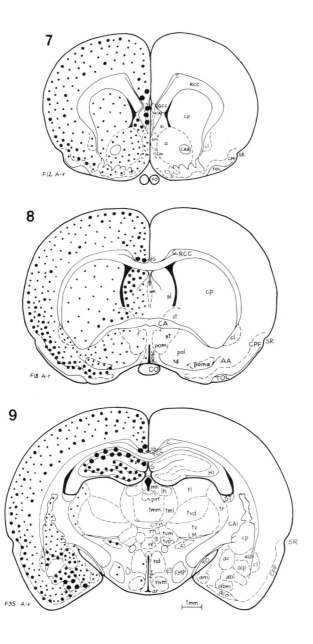

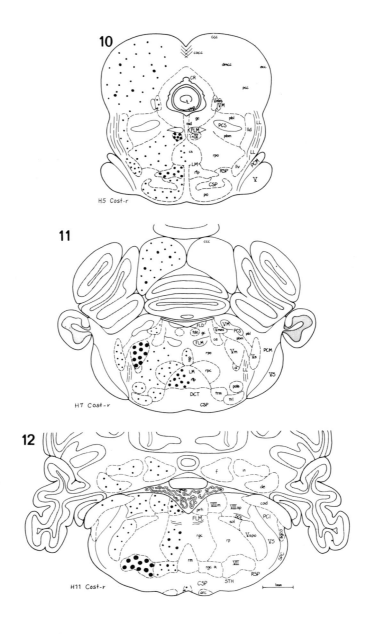

Figs. 4–19 (continued)

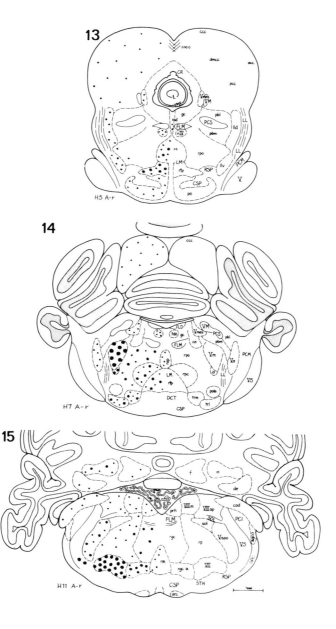

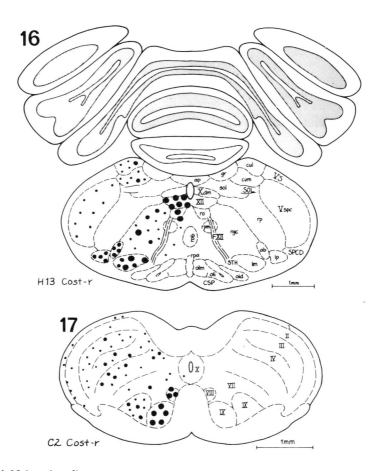

Figs. 4–19 (continued)

In the hypothalamus a few weakly labelled scattered neurons are observed after [³H] aldosterone injection, whereas after [³H] corticosterone no such nuclear labelling is seen under the conditions of the experiments. From the results of the present studies, however, the existence of hypothalamic target neurons for corticosterone cannot be excluded. This lack of nuclear labelling after [³H] corticosterone in all of the regions that show distinct labelling after [³H] aldosterone may be due to true differences in affinity. The general high radioactivity in tissue observed with little or no nuclear concentration may be sufficient to account for glucocorticoid action on certain hypothalamic neurons.

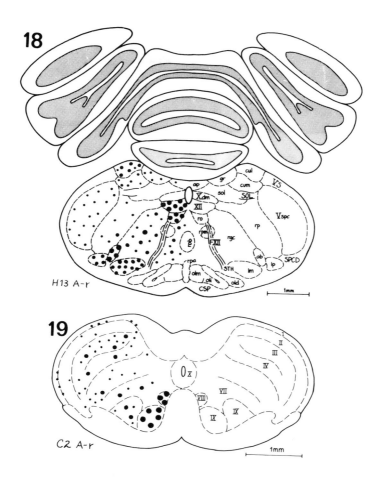

Such action can be postulated to exist from the results of studies with hormonal implants, lesions or the hypothalamus *in vitro*[9–12]. Thus, for example, fast feedback may be mediated by a non-genomic mechanism of action without involving nuclear uptake of hormone.

In the lower brain stem and spinal cord, with both hormones, highest nuclear concentration of radioactivity is seen in motor neurons. Gluco- and mineralocorticosteroid target neurons are widespread and are also found in certain nuclei of the reticular formation, in certain sensory and autonomic nuclei, and in the cerebellum. Even in the spinal cord, no laminar region is free of labelled neurons, with the large motor neurons generally showing highest nuclear retention of radioactivity. Many glial cells throughout the central nervous system, the choroid epithelial cells, ependymal cells and cells of the meninges, showed various intensities of nuclear concentration of radioactivity with all of the adrenal hormones studied. In the brain ventricular lumen, as in lumina of blood vessels, high levels of radioactivity are seen indicating the presence of corticosteroid-binding protein.

CONCLUSION

The observations made in our studies suggest identity of most, if not all, target cells in the central nervous system for gluco- and mineralo-corticosteroids. The extensive distribution of [^{3}H]aldosterone-related target cells in the brain indicates an important role in brain functions not only for "glucocorticoids", as generally assumed, but also for "mineralocorticoids," calling into question, perhaps, some of the distinctions generally made for these two classes of compounds. The apparent involvement of so many brain structures as target sites for adrenal steroids correlates well with the manyfold clinical symptoms seen, for instance, in hypoadrenalism.

The topographic pattern of target cells for adrenal cortical hormones is different from the pattern published by us for [^{3}H]estradiol. There is only minimal overlap with [^{3}H]estradiol in contrast to the androgen [^{3}H]dihydrotestosterone[13,14]. Androgen target neuron accumulations were similar to those of the natural adrenal steroids, for instance, in spinal cord and brain stem motor neurons, in the hippocampus, in the dorsal septum, and in the pallium. This suggests genomic activation of certain identical groups of neurons by androgens and corticosteroids—although probably through different receptors with possible hormonal synergism—is related to effects on motor activity, aggressive behavior as well as certain sensory and autonomic functions.

ACKNOWLEDGEMENT

The work of the authors is supported by PHS Grant NS09914.

REFERENCES

1. Stumpf, W. E. and Roth, L. J. (1964). *Stain Technology* **39**, 219.
2. Stumpf, W. E. and Roth, L. J. (1966). *J. Histochem. Cytochem.* **14**, 274.
3. Stumpf, W. E. and Sar, M. (1965). *In* "Methods in Enzymology", Vol. XXXVI, Hormone Action, Part A. Steroid Hormones, (O'Malley, B. W. and Hardman, J. G. eds.), pp. 135–156, Academic Press, New York.
4. Stumpf, W. E. and Sar, M. (1976). *In* "Receptors and Mechanism of Action of Steroid Hormones, (Pasqualini, J. ed.), pp. 41–84, Marcel Dekker, New York.
5. Stumpf, W. E. and Sar, M. (1973). *In* "Progress in Brain Research", (Gipsen, W. H. *et al.* eds.), pp. 53–71, Elsvier, Amsterdam.

6.   Stumpf, W. E. and Grant, L. D. (1975). (eds.) Anatomical Neuroendocrin-
     ology, 472 pps., S. Karger, Basel.
7.   Rees, H. D. *et al.* (1975). *In* "Anatomical Neuroendocrinology", (Stumpf,
     W. E. and Grant, L. D. eds.), pp. 262–9, S. Karger, Basel.
8.   Anderson, N. S. III and Fanestil, D. D. (1976). *Endocrinology* **98**, 676.
9.   Smelik, P. G. (1965). *Acta Physiol. Pharmacol. Neur.* **13**, 370.
10.   Bohus, B. and Strashimirov, D. (1970). *Neuroendocrinol.* **6**, 197.
11.   Kendall, J. W. *et al.* (1975). *In* "Anatomical Neuroendocrinology"
     (Stumpf, W. E. and Grant, L. D. eds.), pp. 276–83, S. Karger, Basel.
12.   Jones, M. T. *et al.* (1976). *In* "Frontiers of Neuroendocrinology" (Martin, L.
     and Ganong, W. F. eds.), Vol. 4, pp. 195–226, Raven, New York.
13.   Sar, M. and Stumpf, W. E. (1975). *In* "Anatomical Neuroendocrinology"
     (Stumpf, W. E. and Grant, L. D. eds.), pp. 120–133, S. Karger, Basel.
14.   Sar, M. and Stumpf, W. E. (1977). *J. Steroid Biochem.* **8**, 1131.

15

ADRENAL FEEDBACK ON STRESS-INDUCED CORTICOLIBERIN (CRF) AND CORTICOTROPIN (ACTH) SECRETION

Mary F. Dallman

Department of Physiology, University of California, San Francisco, California 94143, U.S.A.

INTRODUCTION

In 1947 Sayers and Sayers demonstrated the overall characteristics of the interactions between stimulus-induced activation of the adrenocortical system and corticosteroid-induced inhibition of adrenocortical responses to noxious stimuli[1]. In summary, these studies demonstrated that the greater the intensity of the stimulus applied to the organism, the greater the adrenal response (adrenal ascorbic acid depletion), and that the larger the dose of corticosteroid administered several hours before stimulation, the smaller the adrenocortical response to a given stimulus (delayed or proportional feedback). Moreover, in one experiment, Sayers and Sayers[1] showed that the adrenal response to injection of epinephrine was inhibited when administration of the drug was preceded by 3 min by an infusion of cortisol, thus demonstrating what has subsequently been termed fast, or rate-sensitive feedback.

This paper will present a limited review of studies on the interrelationships between the intensity and type of stimulus used to provoke adrenocortical activation, and the efficacy and time course of inhibition of the system after pretreatment with corticosteroids (frequently the potent synthetic steroid dexamethasone). Emphasis will be placed on those studies that reveal information about the sites and physiology of corticosteroid modulation of basal and stimulus-induced activity of the adrenocortical system. Finally, recent evidence

149

will be presented that suggests that an adrenal factor in addition to corticosteroids feeds back to modulate secretion of corticoliberin (CRF) and corticotropin (ACTH) in response to afferent stimuli.

CORTICOSTEROID INHIBITION OF ADRENOCORTICAL FUNCTION — TEMPORAL RELATIONSHIPS

Any discussion of studies of corticosteroid-induced inhibition of function in the adrenocortical system must take into account the dosage regimen and duration of treatment as well as the stimuli used to provoke activity in the system since these are important variables determining the results obtained. In addition, much of the experimental work on feedback regulation of CRF and ACTH secretion has used the potent synthetic corticosteroid dexamethasone, with the implicit assumption that its effects do not differ in kind from those of the naturally occurring corticosteroids. This assumption may not be valid since the sites of regional uptake and the degree of nuclear retention of dexamethasone in brain and pituitary differ from those described for corticosterone and cortisol[2]. The use of dexamethasone in studies attempting to determine the primary locus of steroid feedback action may provide results that give undue weight to the pituitary as a major feedback site. Recent results[3,4] have demonstrated that there is a transcortin-like binding protein associated with anterior pituitary cells, and that dexamethasone (which does not bind to transcortin) has greater access to pituitary cell nuclei than does corticosterone or cortisol.

Experiments studying the feedback effects of corticosteroids on the adrenocortical system can be divided into several categories: treatment with multiple large doses of ACTH or corticosteroids for periods longer than 24 h; treatment with multiple large doses of corticosteroids or continuous supply of steroid in the drinking water for 16–24 h; treatment with a single large dose of corticosteroid; treatment with small doses of the naturally occurring steroid with study of the effects 2–4 h later; treatment with small doses of the naturally occurring steroid with study of the effects occurring during the time plasma corticosteroid levels are rising as a result of the injection or infusion. Within each of the categories outlined above, some conclusions can be drawn about the primary site of corticosteroid feedback.

1. Chronic Experiments

When large doses of ACTH or natural or synthetic corticosteroids are administered systemically or locally for periods of 2 or more days without the concurrent application of ACTH-releasing stimuli, the capacity of the adrenocortical system to respond to stimulation is essentially abolished[5–7]. The only stimulus to the adrenocortical system that was demonstrated to cause a corticosteroid response in rats after 14 days of daily treatment with ACTH was endotoxin[7], a stimulus that causes corticosteroid secretion in rats with isolated pituitaries[8]. Daily treatment of hypophysectomized rats for 3 weeks with large doses of ACTH and small doses of cortisol results in markedly decreased CRF content in the medial basal hypothalamus[9]. Similarly, prolonged systemic treatment with high doses of corticosteroids results in decreased numbers of ACTH cells[10] and pituitary ACTH content[11]. When hypothalamic CRF content and pituitary ACTH content were measured 2 weeks after implants of dexamethasone into either the medial basal hypothalamus or the anterior pituitary, it was found that CRF activity falls after hypothalamic implants and increases after pituitary implants, whereas pituitary ACTH content decreases after both treatments[9]. Repeated administration of dexamethasone during 24–42 h results in decreased adrenal weight[6] and decreased adrenocortical responsiveness to ACTH[12]. Taken together, these results suggest strongly that chronic treatment with high doses of corticosteroids effectively abolishes the activity of the adrenocortical system in a heirarchical fashion, by inhibiting afferent input to the CRF neuron, and/or CRF synthesis and secretion, thus removing its trophic effect from the corticotroph, and thence the trophic effect of ACTH from the adrenal.

These results from studies in rats agree with the well-known inhibition of the adrenocortical axis that persists in man for months after withdrawal from chronic treatment with corticosteroids. After cessation of steroid therapy, or removal of hyperactive steroid-secreting tissue, recovery of normal and then supranormal levels of circulating ACTH precedes adrenal recovery and the re-establishment of normal circulating levels of cortisol and ACTH[13].

2. At 2 to 24 h After Treatment with Large Doses of Corticosteroids

The degree of inhibition of the adrenocortical response to ACTH-releasing stimuli that occurs during this period appears to depend on the nature of the stimulus used to excite the system and the mode of steroid pretreatment.

Stimuli to ACTH secretion have been divided into a variety of categories based on those that provoke responses after a given experimental manipulation versus those that no longer increase adrenocortical activity. One such categorization of stimuli has been based on whether a given stimulus activates the adrenocortical system when applied 2–7 h after treatment with maximally effective doses of dexamethasone[14,15]. On the basis of this criterion, stimuli have been divided into those that activate steroid-sensitive, low-threshold neural pathways to the CRF neuron (steroid-sensitive), and those that activate in addition steroid-resistant, high-threshold neural pathways (steroid-resistant). Examples of some corticosteroid-sensitive and corticosteroid-resistant stimuli drawn from the work of several laboratories are shown in Fig. 1. The data represent the results from experiments in three species (man[16], dog[15,17] and rat[14,18–20]), and are in remarkably good agreement across laboratories in the same species, and across species in those cases where comparison is possible.

An alternative explanation for the results shown in Fig. 1 has been advanced by others[1,18,21]. Rather than high-threshold, steroid-resistant pathways, the results are equally well explained theoretically as responses to very strong stimulation of a single, low-threshold pathway, under the conditions that the feedback sites have been saturated by corticosteroids. New evidence from experiments to be presented below suggests strongly that steroid-sensitive and steroid-resistant pathways exist. In addition, Sirett and Gibbs[18] presented evidence that some stimuli that provoked adrenocortical activity when presented 4 h after treat-

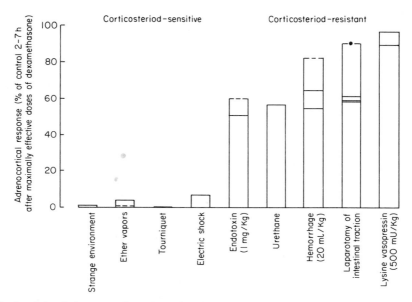

Fig. 1. Stimuli that normally activate the adrenocortical system are divided into those in which the adrenal response is blocked by pretreatment with a single large dose of corticosteroids (corticosteroid-sensitive) and those that still cause a response after pretreatment with a maximally effective dose of corticosteroids (corticosteroid-resistant). The figure is drawn from work from many laboratories and represents data obtained in man (-•-, 16), dogs (- - -, 15, 17) and rats (———, 14, 18, 19, 20).

ment with a maximally effective dose of dexamethasone, did not activate the system when presented 16 h after providing dexamethasone in the drinking water (Fig. 2). In agreement with Sayers and Sayers, these authors concluded that inhibition of ACTH secretion by large doses of dexamethasone is a function of the intensity of the ACTH-releasing stimulus and the time interval between steroid administration and stimulus application. An equally plausible interpretation of these results is that with increasing intervals between the initial administration of corticosteroid (provided that it is supplied continuously, as in the drinking water, or repeatedly, as in multiple injections) the humoral components of the system become progressively incompetent as indicated by the results from chronic experiments outlined in part 1. This interpretation is supported by the results of experiments from three laboratories[19,22,23] which determined the time course of inhibition of the adrenocortical response to stimuli after a single injection of maximally effective doses of corticosteroids to rats. The period of maximal inhibition was achieved between 2–4 h after injection and persisted at that degree of inhibition for 5–9 h before beginning to wear off (Fig. 3). The responses to laparotomy with intestinal traction and adrenal vein cannulation (which may involve a component of intestinal traction) were not entirely inhibited at any time, whereas the response to strange environment was totally inhibited. A comparison of the results of Figs. 2 and 3 suggests strongly

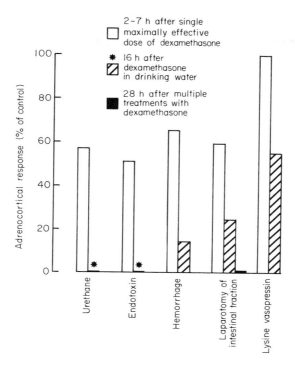

Fig. 2.   The adrenal response to stimuli that after a single maximally effective dose of dexamethasone is progressively inhibited by prolonging the period of ingestion or injection of the steroid. The figure represents data redrawn from Sirett and Gibbs (18,☐ and ▨) and from Engeland *et al.* (6,■).

that continuous or repeated treatment with very high doses of corticosteroids causes a progressive atrophy of the system within 24 h which is not caused by a single injection.

a.   Site of Delayed Feedback

From the results of studies on rat tissue *in vitro*, it is clear that corticosterone, cortisol and dexamethasone act both at the anterior pituitary to inhibit ACTH (synthesis and) secretion[24,25], and at the hypothalamus to inhibit CRF synthesis (and secretion)[26]. It is not possible from such studies to estimate the relative capacity of feedback at the two sites.

Pituitary. The results from two studies, which compared adrenal responses to an ACTH-releasing stimulus with those to a partially purified CRF preparation after pretreatment of rats with increasing doses of cortisol, suggested that pituitary sites are unaffected by cortisol treatment, or saturate at lower doses than brain feedback sites[27,28]. Similar conclusions were drawn from experiments that used dexamethasone as the blocking agent[19,29]. The marked similarities between the

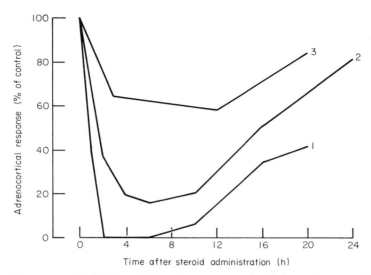

Fig. 3. Time course of inhibition of adrenal responses to stimuli that activate steroid-sensitive (line 3) pathways and steroid-resistant (lines 1, 2) pathways after a single maximally effective dose of corticosteroid at 0 time. The figure is drawn from the data of Smelik (22), Kendall (23) and Takebe *et al.* (19) and shows the time course of inhibition in response to the stimuli of strange environment, (line 1), adrenal vein cannulation (line 2) and laparotomy with intestinal traction (line 3). Increasing the dose of steroid given at time 0 prolongs the duration of the inhibition, but does not increase its magnitude after stimuli that activate steroid-resistant pathways (19).

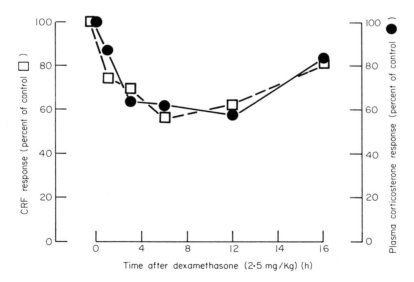

Fig. 4. The time course and degree of inhibition of response in hypothalamic CRF activity (measured at 2 min) and in plasma corticosterone (measured at 20 min) are similar after laparotomy, with intestinal traction presented at the indicated times after treatment of rats with a maximally effective dose of dexamethasone (2.5 mg/kg) at 0 time. Data redrawn from ref. (19).

time course and degree of inhibition of the CRF and plasma corticosterone responses to laparotomy with intestinal traction determined by Takebe *et al.*[19] suggest that the effect of dexamethasone at the pituitary is negligible (Fig. 4).

CRF neuron and central nervous pathways. There are, as yet, no results from feedback studies *in vivo* that can distinguish absolutely between inhibition of the excitatory neural input to the CRF neuron and inhibition of CRF synthesis within the neuron. Pretreatment of rats with cortisol has been shown to abolish the normal increase in hypothalamic CRF activity after ether and sham-adrenal-ectomy[3], a stimulus that is dexamethasone-sensitive[14]. However, treatment with large doses of dexamethasone diminished, but did not block the normal increase in hypothalamic CRF content after laparotomy with intestinal traction[19]. These results suggest that in the former experiment the steroid acted on steroid-sensitive pathways to inhibit input to the CRF neuron, since the latter experiments demonstrated that a normal pattern of CRF response could occur in the face of maximally effective corticosteroid blockade. Other evidence also makes it seem likely that corticosteroids act to inhibit the input to the CRF neuron by afferent neural pathways that are steroid-sensitive. The fact that the adrenocortical response to exposure to ether vapors, sham-adrenalectomy or scald of a hind foot (under deep pentobarbital anesthesia) in the rat is completely inhibited by pretreatment of rats with 2 μg of dexametha-sone/100 g body wt.[14] (unpublished results), whereas the adrenocortical response to stimuli involving general visceral afferents, such as intestinal traction or large hemorrhage, cannot be entirely suppressed by a maximally effective dose of corticosteroids, argues in favor of potent inhibition by steroids of selected sensory afferent pathways. This argument is furthered by the observa-tions that, in the absence of dexamethasone treatment, the magnitudes of the elevations in hypothalamic CRF content at 2 min, and of circulating ACTH as well as corticosterone levels 20 min after administration of the highly dexa-methasone-sensitive stimulus of sham-adrenalactomy and the steroid-resistant stimulus of laparotomy with intestinal traction are similar[31].

b. *Inhibition of ACTH-secretion with Doses of the Naturally Occurring Steroid within the Physiological Range; Stimulus-induced Facilitation of Subsequent Responses*

Infusions of cortisol for 45 min or longer into patients with Addison's disease[32] or into adrenalectomized dogs[33] or of corticosterone into adrenal-ectomized rats[34] reduce the high initial circulating ACTH levels in proportion to the dose of steroid infused. Plasma corticosteroid levels resulting from these infusions were within the range that can be achieved by adrenal secretion.

Several laboratories have now shown that corticosterone, infused intravenously, intraperitoneally or injected subcutaneously to increase plasma corticosterone concentration to levels similar to those observed after acute stimulation of the system, will inhibit the adrenocortical response to those stimuli previously defined by the use of dexamethasone as steroid-suppressible. The responses of rats to ether, sham-adrenalectomy[35], intraperitoneal injection[36], or low doses of histamine[37,38], have all been shown to be inhibited by elevation of plasma corticosterone levels for part or all of the 2 h preceding the stimulus.

These results suggest that corticosteroids secreted in response to an initial stimulus would inhibit the response to subsequent stimuli. There have been repeated attempts to demonstrate such a phenomenon in the rat; all have been unsuccessful (for review see ref. 39). In experiments in which the increase in plasma corticosterone levels in response to restraint was determined and matched in other rats by injections with either corticosterone or ACTH, Dallman and Jones[36] showed that treatment with either corticosterone or ACTH 3 h before intraperitoneal injection inhibits the adrenocortical response to injection, but that prior restraint, with equivalent increases in circulating corticosterone, does not. These authors concluded that the initial stimulus to the adrenocortical system left a facilitatory trace that exerted an equal and opposite effect to the inhibitory effect of the elevated corticosteroid levels. Gann *et al.*[40] later provided evidence of stimulus-induced facilitation or inhibition of subsequent adrenocortical responses in the dog by manipulating the magnitudes of the initial and final stimuli to the adrenocortical system.

In animals with intact adrenals therefore the feedback effects of physiological quantities of injected corticosteroids can be demonstrated, but corticosteroid secretion appears to play no discernible role on the subsequent function of the adrenocortical system. It is clear, however, that repeated bursts of adrenocortical activity affect activity in other endocrine systems, and it may be that repeated elevations in circulating corticosteroid levels alter the patterns of other endocrine responses to repeated stimuli (e.g. ref. 39).

3. Fast or Rate-sensitive Feedback

a. *Characteristics*

By 1962 at least three laboratories had demonstrated that inhibition of the adrenocortical response to ACTH-releasing stimuli occurred within seconds to minutes of the intravenous administration of corticosteroids[1,28,41]. The physiological relevance of these results was questioned because of the exceedingly high transients in corticosteroid levels achieved after a bolus injection, and because no inhibition was demonstrable during the period several minutes to 2 h after such injections[22,42]. Re-examination of the problem in 1969[37], with infusions of corticosterone that never caused plasma levels to exceed the physiological range, revealed that there was inhibition of the adrenocortical response to the stimulus of histamine if the substance was administered as plasma corticosterone levels were rising rapidly, near the onset of the corticosterone infusion. No inhibition of the response to histamine was detected after plasma corticosterone levels had reached a plateau (10 min) and inhibition of the response was detected once again at 2 h, the time of the delayed corticosteroid feedback effect. Since that time Jones *et al.*[43] have demonstrated that the fast-feedback effect of corticosterone requires a rate of change in plasma corticosterone levels of at least 1.3 μg/min/100ml in male rats. The inhibitory effect of increasing steroid levels does not depend on low initial values[34]. In female rats, the requisite rate of rise in plasma corticosterone to effect inhibition of the response to steroid-suppressible stimuli appears to be about 4 μg/min/100ml[44,45]. The difference in the threshold of inhibition between male and female rats may be explained on the basis of the greater binding of corticosterone by transcortin in female rat plasma, which leaves proportionately less free (presumably active) steroid at any given total concentration of corticosterone. In addition to suppressing adrenocortical responses to many of the steroid-sensitive stimuli defined by delayed-feedback studies, rate-sensitive feedback has been shown in one study to inhibit the response in proportion to the strength of the stimulus[44]. Additionally, stimuli that were shown to be steroid-resistant with the use of dexamethasone in the delayed-feedback time-domain, are also not inhibited by a fast-rate corticosteroid signal[44]. Jones and his co-workers[35] have done convincing pharmacological studies using steroid agonists and antagonists to demonstrate that the receptors mediating the fast and slow feedback actions of corticosteroids are different.

b.   Site of Fast-feedback

Studies of tissues *in vitro* have demonstrated fast feedback both at the pituitary to inhibit ACTH release[25,46], and at the hypothalamus to inhibit CRF release and elevate CRF content[26]. Studies testing pituitary–adrenal responsiveness to a CRF preparation *in vivo* showed no effect of fast feedback on the response to CRF using doses of hypothalamic extract that did not cause maximal adrenal activation[28,44]. Results from a study *in vivo* support the conclusion that a rapid rate of rise in plasma corticosterone levels inhibits secretion, but not synthesis of CRF when the steroid is provided *after* application of a steroid-sensitive stimulus to CRF secretion[31]. The results demonstrated that hypothalamic CRF content increased and subsequently ACTH levels decreased suggesting corticosteroid inhibition of the CRF secretory process. However, there is also evidence[44] that rate-sensitive feedback acts at central neural sites proximal to the CRF neuron, since the normal increase in CRF content that occurs 2 min after the steroid-sensitive stimulus of histamine, is prevented when an adequate rate of rise in plasma corticosterone is provided *before* the stimulus. Moreover, it was shown in the same study that after treatment with 6-hydroxydopamine the fast- but not slow-feedback efficacy of corticosterone was abolished, suggesting that the steroid required noradrenergic neural inputs for its feedback action[44].

c.   Effect of Feedback In Vivo *Revealed by* the Stimulus of Adrenalectomy

Normally corticosteroid secretion *follows* the application of a stimulus to the adrenocortical system. The studies reviewed above examined either the effects of steroids injected before the application of an ACTH-releasing stimulus, or the inhibition of ACTH levels elevated by the chronic absence of corticosteroids. To examine the normal physiology of corticosteroid feedback, bilateral adrenalectomy has been used as an acute stimulus to the adrenocortical system and the results of corticosteroid replacement on hypothalamic CRF content and circulating ACTH levels determined[31,47]. Rats subjected to sham bilateral adrenalectomy constituted the reference groups. After bilateral adrenalectomy, circulating ACTH levels increase within minutes and remain elevated above those observed in sham-operated rats from 10–40 min until at least 30 days[5, 31, 47–49]. Replacement with corticosterone injected subcutaneously 2 min after bilateral adrenalectomy restores the patterns of changes in hypothalamic CRF content[31] and circulating ACTH levels[31,47] to those observed after sham-adrenalectomy.

In the absence of corticosterone replacement, changes in hypothalamic CRF content and circulating ACTH levels during the first 2 post-operative hours, resemble those observed in rats subjected to the corticosteroid-resistant stimulus of laparotomy with intestinal traction[31]. Consideration of the observed changes in CRF content and circulating ACTH levels in the presence and absence of corticosterone replacement led to the conclusion that normally the fast-feedback action of corticosterone is to inhibit CRF secretion and the delayed action is to inhibit CRF synthesis[31]. Identical conclusions were reached by Jones *et al.*[26] studying the direct effect of corticosterone on CRF-secretion from the stimulated hypothalamus *in vitro*.

The supposition that new CRF synthesis probably occurs 60–80 min after the application of a steroid-resistant stimulus[31,50] or adrenalectomy is strengthened by the recent finding by Hiroshige *et al.*[50] that the rise in hypothalamic CRF content normally observed 60–80 min after laparotomy with intestinal traction is prevented by pretreatment of rats with the protein synthesis inhibitor cycloheximide[50]. After cycloheximide, the stimulus provoked the initial rapid increase in CRF and ACTH levels but the response was not sustained for more than 10 min.

Under normal conditions both the fast- and delayed-feedback actions of corticosteroids limit the duration and magnitude of CRF and ACTH secreted in response to steroid-sensitive stimuli. In response to steroid-resistant stimuli, or adrenalectomy without corticosteroid replacement, it appears that the capacities of the CRF neuron to synthesize and secrete CRF[26], and the corticotrophe to synthesize and secrete ACTH[48,49] may limit the ability of the adrenocortical system to respond maximally for periods longer than several hours. It appears to require at least 48 h after adrenalectomy to achieve normal CRF[26] and ACTH[48,49] secretory capacity.

INTERACTIONS AMONG CORTICOSTERONE, ADRENAL NUMBER AND STEROID-SUPPRESSIBLE AND -RESISTANT STIMULI

From anatomical studies, Halasz and Szentágothai[51] proposed that a neural feedback from the adrenal to the hypothalamus, inhibited brain–pituitary–adrenal function. Functional evidence for such feedback has recently been obtained by others[31,52].

Recently we[53] have undertaken a formal study of the relationships among the magnitude of corticosteroid feedback signal, the number of adrenal glands borne by the rat (0, bilateral adrenalectomy; 1, unilateral adrenalectomy; 2, sham adrenalectomy) and the magnitude of the ACTH response 3 min after application of stimuli to ACTH secretion. Rats were given corticosterone dissolved in their drinking fluid (0.5% ETOH, 0.5% saline) in doses ranging between 10 and 160 μg of corticosterone per ml. Adrenal surgery was performed 18 h after steroid treatment was initiated, and the steroid-sensitive stimulus of exposure to ether vapors, or the steroid-resistant stimulus of laparotomy with intestinal traction under ether anesthesia was applied on the third day after adrenal surgery. Control and stimulated ACTH levels were measured by radioimmunoassay[31]. Plasma ACTH levels were determined at 3 min after the application of stimuli before plasma corticosterone levels increase, thus avoiding the modifying effects of steroid fast-feedback.

All surgical groups drank similar quantities of corticosteroid water daily, and the volume drunk did not vary across steroid doses. When the volume ingested was determined at 6 h intervals throughout the final 24 h period, it was found that more than 85% of the corticosterone was ingested during the 12 h preceding stress. Plasma corticosterone levels were not different among the three groups at 03 00 h or at 09 00 h for doses of corticosterone ranging between 10 and 160 μg/ml.

Results are shown in Table I and schematically in Fig. 5. Increasing doses of corticosterone resulted in progressive damping of the ACTH response to the steroid-sensitive stimulus. The slopes of the regression lines were significantly different among the groups with 0, 1 or 2 adrenals and, by extrapolation, the dose of corticosterone required entirely to suppress the ACTH response was not different in the three groups. The results show that adrenal number as well as corticosterone feeds back to inhibit ACTH secretion in response to steroid-sensitive stimuli. Additionally, these results suggest that corticosterone acts as a competitive inhibitor of the stimulus-induced ACTH secretion independently of adrenal number.

Increasing doses of corticosterone over the range of 10–80 μg/ml also diminished ACTH responses to the steroid-resistant stimulus; again, the magnitude of the ACTH response varied inversely with adrenal number, showing an inhibitory effect of the adrenal glands that is independent of their capacity to secrete corticosterone. However, after application of the steroid-resistant stimulus, the three sets of lines are not convergent but are rather nearly parallel and, by extrapolation, the dose of corticosterone required entirely to suppress the ACTH response

Table I.   Plasma ACTH levels 3 min after ether (steroid-sensitive) or laparotomy with intestinal traction (steroid-resistant) in rats with 0, 1 or 2 adrenals drinking fluid containing 10 or 40 μg of corticosterone (B)/ml.

	Steroid-sensitive		Steroid-resistant	
Dose of B (μg/ml)	10	40	10	40
Adrenal number[a]				
0	454 ± 53[b]	75 ± 35	532 ± 59	383 ± 57
1	156 ± 83	49 ± 16	155 ± 14	114 ± 19
2	84 ± 22	35 ± 8	130 ± 13	47 ± 6

[a]   0, Bilateral adrenalectomy; 1, unilateral adrenalectomy; 2, sham-adrenalectomy; adrenal surgery was performed 18 h after B was provided *ad lib* in drinking fluid and stress was performed 3 days after surgery.

[b]   Means ($n = 8$ or more) are accompanied by $\pm$ S.E.M.

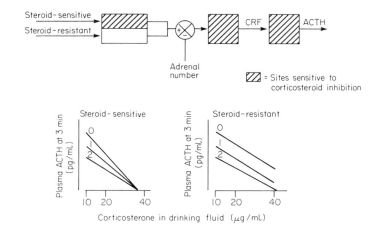

Fig. 5. Patterns of inhibition of ACTH secretion differ after a steroid-sensitive stimulus (ether) and a steroid-resistant stimulus (laparotomy with intestinal traction) in rats with 0, 1 or 2 adrenals drinking corticosterone (10, 20 or 40 mg/ml) *ad lib*. A schematic diagram showing an interpretation of the results is shown at the top of the figure. Increasing amounts of ingested corticosterone progressively inhibit the responses to both stimuli. An adrenal factor in addition to corticosterone determines the magnitude of the response to both stimuli. However, inhibition of the response to the steroid-sensitive stimulus by corticosterone is non-competitive with adrenal number (the 0-ACTH intercept is the same in the three groups). After a steroid-resistant stimulus, there is an interaction between the inhibition of the response by corticosterone and adrenal number (the 0-ACTH intercept depends both on the dose of corticosterone and on adrenal number).

is inversely related to the number of adrenal glands carried by the animal. When the amount of corticosterone is increased to 80 and then to 160 μg/ml the ACTH response to laparotomy with intestinal traction is reduced and then abolished in all three groups of rats.

The data from both sets of experiments suggest that an adrenal factor in addition to corticosterone feeds back to inhibit stress-induced ACTH secretion. From the results of other experiments[52], it seems likely that adrenal afferent nerves mediate the inhibition.

Additional inferences about the sites of corticosteroid and adrenal neural feedback can be drawn when the results of the experiments using steroid-sensitive and steroid-resistant stimuli are compared. Plasma ACTH levels observed 3 min after application of each stimulus are not different in the groups of rats drinking 10 μg of corticosterone/ml. However, the 0-ACTH intercept is approximately 30–40 μg of corticosterone for the steroid-sensitive stimulus, and is independent of the number of adrenal glands in the experimental animal. In contrast, in response to the steroid-resistant stimulus, the extrapolated 0–ACTH intercept is in all cases greater than 40 μg of corticosterone/ml, and the fewer the adrenals, the larger the dose of corticosterone required to inhibit totally the ACTH response. Taken together, these results suggest strongly that the major inhibitory effect of corticosterone on the response to the steroid-sensitive stimulus is proximal to the effect of adrenal number and that the inhibitory effect of corticosterone on the response to steroid-resistant stimuli is distal to the input of the adrenal glands. A possible schematic arrangement which accommodates the results is shown in Fig. 5.

In complete agreement with the inferences drawn from other studies reviewed above, the results of these experiments suggest that the components of the adrenocortical system with greatest sensitivity to corticosteroids are certain neural afferent pathways which, when excited, lead to CRF and ACTH secretion. Other neural afferent pathways (subserving the responses to stimulation of general visceral afferents?) are not sensitive to corticosteroids; however, at sufficiently high doses, corticosteroids act to inhibit the function of the adrenocortical system at the level of the CRF neuron (and consequently, at the corticotroph).

ACKNOWLEDGEMENTS

This work was supported in part by United States Public Health Services Grants AM06704 and NSAM00072 and NASA-Ames University Interchange Agreement NCA20R665-806.

REFERENCES

1. Sayers, G. and Sayers, M. (1947). *Endocrinology* **40**, 265.
2. McEwen, B. S. (1977). *Ann. N. Y. Acad. Sci.* **297**, 568.
3. Koch, B. *et al.* (1975). *Neuroendocrinol.* **18**, 299.
4. de Kloet, R. *et al.* (1975). *Endocrinology* **96**, 598.
5. Buckingham, J. C. and Hodges, J. R. (1974). *J. Endocrinol.* **53**, 213.
6. Engeland, W. C. *et al.* (1975). *Am. J. Physiology* **229**, 1461.
7. Stark, E. *et al.* (1968). *Canad. J. Physiol. Pharmacol.* **46**, 567.
8. Stark, E. *et al.* (1974/5). *Neuroendocrinol.* **13**, 224.
9. Chowers, I. *et al.* (1967). *Neuroendocrinol.* **2**, 193.
10. Siperstein, E. R. and Miller, K. J. (1970). *Endocrinology* **86**, 451.
11. Kraicer, J. *et al.* (1973). *Neuroendocrinol.* **11**, 156.
12. Dallman, M. F. *et al.* (1978). *Am. J. Physiology (in press).*
13. Graber, A. L. *et al.* (1965). *J. Clin. Endocrinol. Metab.* **25**, 11.
14. Dallman, M. F. and Yates, F. E. (1968). *Mem. Soc. Endocrinol. (London)* **17**, 39.
15. Gann, D. S. and Cryer, G. S. (1973). *In* "Brain–Pituitary–Adrenal Inter-relationships", (Brodish, A. and Redgate, E. S., eds.), Karger, Basel.
16. Estep, H. L. *et al.* (1963). *J. Clin. Endocrinol.* **23**, 419.
17. Egdahl, R. H. (1964). *J. Clin. Invest.* **43**, 2178.
18. Sirett, N. E. and Gibbs, F. P. (1969). *Endocrinology* **85**, 355.
19. Takebe, K. *et al.* (1971). *Endocrinology* **89**, 1014.
20. Allen, J. P. *et al.* (1973). *In* "Brain–Pituitary–Adrenal Interrelationships", (Brodish, A. and Redgate, E. S., eds.), Karger, Basel.
21. Yates, F. E. and Brennen, D. (1969). *In* "Hormonal Control Systems", (Stear, E. B. and Kadish, A. H. eds.), American Elsevier, New York.
22. Smelik, P. G. (1963). *Proc. Soc. Exp. Biol. Med.* **113**, 616.
23. Kendall, J. W. (1961). *Proc. Soc. Exp. Biol. Med.* **107**, 926.
24. Fleisher, N. and Rawls, W. E. (1970). *Am. J. Physiol.* **219**, 445.
25. Sayers, G. and Portanova, R. (1974). *Endocrinology* **94**, 1723.

26.   Jones, M. T. *et al.* (1976). *In* "Frontiers in Neuroendocrinology" Vol. 4, (Martini, L. and Ganong, W. F., eds.), Raven Press, New York.
27.   Vernikos-Danellis J. (1965). *Endocrinology* **76**, 122.
28.   Leeman, S. E. *et al.* (1962). *Endocrinology* **70**, 249.
29.   Russell, S. M. *et al.* (1969). *Endocrinology* **85**, 512.
30.   Vernikos-Danellis, J. (1964). *Endocrinology* **75**, 514.
31.   Sato, T. *et al.* (1975). *Endocrinology* **97**, 265.
32.   Wolfsen, A. R. and Odell, W. H. (1973). *In* "Brain–Pituitary–Adrenal Interrelationships", (Brodish, A. and Redgate, E. S. eds.), Karger, Basel.
33.   Cowan, J. S. and Windle, W. J. (1978). *Endocrinology* **103**, 1173.
34.   Rotsztejn, W. H. *et al.* (1975). *Endocrinology* **97**, 223.
35.   Jones, M. T. *et al.* (1974). *J. Endocrinol.* **60**, 223.
36.   Dallman, M. F. and Jones, M. T. (1973). *Endocrinology* **92**, 1367.
37.   Dallman, M. F. and Yates, F. E. (1969). *Ann. N. Y. Acad. Sci.* **156**, 696.
38.   Kaneko, M. and Hiroshige, T. (1978). *Am. J. Physiol.* **234**, R46.
39.   Dallman, M. F. and Wilkinson, C. W. (1978). *In* "Environmental Endocrinology", (Assenmacher, I. and Farner, D. S. eds.), Springer-Verlag, Berlin.
40.   Gann, D. S. *et al.* (1977). *Am. J. Physiol.* **232**, R5.
41.   Gray, W. D. and Munson, P. L. (1951). *Endocrinology* **48**, 471.
42.   Hodges, J. R. and Jones, M. T. (1964). *J. Physiol. (London)* **173**, 190.
43.   Jones, M. T. *et al.* (1972). *J. Endocrinol.* **55**, 489.
44.   Kaneko, M. and Hiroshige, T. (1978). *Am. J. Physiol.* **234**, R39.
45.   Abe, K. and Crichlow, V. (1977). *Endocrinology* **101**, 498.
46.   Smelik, P. G. (1977). *Ann. N. Y. Acad. Sci.* **297**, 580.
47.   Dallman, M. F. *et al.* (1971). *Endocrinology* **91**, 961.
48.   Dallman, M. F. *et al.* (1974). *Endocrinology* **95**, 65.
49.   Ruhmann-Wennhold, A. and Nelson, D. H. (1977). *Ann. N. Y. Acad. Sci.* **297**, 498.
50.   Hiroshige, T. *et al.* (1977). *Ann. N. Y. Acad. Sci.* **297**, 436.
51.   Halász, B. and Szenágothai, J. (1959). *Z. Zellforsch. Mikrosk. Anat.* **50**, 297.
52.   Engeland, W. C. *et al.* (1976). *Fed. Proc.* **35**, Abs. 460.
53.   Dallman, M. F., Wilkinson, C. W., Engeland, W. C. and Shinsako, J. *in preparation.*

16

THE CHARACTERISTICS AND MECHANISM OF ACTION OF CORTICOSTEROID NEGATIVE FEEDBACK AT THE HYPOTHALAMUS AND ANTERIOR PITUITARY

M. T. Jones, B. Gillham*, S. Mahmoud and M. C. Holmes

Sherrington School of Physiology and Department of Biochemistry,
St. Thomas's Hospital Medical School, London SE1 7EH, U.K.*

INTRODUCTION

The earliest work on the influence of corticosteroids on pituitary–adrenocortical activity was by Ingle and associates, who showed that administration of adrenocortical extracts to the intact rat resulted in adrenocortical atrophy, whereas the injection of anterior pituitary as well as adrenocortical extracts did not[1,2]. These results suggested that corticosteroids inhibited corticotropin (ACTH) secretion and that ACTH secretion could be modulated by a negative feedback effect of adrenocortical secretion. Further evidence for such a negative feedback mechanism was subsequently provided by the following observations.

(a)　Adrenalectomy in experimental animals resulted in an elevated blood level of ACTH[3,4,5,6]. Similarly, patients suffering from Addison's disease due to adrenocortical atrophy, also have elevated ACTH levels[7].

(b)　The high plasma ACTH levels resulting from adrenalectomy in experimental animals can be largely reduced by replacement therapy with physiological doses of corticosteroids[8,9]. Similarly replacement therapy reduces blood ACTH levels in Addisonian patients.

(c)　The release of ACTH in response to stress is greatly exaggerated in adrenalectomized animals, or patients suffering from Addison's disease, compared with the response in normal intact state.

The evidence for a negative feedback mechanism being involved and the numerous sites now implicated in this control have created a picture of considerable complexity. First, there appear to be two temporally distinct phases of corticosteroid feedback mechanisms[10], an immediate rate-sensitive feedback (fast feedback) control element associated with the rate of rise in plasma corticosteroid concentration, followed by a delayed feedback which occurs hours later when the plasma corticosterone is declining or low (delayed or slow feedback). The fast-feedback mechanism occurs only during an adequate rate of increase in the plasma corticosteroid level and so has a short duration of action. When the plasma corticosteroid levels reach a plateau, the inhibition disappears (so called "silent period") but without further corticoid administration the delayed feedback appears some 2 h later when the plasma corticosteroid levels are still high or declining. The rate of increase required to reduce the corticotropic (ACTH) response to surgical stress has been defined in the male rat and is about 13 μg/min/1[11,12]. Doubtlessly the rate or rise required will be different in other species and will vary with the stress used. In species where the half-life of corticosteroids is sex-dependent, a higher rate of elevation is required in the sex in which the corticosteroid half-life is shorter[13] (e.g. the female rat).

It is noteworthy that of the many steroids tested (but the list was not an exhaustive one) for fast-feedback activity only corticosterone, cortisol and dexamethasone were active[14]. On the delayed-feedback mechanism a wide variety of steroids exhibit activity[14]. It would appear that different steroid receptor mechanisms mediate the two feedback responses.

SITES OF FEEDBACK ACTION

A number of sites have been proposed for the negative-feedback action of corticosteroids. These include the anterior pituitary, the hypothalamus as well as the amygdala and hippocampus. [^{3}H] Corticosterone is taken up in various parts of the rat brain, particularly the hippocampus and dentate gyrus as well as in the septum[15]. [^{3}H] Corticosterone, unlike the sex steroid hormones, is not concentrated and retained in the hypothalamus, but is present in the anterior pituitary. Autoradiographic studies have therefore provided support for the concept of feedback at all the sites mentioned with the striking exception of the hypothalamus. There is much evidence for a corticosteroid feedback action at the hypothalamus and this suggests that the autoradiographic techniques are not sensitive enough to detect a significant (and important) uptake at this site. In view of the association of the hippocampus in behavioural responses it is quite likely that the effect of corticosteroids at this site is related to behavioural as well as feedback regulation.

Early observations tended to implicate the pituitary as the major point for feedback inhibition. Thus Rose and Nelson[16] found that infusion of cortisol into the pituitary fossa caused adrenal atrophy, whereas infusions into the subarachnoid space was ineffective. Sayers and Portonova[17] reported that cortisol reduces the response of the pituitary to corticoliberin (CRF). However, Vernikos-Danellis[18] found that cortisol injections decreased hypothalamic CRF as well as pituitary and plasma ACTH concentrations. These observations suggest hypothalamic as well as pituitary effects.

Table I. The effect of corticosterone pretreatment *in vivo* or its addition to the incubation medium on basal and acetyl-choline-induced release of CRF from the rat hypothalamus *in vitro*. The release of CRF was induced by stimulation with 3 pg/ml of acetylcholine for 10 min and assayed by corticosterone production *in vitro* in basal hypothalamic-lesioned female rats. The values represent the mean ± S.E.M. of 6 to 12 observations.

Experimental Group	Pretreatment *in vivo*	Pretreatment *in vitro*	Stimulus to CRF secretion	CRF secretion expressed as corticosterone production *in vitro* (µg/100 mg/h)
A	Vehicle s.c. 4 h before death.	NIL	Basal release Ach	2.3 ± 0.3 (9) 5.9 ± 0.5 (12)
B	2 mg corticosterone/100g s.c. 4 h before death	NIL	Basal release Ach	1.6 ± 0.2 (9) 1.9 ± 0.2 (12)
C	Vehicle s.c. 4 h before death	Steroid-free medium changed at 30 min and 90 min before stimulation *in vitro*.	Basal release Ach	2.1 ± 0.3 (6) 5.5 ± 0.4 (12)
D	Vehicle s.c. 4 h before death	100 ng/ml corticosterone for 30 min, steroid-free medium for further 90 min before stimulation *in vitro*.	Basal release Ach	1.5 ± 0.1 (12) 1.7 ± 0.2 (9)

A. Hypothalamus

1.   Delayed Feedback

Implantation of cortisol [19] in rabbits is ineffective when the implant is placed in the anterior pituitary but is extremely effective when placed in the hypothalamus; this argues for a hypothalamic site of delayed feedback. Cortisol injections and dexamethasone implants[20] in the hypothalamus decrease hypothalamic CRF as well as pituitary and plasma ACTH concentrations. More direct evidence for delayed corticosteroid feedback at the hypothalamus comes from experiments carried out using the hypothalamus *in vitro*, following pretreatment *in vivo*, or pre-incubation *in vitro* with corticosteroids before stimulation of CRF release with an excitatory neurotransmitter[21]. Composite results are shown in Table I.

2.   Fast Feedback

Inhibition by corticosterone and cortisol of neurotransmitter-induced release has been demonstrated using the hypothalamus *in vitro*[21,22] and hypothalamic synaptosomes *in vitro*[23]. Changes in hypothalamic CRF induced by stress and

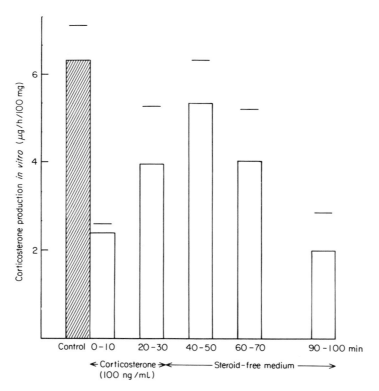

Fig. 1.   The effect of corticosterone (100 ng/ml) on the acetylcholine (3 pg/ml) induced release of CRF. Each histogram gives the mean ± S.E.M. of observations in 9 to 12 animals.

corticosteroid treatment have similarly been interpreted as evidence for fast feedback at the hypothalamus[24].

It has to be mentioned that what has been demonstrated at the hypothalamus *in vitro* is the immediate inhibition of neurotransmitter-induced release of CRF. This is certainly compatible with fast feedback but whether it is truely a rate-sensitive feedback effect has yet to be established. However, Abe and Critchlow[12] demonstrated fast feedback in the rat and found that the inhibition occurred when the hypothalamus was surgically isolated, thus showing that fast feedback lies within the hypothalamo–pituitary complex. As fast feedback at the pituitary is not rate sensitive, it must be concluded that the hypothalamus is the rate-sensitive component of the hypothalamo-pituitary complex. The data in Fig. 1 are compatible with the fast feedback being rate-sensitive since 30 min after addition of the steroid, when there would presumably be an equilibrium between the steroid and its receptor, the inhibition of neurotransmitter-induced release of CRF *in vitro* is only partial. The delayed feedback does not appear until 100 min after the addition of the steroid. However, more rigorous tests are required to establish whether the effect at the hypothalamus is indeed rate-sensitive.

3.   *Possible mechanisms of corticosteroid feedback at the hypothalamus*

In experiments on the fast-feedback mechanism (Table II) it was found that corticosterone significantly ($p < 0.001$) inhibited the release of CRF and at the same time caused an increase in the tissue content of CRF activity ($p < 0.005$).

Table II.   The effect of fast and delayed corticosterone negative feedback on the content of CRF in the rat hypothalamus *in vitro* after stimulation with acetylcholine (Ach) (3 pg/ml) for 10 min. The CRF values are expressed in terms of corticosterone production *in vitro* (μg/h/100 mg) obtained in basal hypothalamic-lesioned female rats. The values represent mean ± S.E.M. The numbers of assay animals are shown in parentheses; 12 hypothalami were used in each group. Values in groups A and B are significantly different in terms of hypothalamic CRF content ($p < 0.01$) and CRF release ($p < 0.001$). Hypothalamic CRF content in groups C and D are not significantly different but CRF release is at $p < 0.001$.

Group	Treatment	CRF content of ½ hypothalamus	CRF release into the medium
A	No feedback	4.5 ± 0.8 (6)	5.8 ± 0.6 (16)
B	Fast feedback (1 ng/ml corticosterone)	6.8 ± 0.6 (9)	2.5 ± 0.3 (18)
C	No feedback	4.3 ± 0.8 (9)	4.7 ± 0.5 (13)
D	Delayed feedback (100 ng/ml corticosterone)	4.4 ± 0.7 (9)	0.9 ± 0.3 (7)

This suggests that the fast-feedback action of corticosterone is mediated *via* the inhibition of CRF release but that there is little or no effect on the synthesis of CRF. Similar results were obtained using cortisol (1 ng/ml) as the fast-feedback signal.

In previous studies we had shown that both noradrenaline and γ-aminobutyric acid (GABA) inhibited CRF release *in vitro*. We therefore tested for the possibility that the fast-feedback action of corticosterone *in vitro* is *via* the release of endogenous noradrenaline or GABA. The results (Fig. 2b), show that corticosterone (10 ng/ml) reduced the acetycholine-induced release of CRF to basal levels and that this inhibition was unaffected by either phentolamine (100 ng/ml) or picrotoxin (100 ng/ml). The antagonists were used in doses that have been shown to be effective in antagonizing the inhibitory action of noradrenaline and GABA *in vitro*[21,22]. These results suggest that the fast-feedback action of corticosterone *in vitro* is not mediated *via* the release of endogenous GABA or noradrenaline.

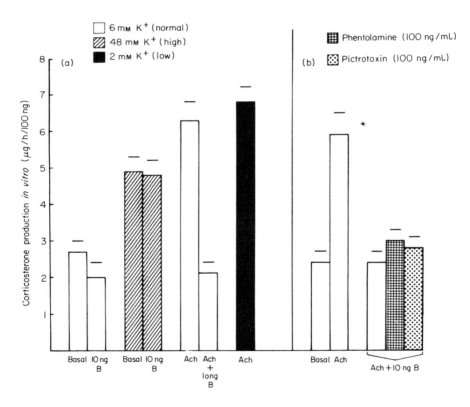

Fig. 2. (a) The effects of acetylcholine (Ach, 3 pg/ml) and corticosterone (B) on the release of CRF from hypothalami incubated in medium containing various concentrations of K^+. (b) The effect of phentolamine (▦) and picrotoxin (▦) on the corticosterone-induced inhibition of the release of CRF in response to acetylcholine. Each histogram gives the mean ± S.E.M. of a minimum of 10 observations.

(a)   *Potassium studies.* Hypothalami, incubated in a medium in which the concentration of K^+ was elevated (12–48mM), showed a higher basal secretion of CRF than hypothalami incubated in medium containing a normal K^+ concentration (6mM). A summary of our studies on the effects of K^+ on CRF secretion are given in Fig. 2(b). Corticosterone in a dose of 10 ng/ml inhibited the acetylcholine-induced release of CRF, but had no effect on the basal release of CRF from the hypothalami incubated in normal medium (6mM K^+) or from the hypothalamic incubated in a medium with a raised K^+ level (48mM K^+). The depolarization of CRF cells with K^+ overcomes the inhibitory action of corticosterone on CRF release and this suggests that the action of corticosterone may be that of membrane stabilization. One possibility is that corticosterone may affect K^+ flux and thus effect hyperpolarization. This was tested by incubating hypothalami in medium with a low level of K^+ (2mM). Hypothalami incubated in such a medium did not show any impaired ability to release CRF in response to acetylcholine (Fig. 2).

(b)   *Calcium studies.* Since Ca^{2+} appears to play a role in stimulus-secretion coupling, we examined the effect of alterations in the Ca^{2+} concentration of the incubation medium on CRF secretion from the hypothalamus. Table III shows that increasing the concentration of Ca^{2+} in the medium from 0 to 6mM increased the release of CRF activity into the medium. The amount of CRF released in the Ca^{2+}-free medium was not significantly different from the baseline of the assay. The presence of Ca^{2+} in the medium is essential for the release of CRF since acetylcholine did not cause any significant release of CRF from hypothalami incubated in Ca^{2+}-free medium. Further support for this hypothesis is provided by experiments in which the Ca^{2+} concentration of the medium was increased from 1.45mM (normal) to 4.0mM as this resulted in an increase in the release of CRF in response to acetylcholine.

It is possible that the enhanced release of CRF in high Ca^{2+} medium might be due to an increased release of endogenous acetylcholine. This seems unlikely, however, since hexamethonium, in a dose (1 μg/ml) that has been shown to be effective[21,22] in blocking the acetylcholine-induced release of CRF *in vitro*, is without effect on CRF release in high-Ca^{2+} medium.

Corticosterone (10 pg/ml) had no effect on the basal release of CRF in medium containing a high concentration of Ca^{2+}. However, when the concentration of corticosterone in the medium was increased to 1 ng/ml there was a highly significant ($p < 0.001$) reduction in the release of CRF. This suggests that the fast-feedback action of corticosterone might be mediated *via* an effect on Ca^{2+} flux. This appears to be confirmed by experiments that showed that the inhibitory action of corticosterone on CRF secretion in high-Ca^{2+} medium can be mimicked by the presence in the medium of 12 mM manganese, which is known to block Ca^{2+} channels (Table III). Further support is provided by experiments that showed that the effects of Ca^{2+} on CRF secretion could be mimicked by the replacement of Ca^{2+} by strontium (Table III). However, corticosterone in the same dose as that used in the Ca^{2+} experiments did not block the CRF secretion in response to a high concentration (6mM) of Sr^{2+}.

In delayed-feedback studies on the hypothalamus *in vitro*, it was found that acetylcholine caused a highly significant release of CRF activity which could be inhibited ($p < 0.001$) by exposure to a delayed-feedback signal 2 h previously

Table III. The influence of Ca^{2+} and Sr^{2+} on the release of CRF and the effect of corticosterone and manganese on the Ca^{2+}-induced changes. CRF was estimated as described in Tables I and II. 6-12 hypothalami were used in each group. *In vitro* corticosterone production in lesioned rats injected with saline was 0.9 ± 0.1 $\mu g/h/100$ mg. All values represent the mean $\pm$ S.E.M.

Group	Alteration in the ionic composition of incubating medium	Stimulus to CRF secretion	CRF secretion expressed as corticosterone *in vitro* ($\mu g/h/100$ mg)
A	Ca^{2+}-free	Basal Ach	1.4 ± 0.3 (6) 1.4 ± 0.4 (6)
B	1.45 mM Ca^{2+} (Normal)	Basal Ach	1.9 ± 0.1 (12) 5.3 ± 0.5 (9)
C	6.0 mM Ca^{2+} (High)	Basal Basal + corticosterone (10 pg/ml) Basal + corticosterone (1 ng/ml) Basal + 1 μg hexamethonium Ach	4.6 ± 0.5 (9) 4.7 ± 0.7 (9) 2.0 ± 0.3 (12) 4.8 ± 0.4 (6) 9.1 ± 0.9 (9)
D	6.0 mM Ca^{2+} + 12 mM Mn^{2+}	Basal	1.6 ± 0.4 (9)
E	Sr^{2+} 6 mM	Basal Basal + corticosterone (1 ng/ml)	8.6 ± 1.0 (6) 5.8 ± 0.6 (6)

(Table II). However, the corticosterone did not significantly alter the CRF content, suggesting that corticosterone inhibits the formation as well as the release of CRF. These delayed-feedback effects fit the classical concept of a steroid–receptor complex acting *via* the genome to affect the biosynthesis of a peptide hormone or its precursor.

B.   Anterior Pituitary

Of the many techniques available for the study of corticosteroid feedback at the anterior pituitary, we used the basal hypothalamic-lesioned rat, pretreated with vehicle or a steroid and stimulated to release ACTH in response to the injection of hypothalamic extract (HE-CRF) or 5-HT-stimulated CRF (5-HT-CRF). The major drawback of this system is its lack of practicability owing to the tedium of the operation and an overall mortality of 10%. In addition, there is always the danger of damage, because the lesioning disrupts pituitary blood flow. However, the latter problem seems potential rather than real in our experiments and indeed Porter *et al.*[25] have shown the pituitary has a normal flow at the time when we use the animals (i.e. 2 days after lesioning). The 5-HT-stimulated CRF was obtained by adding 10 ng/ml to 6–9 hypothalami *in vitro* (three per tube containing 1 ml of CSF-like medium) and 0.5 ml was injected i.v. into the lesioned animals.

1.   Fast Feedback

In these studies the rats were treated with vehicle or a steroid in a dose of 100 μg/100 g s.c. 20 min before the injection of HE- or 5-HT-CRF. Table IV

Table IV.   The effect of corticosterone pretreatment in lesioned rats on the response to either hypothalamic extracts (HE) or 5-HT CRF. Each value represents the mean ± S.E.M. of five to nine animals. Whole hypothalamic extract in 1.0 ml of 0.1 M HCl, neutralized and 0.5 ml injected i.v. into each lesioned rat. 5-HT-CRF was obtained as described previously (21) and 0.5 ml was injected i.v.

Group	ACTH stimulus	Time of HE injection after corticosterone pretreatment	Corticosterone production *in vitro* (μg/h/100 mg)
A	0.5 H.E. i.v.	0	10.5 ± 0.7 (6)
		10 min	11.3 ± 0.5 (9)
		20 min	2.9 ± 0.3 (9)
		40 min	10.7 ± 0.6 (9)
		50 min	1.4 ± 0.2 (6)
		100 min	0.9 ± 0.1 (9)
B	0.5 ml 5-HT-CRF i.v.	0	8.5 ± 0.3 (6)
		10 min	7.9 ± 1.0 (5)
		15 min	3.5 ± 1.0 (6)
		20 min	2.3 ± 0.7 (6)
		40 min	8.0 ± 1.2 (6)
		100 min	1.5 ± 0.7 (8)

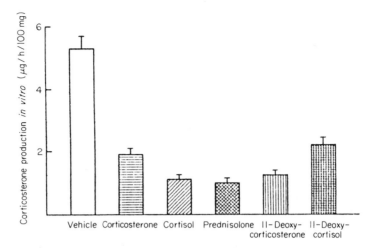

Fig. 3. The increase in corticosterone production *in vitro* (reflecting ACTH secretion) after crude CRF injection i.v. in basal hypothalamic-lesioned rats. Rats were injected with vehicle or the steroids in a dose of 100 μg/100 g 20 min before i.v. CRF administration. Each histogram is the mean ± S.E.M. of six or more observations.

shows that the administration of 500 μg corticosterone subcutaneously to basal hypothalamic-lesioned rats leads to significantly reduced response to CRF derived from either source. The ACTH release induced by both CRF stimuli was inhibited 20 min after injection but the effect had disappeared by 40 min. However, 100 min after administration of the steroid there was a further inhibition of the CRF response. This demonstrates the biphasic inhibitory response to corticosteroid occurs at the pituitary as well as at the hypothalamic level. However, it is important that too much is not made of gross similarities between the two tissues feedback sites for there are a number of ways in which the mechanisms at the two sites differ and these will be explained later. As shown in Fig. 3, corticosterone, cortisol, prednisolene, 11-deoxycorticosterone and 11-deoxycortisol significantly ($p < 0.001$) inhibited ACTH release. In contrast to the reduction provided by corticosterone and cortisol, progesterone and pregnenolone did not influence the corticotrophic response to CRF.

In an attempt to assess the possible relevance of fast feedback at the anterior pituitary, experiments were performed in which CRF was injected into lesioned animals bearing one or two adrenals when the magnitude of the corticotrophic response (as indicated by corticosterone production *in vitro*) was determined. With animals bearing one adrenal, subsequent corticosterone production *in vitro* by that gland is greater than in comparable experiments when one adrenal is removed from animals with two (Fig. 4). This difference may derive from differences in either pituitary or adrenal sensitivity between the two groups of animals. The possibility of differences in adrenal sensitivity occurring under these circumstances was eliminated when it was found that injection of Tetracosactrin (4 ng/100 g body weight) i.v. caused the release of 5.5 ± 0.5 μg/h/100 mg *in vitro*

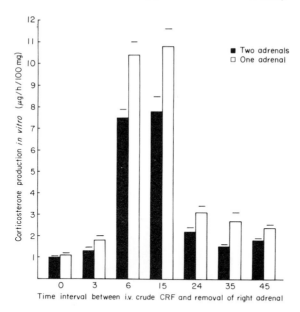

Fig. 4.   Increase in corticosterone production *in vitro* at various times after i.v. injection of crude CRF (½ hypothalamic equivalent) into basal hypothalamic-lesioned animals with one adrenal (□) or two adrenals (■). Each histogram is the mean ± S.E.M. of six or more observations.

when the adrenal was removed from animals bearing only one gland and 4.9 ± 0.3 when the gland was one of two from the animal, these differences in responsivity not being significant. A difference in pituitary response might be ascribed to a more rapid or a more profound rise in plasma corticosterone before the excision of the adrenal for incubation *in vitro* in the case of animals with two adrenals. These results imply that fast feedback is responsive to the amount that is normally secreted by adrenal glands.

   Is fast feedback at the pituitary rate sensitive? Changes in plasma corticosterone concentrations in animals with two adrenals showed that the levels reached a plateau by 10 min and thereafter the concentration falls (preinjection concentration = 2 ± 2; 5 min = 28 ± 3; 10 min = 42 ± 1.5; 20 min = 37 ± 1.7; 30 min = 31.0 ± 2.1 μg/100 ml). However, the ACTH response was not inhibited at 5 min. — the time at which the rate of increase in plasma corticosterone was most rapid, but it was inhibited at 10,20 and 30 min. Thus inhibition at the pituitary level is seen when the concentration has reached a plateau and even when the plasma corticosterone concentration is falling (i.e. at 30 min) but not at the time when corticosterone is rapidly increasing (5 min). This means that fast feedback is not rate sensitive at this site, which is in contrast with observations in response to stress in the normal animal where the fast feedback shows rate sensitivity. It must be concluded that the rate sensor is above the pituitary level.

2.   *Delayed Feedback*

The delayed-feedback action of corticosterone is not apparent until 1 h or longer after the steroid injection and the degree and duration of inhibition depends on the dose given[10]. In experiments designed to test for the delayed-feedback action of corticosteroids, these were given subcutaneously in arachis oil to basal hypothalamic-lesioned rats and the corticotrophic responses to CRF injection was tested 4 h after treatment with the steroid. (The CRF was injected 48 h after lesioning.) The steroids that inhibited ACTH release include corticosterone, cortisol, 11-deoxycorticosterone, 11-deoxycortisol, dexamethasone,

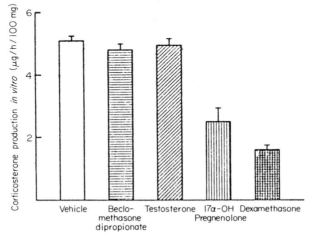

Fig. 5.   Corticosterone production *in vitro* in basal hypothalamic-lesioned rats in response to crude CRF (½ hypothalami equivalent) treated s.c. 4 h before with vehicle or steroid (5 mg/100 g). Each histogram represents the mean ± S.E.M. of six or more observations.

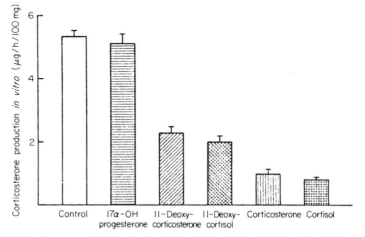

Fig. 6.   Corticosterone production *in vitro* in basal hypothalamic-lesioned rats in response to crude CRF (½ hypothalamic equivalent) after treatment s.c. 4 h before with vehicle or steroid (5 mg/100 g). Each histogram represents the mean ± S.E.M. of six or more observations.

Table V. Differences between fast- and delayed-feedback mechanisms at the hypothalamus and anterior pituitary. C, corticosterone; DOC, 11-deoxycorticosterone; S, 11-deoxycortisol; P, progesterone; 17 α-OH-P, 17-α-OH-progesterone; 17 α-OH-PN, 17-α-OH-pregnenolone; BD, beclamethasone diproprionate.

Nature of feedback	Hypothalamus	Anterior pituitary
Fast feedback (FFB)	(1) DOC, an antagonist (i.e. antagonizes the FFB action of C)	(1) DOC, an agonist
	(2) S, an antagonist	(2) S, an agonist
	(3) P, an antagonist	(3) P, an agonist
	(4) 17 α-OH-P, an antagonist	(4) 17 α-OH-P, no effect
	(5) FFB probably rate sensitive	(5) FFB does not show rate sensitivity
Delayed feedback (DFB)	(1) 17 α-OH-P, an antagonist (i.e. antagonizes the DFB action of C)	(1) 17 α-OH-P, no effect
	(2) 17 α-OH-PN, no effect	(2) 17 α-OH-PN, an agonist
	(3) BD, an agonist inhibiting CRF secretion at 4 h after pretreatment *in vivo*	(3) BD, no effect at 4 h but does at 24 h
	(4) P, no effect	(4) P, an agonist

and 17 α-OH-pregnenolone (Figs. 5 and 6). By contrast 17 α-OH-progesterone, beclamethasone diproprionate and also testosterone showed no inhibitory effect in the lesioned animals. It is especially noteworthy that 17 α-OH-progesterone has been shown to block the delayed-feedback action of corticosterone at the hypothalamus[21], but all attempts to show a cognate effect at the anterior pituitary failed. So this lack of effect of 17 α-OH-progesterone demonstrates that the delayed-feedback mechanisms at the hypothalamus and anterior pituitary are different. This and other differences between fast feedback and delayed feedback at the two sites are summarized in Table V.

RELATIVE IMPORTANCE OF THE HYPOTHALAMUS AND ANTERIOR PITUITARY AS FEEDBACK SITES

One approach to this question is the study of the effect of steroids at the two sites and then correlate these findings with what happens in the intact animal in response to stress.

A. Fast Feedback

Some steroids have very different effects at the two sites. Thus 11-deoxycorticosterone and 11-deoxycortisol antagonize the fast-feedback action of corticosterone at the hypothalamus but are agonists at the anterior pituitary (i.e. suppress ACTH release). If the pituitary were the more important site of action for these steroids then the stress response would be suppressed, whereas the stress response would be exaggerated if the hypothalamus were the more important. The corticotropic response to the stress of sham bilateral adrenalectomy in intact animals pretreated with 11-deoxycorticosterone or 11-deoxycortisol is exaggerated[14], thus indicating that for the rapidly effective feedback the anterior pituitary is of little importance. The antagonism of the fast-feedback action of corticosterone by these 11-deoxycorticosteroids is of considerable theoretical importance because these data indicate that occupation of hypothalamic receptor sites by corticosterone must occur in the course of the stress response and this can be prevented by steroids that also bind but produce no effect. Another observation points to the relative dominance of fast feedback at the hypothalamus. In this case, prednisolone was shown to be agonistic at the pituitary, but had no effect at the hypothalamus *in vitro* or in intact animals subjected to surgical stress. A word of caution is necessary, however, for it must be remembered that we are dealing here with surgical stress and the importance of the different sites may depend on the nature of the stress used since different neural and humoral pathways will be involved. Therefore inferences based on the present findings should be restricted to surgical stress.

The hypothalamus is "upstream" in relation to the pituitary and so it should not be altogether suprising if CRF does override feedback at the pituitary. That such an effect can occur is demonstrated in Table VI where increasing doses of hypothalamic-extract overcomes the feedback action of deoxycorticosterone in the lesioned animal.

Table VI. The effect of increasing the dose of hypothalamic extract on the fast-feedback action induced by 11-deoxycorticosterone (DOC) at the anterior pituitary. Each value represents the mean ± S.E.M. of the numbers of animals given in parentheses.

Pretreatment	Amount of hypothalamic extract i.v.	Corticosterone production *in vitro* (μg/h/100 mg)
Vehicle s.c. 20 min	½ HE	5.8 ± 0.5 (8)
Vehicle s.c. 20 min	1½ HE	12.5 ± 0.6 (7)
DOC (100 μg) s.c. 20 min	½ HE	1.7 ± 0.1 (7)
DOC (100 μg) s.c. 20 min	1½ HE	6.9 ± 0.3 (9)

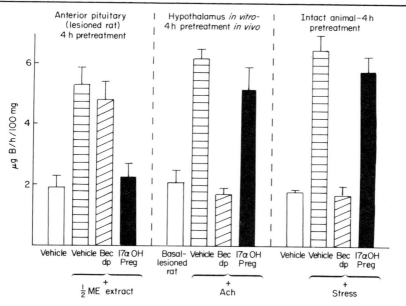

Fig. 7. The effects on the stress response and the responsiveness of the anterior pituitary and hypothalamus induced by 4 h pretreatment with beclamethasone diproprionate (Bec. dp.) or 17 α-OH-pregnenolone (17 α OH preg). Each steroid was given in a dose of 10 mg/100 g s.c. Data in the left panel represents those obtained when the steroids were injected into basal-hypothalamic-lesioned rats and the response to ½ median eminence extract (½ ME) was tested. The centre panel represents data obtained when hypothalami were removed from pretreated rats and challenged to release CRF in response to acetylcholine (Ach, 3 pg/ml). The right panel represents the findings when pretreated rats were subjected to the stress of sham bilateral adrenalectomy. All columns represent the mean ± S.E.M. of six or more observations.

B.   Delayed Feedback

We have little information of the relative importance of the two sites for the delayed-feedback system: only two steroids show differential effects on delayed feedback. These are 17 α-OH-pregnenolone and beclamethasone diproprionate. The former shows delayed feedback at the pituitary and none at the hypothalamus, whereas the latter drug inhibits CRF release at 4 h after pretreatment but no effect is seen at anterior pituitary until 24 h. When animals pretreated 4 h previously with these drugs are subjected to surgical stress, the response is normal in the case of 17 α-OH-pregnenolone and completely inhibited in the case of beclamethasone diproprionate (Fig. 7). It would seem that after a single administration, the hypothalamus is a more important feedback site than the pituitary – but again this may only apply to consideration of surgical stress. We have no data to indicate the relative importance of the sites when dealing with the normal feedback steroid of the rat, i.e. corticosterone.

INTERACTIONS BETWEEN FAST AND DELAYED FEEDBACK MECHANISMS

The mechanisms and dynamics of the two feedback systems are different, and it is a matter of considerable interest to know how they interact to provide an efficient homoeostatic control system.

The two mechanisms are activated by the same corticosteroids under physiological conditions, these steroids being cortisol and/or corticosterone. The data in Table VII goes some way to demonstrate the importance of the interaction for they show that the hypersecretion of ACTH in response to stress, is reduced to normal (intact) values only when both kinds of feedback are used. Table VII shows the effect of corticosterone replacement therapy (in both 3 day adrenalectomized and sham-operated rats) on the basal and ether-induced release of radioimmunoassayable ACTH. The result of adrenalectomy is to cause an increase in both basal and stress-induced secretion of ACTH as compared with sham-operated animals. Although a delayed-feedback signal (200 μg and 10.00 h and 20.00 h) serves to normalize basal secretion of ACTH, such a dose fails to normalize the stress response. When given alone, neither a fast-feedback signal (150 or 550 μg 20 min before stress) nor a chronic delayed-feedback signal (350 μg, last injection 2 h before stress) are able to normalize the stress response. However, when animals are treated with a delayed-feedback (220 μg b.d.) and a fast-feedback (150 μg) dose, a normal basal ACTH level and also a normal stress response is seen. Thus both signals are required for a normally responsive hypothalamo–pituitary axis. Of course, ACTH secretion can be normalized by using higher doses of corticosteroids as a delayed-feedback signal alone, but such doses are well in excess of the amounts of steroids the animals are able to secrete. The important point about the data contained in Table VII is that the total dose of a steroid given as fast- and delayed-feedback signals is 550 μg, within the physiological range of the rat. This argues that the two feedback mechanisms constitute an integrated system that has evolved as an economical means of regulation in that it allows the stress response to occur and to be modulated by

Table VII. The interaction between fast- and delayed-feedback mechanisms in the rat. All the animals used were adrenalectomized 3 days before the experiment, except for two groups that were sham-operated at that time. Animals that received corticosterone before measurements of the basal or the stress-induced release of ACTH, were given acute steroid therapy (20 min before stress), or chronic steroid therapy (at 2.00 h and 10.00 h, last dose 2 h before stress), or a combination of both treatments.

Group	Treatment	Replacement category	Plasma ACTH (pg/ml)	
			Basal	Stress[a]
Sham-operated	saline	None	38.4 ± 3.8	247.5 ± 37.7
Adrenalectomized	saline	None	277.4 ± 13.2	707.6 ± 99.0
Adrenalectomized	acute B (150 g)	Acute	—	657.7 ± 56.2
or	acute B (550 g)	Acute	—	524.5 ± 28.3
Adrenalectomized	chronic B (200 g)	Chronic	75.8 ± 21.0	467.8 ± 95.8
or	chronic B (350 g)	Chronic	—	476.3 ± 35.7
Adrenalectomized	acute B (150 g)	Acute and		
and	chronic B (200 g)	Chronic	45.8 ± 9.6	273.5 ± 26.5

[a] Stress was caused by ether inhalation.

amounts of corticosteroids that are insufficient to produce hypercorticism. Following this line of argument, it might be suggested that the delayed-feedback mechanism serves to reduce the responsiveness of the system to a level that can be modulated, on a moment-to-moment basis, by the fast-feedback mechanism. Examples of the operation of such moment-to-moment control may be the episodic drive in the axis and the condition of acute stress.

CONCLUSION

Corticosteroids exert a fast and a delayed feedback at both the hypothalamus and the anterior pituitary. The fast-feedback mechanism acts on the hypothalamus by inhibiting CRF secretion by stabilizing the membrane and blocking Ca^{2+} flux. Delayed feedback acts by inhibiting CRF synthesis as well as release. The hypothalamus is the more important site of fast feedback under conditions of surgical stress. The two feedback mechanisms constitute an integrated system that has evolved as an economical means of regulating ACTH secretion.

REFERENCES

1. Ingle, D. J. (1937). *Anat. Rec.* **71**, 363.
2. Ingle, D. J. (1938). *Science* **86**, 245.
3. Sydnor, K. L. and Sayers, G. (1954). *Endocrinology* **55**, 621.
4. Ruhmann-Wennhold, A. and Nelson, D. H. (1977). *Ann. N.Y. Acad. Sci.* **297**, 498.
5. Matsyama, H. *et al.* (1971). *Endocrinology* **88**, 696.
6. Mims, R. B. (1973). *Horm. Metab. Res.* **5**, 368.
7. Bethune, J. E. *et al.* (1956). *J. Clin. endocr. Metab.* **16**, 913.
8. Dallman, M. F. *et al.* (1972). *Endocrinology* **91**, 961.
9. Dallman, M. F. and Jones, M. T. (1973). *Endocrinology* **92**, 1367.
10. Dallman, M. F. and Yates, F. E. (1969). *Ann. N.Y. Acad. Sci.* **156**, 696.
11. Jones, M. T. *et al.* (1972). *J. Endocrinol.* **55**, 487.
12. Abe, K. and Critchlow, V. (1977). *Endocrinology* **101**, 489.
13. Kaneko, M. and Hiroshige, T. (1976). *Abs. V. Int. Cong. Endocrinol.* p. 132.
14. Jones, M. T. *et al.* (1974). *J. Endocrinol.* **60**, 223.
15. McEwen, B. S. (1977). *Ann. N.Y. Acad. Sci.* **297**, 568.
16. Rose, S. and Nelson, J. (1956). *Aust. J. Exp. Biol. Med. Sci.* **34**, 77.
17. Sayers, G. and Portanova, R. (1974). *Endocrinology* **94**, 1723.
18. Vernikos-Danellis, J. (1965). *Endocrinology* **72**, 574.
19. Smelik, P. G. and Sayers, V. H. (1962). *Acta. Endocrinol.* **41**, 561.
20. Chowers, I. *et al.* (1967). *Neuroendocrinol.* **2**, 193.
21. Jones, M. T. *et al.* (1974). *In* "Frontiers of Neuroendocrinology" (Ganong, W. F. and Martini, L. eds.), p. 194, Raven Press, N.Y.
22. Jones, M. T. and Hillhouse, E. W. (1976). *J. Steroid. Biochem.* **7**, 1189.
23. Edwardson, J. A. and Bennett, G. W. (1974). *Nature* **251**, 425.
24. Sato, T. *et al.* (1975). *Endocrinology* **97**, 265.
25. Porter, J. C. *et al.* (1971). *In* "Frontiers of Neuroendocrinology", (Martini, L. and Ganong, W. F. eds.), p. 145, Oxford University Press.

OBSERVATIONS ON FEEDBACK REGULATION OF CORTICOTROPIN (ACTH) SECRETION IN MAN

J. R. Daly, S. C. J. Reader, J. Alaghband-Zadeh* and P. Haisman**

*The University of Manchester, Department of Chemical Pathology,
Hope Hospital, Salford, M6 8HD, U.K.
and the Departments of Chemical Pathology, *Charing Cross Hospital Medical
School, London, W6 8RF, and **Central Middlesex Hospital,
London NW10 7NS, U.K.*

INTRODUCTION

Negative feedback inhibition of the hypothalamo–pituitary–adrenal (HPA) axis has been described as one of the three main physiological determinants of cortisol secretion, the others being the circadian rhythm and response to stress. However, the physiological importance of feedback in the minute-to-minute regulation of HPA function in man has not been proved.

It was first demonstrated over 40 years ago that adrenal glands transplanted into adrenalectomized animals rapidly regenerated, but that no such regeneration occurred if one adrenal had been left intact in the recipient animal[1,2]. It was also found that oral "cortin" suppressed the regeneration of enucleated adrenals[3] and caused adrenal atrophy in the intact rat[4]. Shortly afterwards, it was shown that prolonged corticosteroid administration inhibited stress-induced overactivity of the adrenal cortex[5]. With the development of bioassays for corticotropin (ACTH) it was shown that adrenalectomy resulted in a marked sustained rise in blood ACTH[6].

Evidence that feedback was relevant to man came a few years after the discovery by Hench et al. [7] that corticosteroids were of therapeutic benefit in non-endocrine disease. Cases of collapse, sometimes fatal, were reported during or after surgery in patients who were receiving, or had at some time received, corticosteroids. These reports have been reviewed by Bayliss[8]. It was demonstrated that patients with Addison's Disease had very high circulating levels of ACTH[9] and innumerable workers found that the plasma cortisol falls and stress responsiveness is impaired after prolonged corticosteroid administration.

This weight of evidence, however, referred exclusively to non-physiological situations or administration of steroids in pharmacological doses, and the belief that the feedback mechanism was involved in the physiological regulation of HPA activity was, although plausible, an unjustified inference. Further, the evidence itself did not go unchallenged. Hodges and Vernikos[10] pointed out that the rise in plasma ACTH in adrenalectomized rats was not apparent until the second postoperative day. The reports of adrenocortical failure during surgery were subjected to devastating criticism[11,12]. Weitzman *et al.*[13] demonstrated that cortisol was secreted episodically, but they were unable to discover any constant relationship between any plasma cortisol concentration and the magnitude and timing of subsequent secretory episodes. Infusion of low doses of cortisol for several hours produced plasma concentrations within the physiological range, but these were sustained throughout the infusion in a manner that was not likely to occur spontaneously. This resulted in inhibition of cortisol secretion for several hours, but the circadian pattern after this period of inhibition was unchanged[14]. The authors concluded that maintenance of a plasma cortisol concentration of sufficient duration and magnitude suppresses ACTH, but that the attainment of a specific plasma concentration for periods of less than 1 h, such as occurs spontaneously, has no such effect. Consequently, there is now considerable scepticism about the physiological significance of feedback, most recently expressed by James *et al.*[15].

In parallel with this increasing scepticism, further experimentation, mostly in the rat, is now strengthening the case for feedback mechanism having physiological importance after all. Dallman *et al.*[16] using a more sensitive ACTH assay than that previously available to Hodges[10], showed that plasma ACTH levels do in fact rise promptly postadrenalectomy and persist above normal before extreme elevation develops on the second postoperative day, and Hodges has now confirmed this[17]. Recent sophisticated work has demonstrated not only that physiological doses of corticosteroids have an inhibitory effect *in vitro* on both ACTH and corticoliberin (CRH) secretion but also that feedback appears to have two distinct components, one immediate, rate-sensitive and saturable, and the other delayed and dose-dependent[18-25].

The present paper describes a series of experiments undertaken in an attempt, as yet tentative, incomplete and far from conclusive, to elucidate some of these problems in the human subject.

SUBJECTS AND METHODS

Plasma corticosteroids were measured by a fluorimetric technique[26], ACTH by cytochemical bioassay[27], later modified[28,29] and described in detail by Daly *et al.*[30]. Blood was withdrawn into heparinized tubes and centrifuged immediately. Samples were stored at $-70°C$ for ACTH determination and at $4°C$ for cortisol.

Subjects, unless otherwise stated, were healthy members of the scientific staff of the departments concerned and thus were not stressed by the procedures. Wherever serial samples were taken an indwelling cannula was used. The technique used for blood collection during sleep has been previously described[31]. For the cortisol-infusion studies a constant-rate syringe pump was used, sampling being from the opposite arm. After insertion of the cannulae a 1 h 'pre-infusion' period allowed the subject to settle down. Saline was infused during this period and then either saline or an appropriate concentration of cortisol infused. Saline was infused for the controls so that the analyst should not know which experiments were controls, and which involved cortisol infusion. The total volume infused never exceeded 50 ml in 10 h.

EXPERIMENTAL AND RESULTS

Experiment 1.   Initially it was decided to check whether a single bolus i.v. injection of 5 mg of cortisol, causing a brisk but brief rise in plasma cortisol to about 49 μg/100 ml (1352 nmol/1) would cause a fall in plasma ACTH. The result is shown in Fig. 1. ACTH fell promptly to below 1 ng/l.

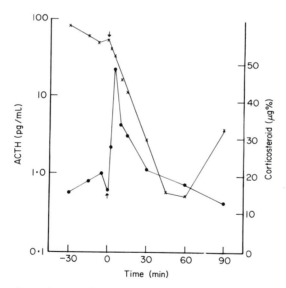

Fig. 1.   Results of experiment 1; X, ACTH; ●, corticosteroid.

Experiment 2.   Perlow *et al.*[14] referred to the apparent inverse relationship between plasma ACTH and cortisol concentration as supporting the negative-feedback theory. To determine whether such a relationship could be observed, cortisol and ACTH concentrations were measured on plasma samples collected at 08.00 and 20.00 h from 14 convalescent hospital in-patients without neurological or endocrine disease. The results are shown in Fig. 2. Between 08.00 and 20.00 h there appears a positive correlation between ACTH and cortisol levels, in that both are high at 08.00 (mean ACTH 69.8 ng/l, cortisol 17.7 μg/100 ml (488 nmol/l)) and low at 20.00 h (mean ACTH 23.8 ng/l, cortisol 6.8 μg/100 ml (188 nmol/l)). However, at each separate time a negative correlation is evident.

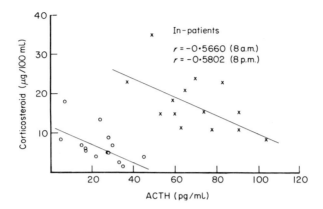

Fig. 2.   Results of experiment 2.

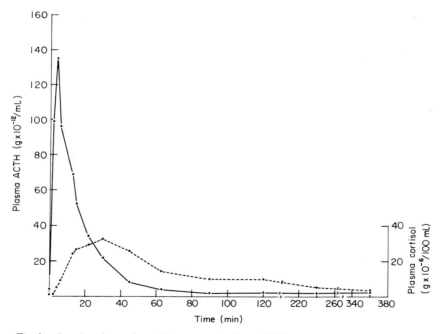

Fig. 3.   Results of experiment 3; – – –, cortisol; –, ACTH.

Experiment 3.   Our initial interpretation that experiment 2 supported the negative feedback was perhaps naive, as shown by this experiment in which an attempt was made to construct a model of a pulse of ACTH secretion by giving 750 ng of α^{1-24}-ACTH in a single i.v. bolus to a dexamethasone-suppressed subject. The plasma cortisol peak follows that of ACTH by some 25 min (Fig. 3). It can be seen that according to the moment of sampling during a secretory episode one might find high ACTH and low cortisol, high ACTH and high cortisol, low ACTH and high cortisol or low ACTH and low cortisol.

Experiment 4.   Blood was sampled for ACTH and cortisol every 20 min from 1 h after sleep onset (at 23.30 h) until awakening (at 07.00 h). This included the period of maximum circadian HPA activity[13]. The mean levels of both cortisol and ACTH rise steadily together throughout (Fig. 4), and in general cortisol seem to reach a peak about 20 min after peaks of ACTH. The pattern here displayed seems compatible with the view that falling cortisol levels initiate a further ACTH pulse, but as sampling (every 20 min) was less frequent than the plasma disappearance half-time of ACTH (8–10 min) it is possible that some peaks of ACTH went undetected.

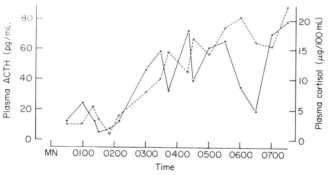

Fig. 4.   Results of experiment 4; ●——●, ACTH; ○-------○, cortisol.

Experiment 5.   Blood was sampled for ACTH and cortisol every 15 min between 11.00 (time O) and 16.00 h (300 min), a period of relative quiescence of the axis. Results are shown in Fig. 5. The plasma cortisol remains fairly steady throughout the experiment, but ACTH pulses of moderate amplitude (around 20 ng/l) persist. This could indicate a 'hunting mechanism' apparent in some servo systems, but otherwise there seems no relationship between changes in plasma ACTH and the level of cortisol.

Experiment 6.   In this experiment cortisol was substituted for saline and infused at a steady rate of 3 mg/h for 5 h (Fig. 6). ACTH fell promptly after the start of the infusion, reaching very low levels which persisted throughout the second hour. Thereafter the plasma ACTH rose to preinfusion levels, and these persisted until the end of the experiment. A puzzling feature is the observation that despite the recovery in ACTH level there is no corresponding rise in plasma cortisol. There is no way of knowing from this experiment what proportion of the plasma cortisol level was contributed by endogenous secretion and what by the infusion.

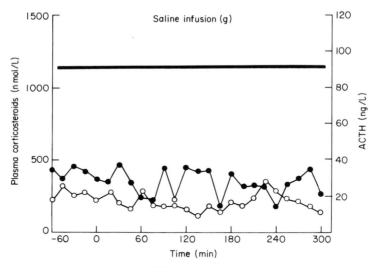

Fig. 5.   Results of experiment 5; •, ACTH; ○, corticosteroids.

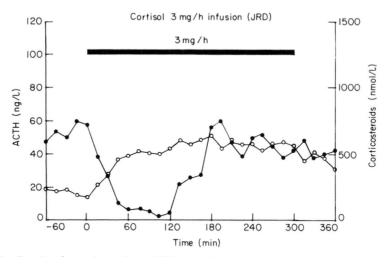

Fig. 6.   Results of experiment 6; •, ACTH; ○, corticosteroids.

Experiment 7.   Cortisol was again infused at a rate of 3 mg/h but at the end of the 5 h infusion the rate was doubled to 6 mg/h for a further 5 h (Fig. 7). Again there was an almost immediate fall in ACTH, which recovered after the second hour of infusion. Following the doubling of the infusion rate the ACTH again fell but once more recovered after about 3 h at the higher rate. The amplitude of the ACTH pulses on recovery was much greater than in the previous experiment.

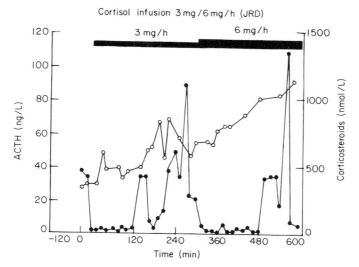

Fig. 7.   Results of experiment 7; •, ACTH; ○, corticosteroids.

DISCUSSION

The experimental design used here is not beyond criticism. For practical reasons blood sampling was usually once every 15-20 min which is substantially longer than the plasma half-time of ACTH (8-10 min). Consequently, peaks of ACTH may have been missed or rhythmic patterns distorted. There are other difficulties when trying to relate plasma ACTH and cortisol levels in man. ACTH may induce a log-dose response at the adrenal. Sampling was remote from the adrenal circulation and hence may not accurately reflect either the rate of ACTH entering the adrenal or of cortisol leaving it, and variations in adrenal blood flow are undetectable. The method used for cortisol determination is not altogether specific[32,33] and measures total not free (i.e. non-protein bound) cortisol, which is the fraction presumably responsible for mediating feedback effects.

Nevertheless, despite these difficulties it appears clear that small rises in plasma cortisol result in a virtually immediate decline in plasma ACTH. Further, the data are compatible with the fast, rate-sensitive feedback observed in rats, as it appears that a rise in cortisol level, and not the level itself, inhibits ACTH secretion. However, the experiments are not directly comparable as it was the response to stress that was inhibited by fast feedback in the rat, not the basal ACTH secretion.

In conclusion, we believe our data support the possibility of negative feedback playing a role in the physiological regulation of ACTH secretion in man. Certainly the mechanism is sufficiently sensitive for it to do so. Our study of the circadian rise of ACTH and cortisol during sleep does not refute the possibility. Attempts to confirm it, and determine whether both fast and delayed feedback exist in man, are the subjects of further experiments.

188   *J. R. Daly et al.*

ACKNOWLEDGEMENTS

We are grateful to Mr. Graham Carter, M.Sc., and the staff of the endocrine laboratory, Charing Cross Hospital, for plasma cortisol measurements. Financial support is gratefully acknowledged from the Medical Research Council of Great Britain and the Clinical Research Committee of Charing Cross Hospital.

REFERENCES

1. Wyman, L. C. and tum Suden, C. (1937). *Endocrinology* **21**, 523.
2. Ingle, D. J. and Higgins, G. H. (1937). *Proc. Staff Meetings Mayo Clinic* **12**, 204.
3. Ingle, D. J. and Kendall, E. C. (1937). *Proc. Staff Meetings Mayo Clinic* **12**, 505.
4. Ingle, D. J. and Kendall, E. C. (1937). *Science* **86**, 245.
5. Selye, H. and Dosne, C. (1942). *Endocrinology* **30**, 581.
6. Sayers, G. (1950). *Physiological Reviews* **30**, 241.
7. Hench, P. S. *et al.* (1949). *Proc. Staff Meetings Mayo Clinic* **24**, 81.
8. Bayliss, R. I. S. (1958). *Brit. Med. J.* **2**, 935.
9. Besser, G. M. *et al.* (1971). *Brit. Med. J.* **1**, 374.
10. Hodges, J. R. and Vernikos, J. (1960). *J. Physiol.* **150**, 683.
11. Cope, C. L. (1966). *Brit. Med. J.* **2**, 847.
12. Roberts, J. C. (1970). *Surg. Clin. Nth. Amer.* **50**, 363.
13. Weitzman, E. D. *et al.* (1971). *J. Clin. Endocrinol. Metab.* **33**, 14.
14. Perlow, M. *et al.* (1974). *J. Clin. Endocrinol. Metab.* **39**, 790.
15. James, V. H. T. *et al.* (1978). *J. Steroid Biochem.* **9**, 429.
16. Dallman, M. F. *et al.* (1972). *Endocrinology* **91**, 961.
17. Buckingham, J. C. and Hodges, J. R. (1974). *J. Endocrinol.* **63**, 213.
18. Dallman, M. F. and Yates, F. E. (1969). *Ann. N.Y. Acad. Sci.* **156**, 696.
19. Kraicer, J. and Milligan, J. V. (1970). *Endocrinology* **87**, 371.
20. Jones, M. T. *et al.* (1972). *J. Endocrinol.* **55**, 489.
21. Jones, M. T. *et al.* (1974). *J. Endocrinol.* **60**, 223.
22. Buckingham, J. C. and Hodges, J. R. (1975). *J. Endocrinol.* **67**, 411.
23. Buckingham, J. C. and Hodges, J. R. (1977). *J. Endocrinol.* **72**, 187.
24. Jones, M. T. *et al.* (1977). *J. Endocrinol.* **73**, 405.
25. Jones, M. T. *et al.* (1977). *J. Endocrinol.* **74**, 415.
26. Spencer-Peet, J. *et al.* (1965). *J. Endocrinol.* **31**, 235.
27. Chayen, J. *et al.* (1972). *Clin. Endocrinol.* **1**, 219.
28. Daly, J. R. *et al.* (1974). *Clin. Endocrinol.* **3**, 311.
29. Alaghband-Zadeh, J. *et al.* (1974). *Clin. Endocrinol.* **3**, 319.
30. Daly, J. R. *et al.* (1977). *Ann. N.Y. Acad. Sci.* **297**, 242.
31. Motson, R. W. *et al.* (1977). *Clin. Endocrinol.* **8**, 315.
32. James, V. H. T. *et al.* (1967). *J. Endocrinol.* **37**, xxvii.
33. Daly, J. R. *et al.* (1968). *Proc. Assoc. Clin. Biochem.* **5**, 73.

18

THE EFFECT OF INTERMEDIATES IN CORTISOL SYNTHESIS ON ITS FEEDBACK CONTROL IN MAN

R. V. Brooks*, G. Jeremiah*, Clara Lowy†, P. H. Sönksen† ,and M. Wheeler*

Departments of Chemical Pathology and Medicine†, St. Thomas's Hospital
Medical School, London SE1 7EH, U.K.*

INTRODUCTION

The work of Jones and his colleagues[1] has demonstrated that certain intermediates in cortisol synthesis exert an antagonistic effect on the negative feedback control exerted by glucocorticoid on its own secretion in the rat. If such a system were also to obtain in man, it would provide an explanation for certain apparently anomalous observations that have been made in cases of congenital adrenal hyperplasia.

The anomalous observations are as follows (a) Cope[2] described a case of congenital adrenal hyperplasia of the 21-hydroxylase block type in which the production rate of cortisol was increased. One would expect that with a partial block in one of the enzymic stages of cortisol synthesis, the production rate of cortisol would be either low or, if the compensatory response were adequate, within normal limits[3].

If, however, 17-hydroxyprogesterone were to exert an antagonistic effect on the cortisol feedback, the greatly raised concentration of this intermediate in the blood of the untreated patient might aggravate the already deficient negative feedback signal of cortisol by occupying and blocking the hypothalamic receptors. This would result in greater secretion of corticotropin (ACTH) than that caused by the cortisol deficiency alone.

(b) It is a fairly common observation that some patients with hitherto untreated congenital adrenal hyperplasia may need a high dose of glucocorticoid to be given initially in order adequately to suppress adrenal secretion. Once control is achieved, it is usually found that a more physiological dose is adequate to maintain suppres-

189

sion. This too could be explained by an antagonistic effect of 17-hydroxyproges-
terone on the negative feedback. However, once control is obtained with the high
dose, the concentration of abnormal precursor falls, the receptors are unblocked
and the sensitivity to a normal maintenance dose is restored.

(c) Escape from control in patients treated for congenital adrenal hyperplasia
can occasionally occur on a dose of glucocorticoid that has previously been
observed to be adequate. This has occurred with two of our patients and control
has not been regained while continuing on the same maintenance dose. To regain
control it is necessary to increase the dose considerably for a few days. The
escape from control may be due to an episode of stress or a brief lapse in medication. In either case, control with the normal maintenance dose can only be
restored after suppressing the intermediates with a higher dose. This paper
describes an attempt to test this hypothesis.

ADMINISTRATION OF 17-HYDROXYPROGESTERONE

The rates of secretion of 17-hydroxyprogesterone by adult patients with
congenital adrenal hyperplasia are often in excess of 1 mmol/day. Therefore to
stimulate the feedback interference from this source it would be necessary to
administer about 300 mg of 17-hydroxyprogesterone/24 h. This is difficult
because of the intermediate polarity of this steroid: not soluble enough in
aqueous media or aqueous alcohol to permit intravenous infusion nor soluble
enough in arachis oil (even containing 10% benzyl alcohol) for intramuscular
injection. The steroid was therefore micronized to small particles to make a
suspension in sterile arachis oil which was injected as a sludge through a thick
needle. Six 100 mg injections over a period of 3 h resulted in peak concentrations of 17-hydroxyprogesterone of about 300 nmol/l, but the concentration
fell to about half this amount after 24 h. Sublingual absorption was also examined
as a possible alternative mode of administration. Sucking three 100 mg lozenges
of 17-hydroxyprogesterone over a period of 1 h gave a concentration of only
30 nmol/1 at the end of 1 h and 300 nmol/1 at 2 h. This declined rapidly to
50 nmol/1 at 4 h. The rather slow rate of increase of concentration in this test
suggested that little oral absorption was taking place and that most of it enters
through the intestine with probably a large fraction being metabolized as it
passes through the liver. It was nevertheless decided to combine the intramuscular
injection of the micronized 17-hydroxyprogesterone with oral administration of
the lozenges in an attempt to achieve adequate plasma concentrations of the
steroid.

The subject for this investigation was a 38-year-old woman with congenital
adrenal hyperplasia which had proved difficult to control since treatment started
in 1952. She demonstrated both the need for a large initial dose of glucocorticoid
to achieve control as well as escape on a regular dose which had proved previously
to be adequate. This was a total dose of 1 mg of dexamethasone per day, 0.75 mg
being given at 22.00 h and 0.25 mg at 08.00 h. This dose had been adequate to
maintain suppression while the patient was in hospital, but she had escaped more
than once at home and Fig. 1 shows the results when she was admitted to hospital
after such an escape. The plasma 17-hydroxyprogesterone concentrations

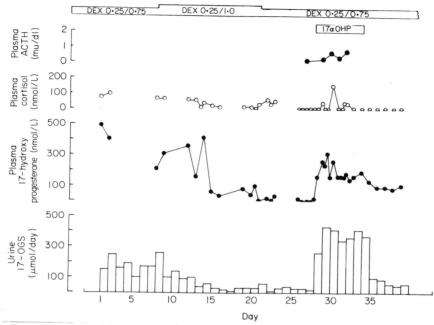

Fig. 1.   Suppression of adrenocortical secretion in a patient with congenital adrenal hyperplasia (21-hydroxylase defect). Effect of 17-hydroxyprogesterone administration (6 × 100 mg i.m. in arachis oil on days 28 and 29 and 3 × 100 mg lozenges before each dose of dexamethasone on days 28–32).

(400–500 nmol/1) and urinary 17-oxogenic steroids (150–300 μmol/day) were very high. Despite careful supervision of the medication after the patient was admitted to hospital, control was not regained on this dose of dexamethasone, which would have been quite enough to suppress the adrenocortical secretion of a normal subject. Increasing the 22.00 h dose to 1 mg resulted in control being attained as shown by the suppression of both the plasma 17-hydroxyprogesterone and the urinary 17-oxogenic steroids to low levels. This control was maintained despite resumption of the lower dose of dexamethasone.

   At this point, the patient was given 17-hydroxyprogesterone the object being to antagonize the inhibition by the dexamethasone and so tip the patient out of control. The steroid was given by injection (6 × 100 mg 17-hydroxyprogesterone in arachis oil on days 28 and 29) and by three 100 mg lozenges of 17-hydroxy-progesterone before each dose of dexamethasone on days 28, 29, 30, 31 and 32. The concentrations of 17-hydroxyprogesterone in the plasma (200–300 nmol/1) were in the range seen in congenital adrenal hyperplasia, but were lower than those found a few weeks earlier in this patient when she was out of control. There was no significant sustained rise in plasma ACTH or cortisol and after the 17-hydroxyprogesterone administration was stopped, the plasma 17-hydroxy-progesterone and urinary 17-oxogenic steroids slowly declined. It must be concluded from this experiment that either the hypothesis is incorrect or that the experiment was unsuccessful in that the concentrations of 17-hydroxy-progesterone in the blood, achieved as a result of administering the steroid, were not high enough.

EFFECT OF 11-DEOXYCORTISOL

11-Deoxycortisol is also difficult to administer but this problem was circumvented by using the 11β-hydroxylase inhibitor Metyrapone to produce an excess of 11-deoxycortisol endogenously. The effect of metyrapone given 6 hourly and 2 hourly, on the cortisol secretion rate and the excretion of free cortisol in the urine was examined. The purpose of this study was twofold. First, if 11-deoxy-cortisol can interfere with the cortisol feedback one might expect metyrapone to cause an increase in cortisol production; secondly, the success that some investigators have had in the medical treatment with metyrapone of patients with

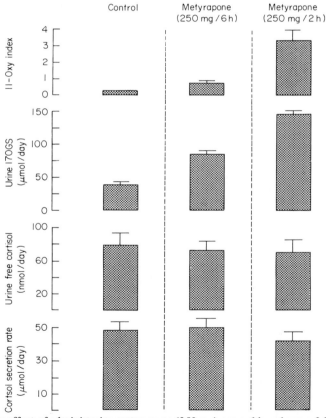

Fig. 2. The effect of administering metyrapone (250 mg) every 6 h and every 2 h (omitting the 02.00 h dose) on the urinary steroids of four normal subjects. Each histogram represents the mean value for the four patients and the horizontal bar indicates the S.E.M.

Cushing's disease[4] suggests a decrease of cortisol secretion in these subjects; we wanted to measure the effect on cortisol secretion in normal subjects.

The study was carried out on four healthy normal subjects over three 2-day periods; a control period, 2 days on metyrapone 250 mg 6 hourly and then a further 2 days on metyrapone 250 mg 2 hourly, excluding the 02.00 h dose. For the two treatment periods the metyrapone was started on the preceding day at 18.00 h to ensure an adequate 'run in' period before the measurements were taken.

Fig. 2 shows the mean 11-oxygenation index, the urinary 17-oxogenicosteroids (17-OGS), urinary free cortisol and cortisol secretion rate for the four normal subjects for the three periods of the study. The 11-oxygenation index is a direct reflection of the average effectiveness of the 11-hydroxylation block over the period of urine collection (48 h)[5]. There is a 3-fold increase in the index on the 6 hourly treatment regime and a 13-fold increase during 2 hourly treatment. The response of the hypothalamo–pituitary–adrenal system to this block is indicated by the rise in urinary 17-oxogenic steroids over the treatment periods representing the increased secretion of C_{21} steroids. The adequacy of this response to the block

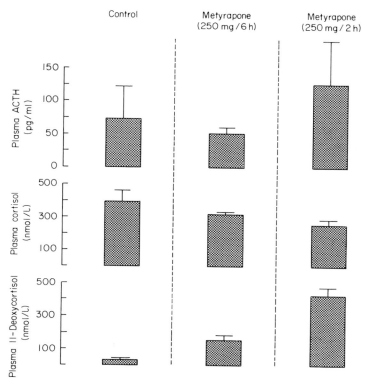

Fig. 3.   The effect of administering metyrapone (250 mg) every 6 h and every 2 h (omitting the 02.00 h dose) on the concentration of ACTH cortisol and 11-deoxy-cortisol of plasma taken at 09.00 h from four normal subjects. Each histogram represents the mean value for the four subjects and the horizontal bar indicates the S.E.M.

is indicated by both the urinary free cortisol, which is remarkably constant in the three periods of study, and by the cortisol secretion rate which indicates only a slight overall fall in the mean secretion during the 2 hourly administration of metyrapone.

The mean plasma concentrations of ACTH, cortisol and 11-deoxycortisol at 09.00 h for the group of four normal subjects are shown in Fig. 3. The blood samples for these determinations were drawn 3 h after the last administration of metyrapone during the 6 hourly regime and 1 h after the last dose during the 2 hourly treatment. The ACTH concentration measured by radioimmunoassay shows a large variation, but there appears to be an increase during the 2 hourly period of administration of metyrapone. The mean concentration of 11-deoxycortisol shows the expected progressive rise, but the cortisol concentration declines on the two treatment periods. This contrasts with the relatively constant excretion of cortisol in the urine in the three experimental periods. This paradox is explained by the observation of Bruno and his colleagues[6] that the disappearance half-life of cortisol in three normal subjects rapidly decreased from a range of 65–78 min to 22–28 min during the administration of metyrapone. This shortening of the half-life appears to be due to a displacement of the steroid from binding proteins in the plasma so that a larger percentage is in the free fraction[7].

CONCLUSIONS

Had the 11-deoxycortisol exerted an antagonism to the feedback inhibition exerted by cortisol, one would have expected to see an increase both in the excretion of cortisol in the urine and in the cortisol secretion rate during treatment with metyrapone. This did not occur and indeed the hypothalamo–pituitary compensation for the block on cortisol synthesis seems to have been very exact and does not suggest any alteration in the sensitivity of the cortisol negative feedback. However, it is possible that metyrapone may be exerting an additional action and the hypothesis should be tested also by the administration of exogenous 11-deoxycortisol.

STUDIES ON CUSHING'S SYNDROME

The completeness of the compensation during treatment of normal subjects with metyrapone at 2 hourly intervals seemed strange in view of the success in treating pituitary–dependent Cushing's syndrome with metyrapone reported by Jeffcoate et al.[4]. The hyperplastic adrenal in this condition is very responsive and gives an exaggerated 17-oxogenic steroid response to metyrapone[8]. Orth[9] has questioned the value of metyrapone as primary therapy in pituitary-dependent Cushing's syndrome. Indeed the failure of surgical subtotal adrenalectomy[10] might lead one to doubt the efficacy of partial enzyme blockage.

Fig. 4 shows the cortisol secretion rate, urinary free cortisol and 17-oxogenic steroids when three patients with Cushing's syndrome were examined by the same experimental protocol. Patient BE had an adrenal adenoma and it is not

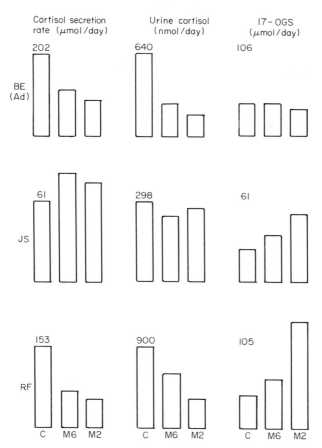

Fig. 4.   Effect of administering metyrapone (250 mg) every 6 h (M6) and every 2h (omitting the 02.00 h dose) (M2) on the cortisol secretion rate, urinary free cortisol and 17-oxogenicsteroids of three patients with Cushings syndrome. Patient BE had an adrenal adenoma, JS and RF had pituitary-dependent Cushings syndrome. The figures for the control values are indicated on the top of the histogram (C).

surprising that the 17-oxogenic steroids did not increase during treatment with metyrapone, whereas both the urinary free cortisol and cortisol secretion rate showed substantial reductions. Patients JS and RF both had pituitary-dependent Cushing's syndrome and although JS showed no reduction of either cortisol secretion rate or urinary-free cortisol, in RF both were well suppressed, the cortisol secretion rate during the 2 hourly treatment being only 55 μmol/day, well within normal limits. It would therefore seem that some patients with Cushing's disease are more susceptible to the action of metyrapone than are normal subjects.

REFERENCES

1. Jones, M. T. *et al.* (1974). *J. Endocrinol.* **60**, 223.
2. Cope, C. L. (1959). *Brit. Med. J.* **1**, 815.
3. Liddle, G. W. and Melmon, K. L. (1974). *In* "Textbook of Endocrinology", (Williams, R. H. ed.), pp. 233–322, W. B. Saunders, Philadelphia.
4. Jeffcoate, W. J. *et al.* (1977). *Brit. Med. J.* **2**, 215.
5. Edwards, R. W. H., *et al.* (1964). *J. Endocrinol.* **30**, 181.
6. Bruno, O. D. *et al.* (1971). *J. Clin. Endocr. Metab.* **32**, 260.
7. Kehlet, H. and Binder, C. (1976). *Acta. Endocr. Copenh.* **81**, 787.
8. Besser, G. M. and Edwards, C. R. W. (1972). *Clin. Endocr. Metab.* **1**, 451.
9. Orth, D. N. (1978). *Ann. Intern. Med.* **89**, 128.
10. Prunty, F. T. G. (1964). Chemistry and Treatment of Adrenocortical Diseases, pp. 190–193, Thomas Springfield, Illinois.

19

SECRETORY PATTERNS OF 18-OH-DOC AND RELATED STEROIDS AND THEIR POSSIBLE ROLE IN HYPERTENSION

M. K. Birmingham, J. T. Oliver, A. Bartova, P. Frei and S. Levy

Allan Memorial Institute of Psychiatry, McGill University, Montreal, Pharma Research Ltd., Pointe Claire, and Queen Mary Veteran's Hospital, Montreal, Quebec.

INTRODUCTION

The historic discovery by Simpson and Tait[1] of aldosterone, an adrenocortical steroid of novel structure with powerful effects on electrolyte metabolism, has focussed interest on 18-oxygenated steroids and their potential physiological significance that remains alive today. In animals with a differentiated adrenal cortex, members of this group of steroids may originate in the zona glomerulosa or the zona fasciculata, attributes that might be expected to implicate them in a diversity of controlling mechanisms. In the rat the most prominent 18-oxygenated steroid and at times its most prevalent adrenocortical hormone is 18-hydroxy-deoxycorticosterone (18-OH-DOC), identified as a natural adrenocortical secretory product by two laboratories in 1960[2,3].

That 18-OH-DOC is under the control of corticotropin (ACTH), but exhibits mineralocorticoid properties, was established for the rat even before its chemical structure had been identified[4,5], attributes that were at odds with the classical concept that associated ACTH with glucocorticoids, and confined mineralocorticoids to the zona glomerulosa. That the human adrenal can also form 18-OH-DOC was first demonstrated conclusively by the rigorous identification of this compound derived from radioactive precursors by De Nicola and Birmingham[6] and subsequently by the isolation of endogenous steroid from adrenal vein blood by Melby *et al.*[7]. In the human furthermore, plasma levels of 18-OH-DOC are exquisitely sensitive to ACTH and exhibit increases of an order of magnitude greatly in excess of the relative rise evoked by ACTH in the levels of plasma cortisol[8,9,10]. In view of the now established hypertensive potential of 18-OH-DOC, to be discussed below, this feature should be stressed since it suggests that 18-OH-DOC might be an aetiological agent in forms of hypertension associated with excess release of ACTH, such as occur in Cushing's Syndrome and other endocrinopathies, and could prevail under conditions of psychogenic and environmental stress. In the latter context the extensive review by Henry and Cassell may be cited, which points to an overriding contribution of environmental and psychosocial over dietary and genetic factors to the incidence of hypertension[11].

PHYSIOLOGICAL STIMULI AND 18-OH-DOC SECRETION

18-OH-DOC, however, originates in the zona glomerulosa as well, as is apparent from studies *in vitro* with the capsular portion of the rat adrenal gland[12,13,14], which forms this steroid in amounts greatly exceeding those anticipated from the contaminating presence of zona fasciculata cells. This suggests that 18-OH-DOC might also be involved in forms of hypertension resulting from changes in fluid volume and electrolyte composition, which control the secretion of aldosterone, the only steroid known to arise exclusively within the zona glomerulosa, at least in the rat. The elegant studies by Moore et al.[14] on cell suspensions derived from capsular and decapsulated portions of the rat adrenal gland corroborate this and indeed have demonstrated a dual control for the secretion of ACTH, depending on its zonal origin: angiotensin II and potassium, agents that stimulate the secretion of aldosterone, stimulate the production of 18-OH-DOC from zona glomerulosa cells, whereas ACTH increases the production from both zones, but is far more effective on fasciculata cells. The dual control of 18-OH-DOC and its sensitivity to ACTH and circadian fluctuation[8,9], may account in part for the controversial results obtained in man and intact animals in studies designed to evaluate effects of angiotensin, posture and changes in sodium intake[9,15]. Restriction of sodium intake has now been shown by Williams et al. to elevate the levels of circulating 18-OH-DOC in man to the same extent as those of aldosterone[14], and Mason et al. have found that angiotensin II evokes a dose-dependent elevation of plasma 18-OH-DOC in human subjects, provided they are subjected to a continuous infusion of ACTH[10].

18-OH-DOC AND HYPERTENSION

Indirect evidence for an involvement of 18-OH-DOC in hypertension is, if not conclusive, highly suggestive. It is based on studies *in vivo* and *in vitro* with animal models, including rats subjected to adrenal regeneration which, under suitable conditions, develop the syndrome of adrenal regeneration hypertension, and certain genetic strains of rats, i.e. animals exhibiting the salt-sensitive form of hypertension or changes in juxtaglomerular index, as well as on clinical findings, all of which have been the subject of detailed reviews[16,17,18]. In man the precise allocation of 18-OH-DOC to one of the many niches into which hypertensive disease has now been compartmentalized, perhaps with undue rigour, is still a matter of debate. Thus elevated 18-OH-DOC levels are confined to low renin hypertension by Genest *et al.*[18], but to normal renin hypertension by Williams *et al.*[8]. Again attention may be drawn to the lability of circulating levels of the steroid which, together with fluctuating renin levels, could obscure relationships often adduced by single sampling techniques.

In the Brattleboro rat, a strain that almost completely lacks the ability to secrete vasopressin, Vinson *et al.* have noted a striking formation of corticosterone[19], the output of which is usually highly correlated with that of 18-OH-DOC, although marked discrepancies between the production of the two steroids have also been noted, i.e. in rats harbouring a mammotrophic tumour[20] and in early stages of adrenal regeneration[21]. The observation of Vinson *et al.* suggests that neurohypophysial peptides might act as trophic agents for the elaboration of 18-OH-DOC, a possibility that could also account for the early unpublished observations by Lantos and Tramezzani of a disproportionate increase in the secretion by suckling rats of an unknown adrenal steroid that later proved to be 18-OH-DOC.

Direct evidence that 18-OH-DOC can in fact elevate blood pressure in experimental animals was first established for the rat by Oliver *et al.*[22] with subcutaneous doses of 200 μg, an amount that can be secreted by this species in minutes, and by Rapp *et al.*[23] who utilized a higher dose of 1 mg, which still may be considered to be in the physiological range for the rat. Hypertensive effects at these dose levels have also been noted by Hall *et al.*[24]. The hypertensive effect occurred only in animals receiving saline and was accompanied by elevated sodium, but not by a depression of potassium levels in the plasma.

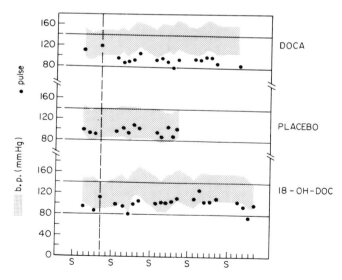

Fig. 1.   Blood pressures and heart rates of intact dogs implanted s.c. with 75 mg DOCA (3.3 mg/kg body wt.), 18-OH-DOC (4.6 mg/kg body wt.) or vehicle consisting of 2 parts bees' wax, 1 part poly(ethylene glycol) 1540, and 1 part poly(ethylene glycol) 4000 (Exp. 1). Measurements were taken daily from Monday to Friday; S, Sunday.

Hypertension has also been elicited with 18-OH-DOC by us in dogs (see discussion by Oliver in ref. 18) and in combination with other steroids by Fan *et al.* in sheep[25]. Our studies on dogs have now been extended. We found that the nature of the blood pressure responses to both 18-OH-DOC and DOC, and accompanying effects on fluid intake and circulating cation levels varied in intact dogs maintained on saline and implanted with steroid pellets containing 75 mg of steroid. The reason for this is not known but could include differences in the composition of the vehicle. Thus in one experiment the hypertensive potency of 18-OH-DOC equalled that of 11-deoxycorticosterone acetate (DOCA) (Table I and Fig. 1), and in a second, 18-OH-DOC evoked a statistically highly significant and a more sustained increase in blood pressure than DOCA or aldosterone (Fig. 2, see also legend), but the maximum elevation in blood pressure attained with DOC was much greater than that observed with 18-OH-DOC or with aldosterone. Heart rates were lowered with DOCA and aldosterone and significantly raised (Table I) or

Table I. Cardiovascular changes induced in intact dogs by implantation of DOCA and 18-OH-DOC. (Exp. 1). Intact dogs maintained on 0.9% saline received subcutaneous implants of pellets composed of 2 parts bees' wax, 1 part poly(ethylene glycol) 1540 and 1 part poly(ethylene glycol) 4000 and containing 75 mg of DOCA or 18-OH-DOC in the steroid-treated animals. Blood pressure was determined in unrestrained dogs by biotelemetry with a Königsberg transducer implanted at the bifurcation of the left subclavian artery with the aorta. Recordings were taken over a minimum of 2 h daily for a period of 4 to 6 weeks. The steroids were implanted only after the blood pressure had become stabilized, 1 to 2 weeks after insertion of the pressure probe. The values for blood pressures and heart rates represent means ± S.E. of 10 to 25 consecutive readings taken at 10 min intervals. Differences equalling or exceeding 8 for blood pressure and 17 for heart rate are statistically significant.

| | BLOOD PRESSURE (mm Hg) | | | | | |
| | Vehicle | | DOCA (3.3 mg/kg) | | 18-OH-DOC (4.6 mg/kg) | |
Before implantation	Syst.	Diast.	Syst.	Diast.	Syst.	Diast.
Before implantation	141 ± 4	84 ± 4	143 ± 2	90 ± 1	148 ± 2	89 ± 2
Day 7	142 ± 2	86 ± 3	163 ± 2	115 ± 2	169 ± 2	114 ± 3
Day 14	142 ± 2	85 ± 2	168 ± 3	114 ± 3	165 ± 1	108 ± 2
Day 21	—	—	162 ± 2	107 ± 2	157 ± 1	106 ± 2
Day 28	—	—	—	—	140 ± 2	93 ± 2
	HEART RATE					
Before implantation	94 ± 5		82 ± 3		87 ± 4	
Day 7	101 ± 3		104 ± 6		106 ± 5	
Day 14	104 ± 3		94 ± 4		112 ± 4	
Day 21	—		89 ± 4		111 ± 3	
Day 28	—		—		97 ± 3	

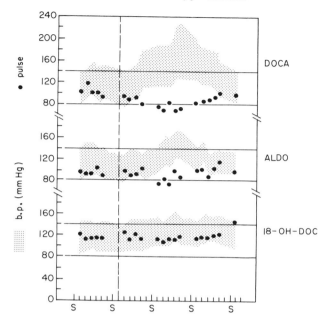

Fig. 2. Blood pressures and heart rates of intact dogs implanted s.c. with 75 mg DOCA (3.2 mg/kg body wt.), aldosterone (4 mg/kg body wt.) or 18-OH-DOC (7.5 mg/kg body wt.), suspended in equal parts of poly(ethylene glycol) 1540 and poly(ethylene glycol) 4000 (Exp. 2). The weekly averages for the mean daily blood pressures, determined five times a week, on the week preceding the implantation and on the three following weeks were for 18-OH-DOC 146 ± 1.2, 146 ± 2.8, 154 ± 3.0* and 155 ± 2.0** (systolic), 92 ± 1.1, 91 ± 2.2, 104 ± 2.8** and 104 ± 1.9*** (diastolic); for aldosterone 145 ± 2.2, 134 ± 2.4, 162 ± 5.5* and 142 ± 5.2 (systolic), 88 ± 1.4, 88 ± 2.4, 111 ± 4.2*** and 99 ± 4.9 (diastolic); for DOCA, 144 ± 3.3, 153 ± 8.5, 201 ± 9.9*** and 178 ± 6.3** (systolic), 88 ± 2.6, 90 ± 6.2, 116 ± 3.4*** and 112 ± 4.3*** (diastolic). The corresponding weekly averages for the mean daily heart rates were for 18-OH-DOC 115 ± 1.4, 118 ± 3.2, 112 ± 2 and 118 ± 1.7, for aldosterone 83 ± 4.3, 96 ± 3.1*, 83 ± 4.3 and 103 ± 4.3*; for DOCA 102 ± 4.5, 89 ± 2.6*, 74 ± 2.7***, and 90 ± 3.0. Asterisks denote significant differences from preimplantation values (*$p < 0.05$, **$p < 0.01$, *** $p < 0.001$).

unaffected (Fig. 2) with 18-OH-DOC. Saline intake was increased significantly by 18-OH-DOC in one experiment (Table II and Fig. 3) and completely unaffected in the second (Fig. 4). Aldosterone increased saline intake, but not as drastically as DOCA, which raised it to a maximum of 16 litres, and peak consumption with aldosterone occurred before the maximum rise in blood pressure, rather than coinciding with it. The relationship between saline consumption and the hypertensive response thus differed for each of the three steroids examined, suggesting that different underlying mechanisms are conducive to or modulate the hypertensive response. Hepp *et al.* found that the synthetic mineralocorticoid 9 α-fluorocortisol elevated blood pressure independently of an increase in saline intake, an effect ascribed by these authors to a glucocorticoid-type hypertension[26].

Table II. Saline intake and serum electrolytes in intact dogs implanted with DOCA and 18-OH-DOC. (Exp. 1). The vehicle consisted of subcutaneous pellets composed of 2 parts bees' wax, 1 part poly(ethylene glycol) 1540, 1 part poly(ethylene glycol) 400. Values represent means ± S. E. of the number of measurements taken per week, indicated in parenthesis.

	VEHICLE				DOCA, (3.3 mg/kg)				18-OH-DOC, (4.6 mg/kg)			
	0.9% saline intake (l)	serum Na$^+$ (mEq./l)	serum K$^+$ (mEq./l)	Na$^+$/K$^+$	0.9% saline intake (l)	serum Na$^+$ (mEq./l)	serum K$^+$ (mEq./l)	Na$^+$/K$^+$	0.9% saline intake (l)	serum Na$^+$ (mEq./l)	serum K$^+$ (mEq./l)	Na$^+$/K$^+$
1st week	2.55 ± 0.36 (7)	158 ± 3 (3)	4.73 ± 0.14 (3)	33.4 ± 0.9 (3)	2.88 ± 0.36 (7)	159 ± 2 (3)	5.27 ± 0.07 (3)	30.1 ± 0.7 (3)	3.56 ± 0.61 (7)	166 ± 6 (3)	4.93 ± 0.27 (3)	34.2 ± 1.70 (3)
2nd week	2.31 ± 0.18 (7)	156 ± 2 (3)	5.07 ± 0.18 (3)	30.8 ± 0.7 (3)	3.06 ± 0.34 (7)	157 ± 2 (3)	4.83 ± 0.23 (3)	32.7 ± 1.9 (3)	4.21 ± 0.34[c] (7)	155 ± 1 (3)	4.87 ± 0.18 (3)	32.0 ± 0.95 (3)
3rd week	2.64 ± 0.34 (7)	157 ± 4 (3)	5.23 ± 0.09 (3)	29.9 ± 0.3 (3)	5.28 ± 0.60 (7)	158 ± 1 (3)	4.23 ± 0.11[b] (3)	37.2 ± 0.2[b] (3)	4.71 ± 0.73 (7)	158 ± 4 (3)	5.70 ± 0.20[a] (3)	27.8 ± 0.86[a] (3)
4th week	2.74 ± 0.27 (7)	151 ± 5 (2)	5.05 ± 0.15 (2)	29.9 ± 0.1 (2)	5.44 ± 0.36 (7)	156 ± 1 (2)	4.40 ± 0.60[b] (2)	36.3 ± 5.3[b] (2)	3.63 ± 0.49 (7)	154 ± 2 (2)	5.40 ± 0.10[a] (2)	28.6 ± 1.00[a] (2)
5th week	—	—	—	—	1.88 ± 0.22 (7)	154 ± 1 (3)	5.23 ± 0.16 (3)	29.6 ± 1.1 (3)	3.06 ± 0.24 (7)	154 ± 2 (3)	5.80 ± 0.11 (3)	27.0 ± 1.20 (3)

[a] Serum potassium levels of the 18-OH-DOC-treated dog rose significantly, and were significantly elevated, by paired daily comparisons with the levels of vehicle-implanted dogs during the third plus fourth week, and the Na$^+$/K$^+$ ratios were significantly lowered.

[b] A highly significant drop in potassium levels occurred during the third and fourth week in the DOCA-treated dog to a low of 3.8 mEq./l, followed by an abrupt rise to 5.2 mEq./l. Correspondingly the Na$^+$/K$^+$ ratios rose to a high of 41.6, and then dropped abruptly to 31.0.

[c] Saline intake was discontinued during the fifth and sixth weeks and reinstated during the seventh week. During the second week, the 18-OH-DOC-treated dog drank significantly more fluid than the control and DOCA-treated dog and exceeded its own fluid intake of the seventh week.

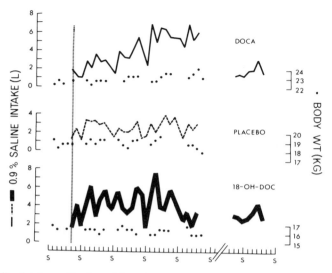

Fig. 3. Saline intake and body weights of intact dogs implanted with steroid-containing pellets or vehicle as described in legends to Tables and Fig. 1 (Exp. 1).

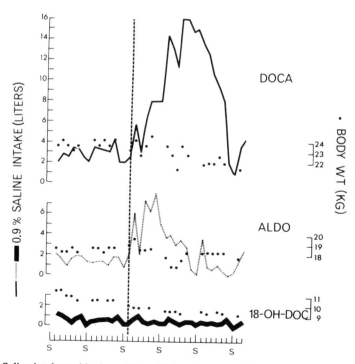

Fig. 4. Saline intake and body weights of intact dogs containing steroid pellets as described in legend to Fig. 2 (Exp. 2).

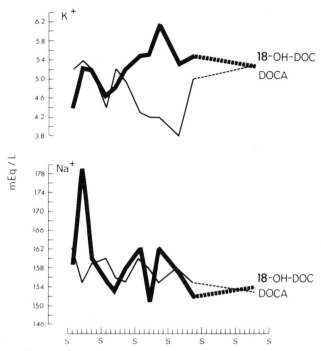

Fig. 5. Serum K$^+$ and Na$^+$ concentrations in intact dogs of Exp. 1. (see legend to Fig. 1). Serum constituents were measured with an autoanalyzer (technicon SMA 12/60), on samples collected three times a week.

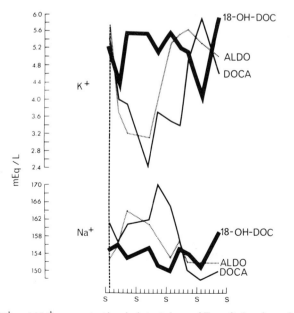

Fig. 6. Serum K$^+$ and Na$^+$ concentration in intact dogs of Exp. 2. (see legend to Fig. 2).

Both DOCA and aldosterone markedly elevated serum sodium and lowered serum potassium levels in Exp. 2, mirroring changes in saline intake (Fig. 4). In Exp. 1, however, serum sodium levels of the dogs exposed to DOCA were not raised, although during the fourth week the values for both the DOCA and 18-OH-DOC treated dogs were above those of the control dog which had declined to 151 mEq./l on day 21 and 146 mEq./l on day 25 (corresponding values for DOCA 155 and 158 mEq./l, for 18-OH-DOC 162 and 157 mEq./l). DOCA lowered the potassium levels in both experiments (Table II, Figs. 5 and 6). In distinct contrast to DOCA and aldosterone, serum potassium levels were raised (Table II, Fig. 5) or unaffected (Fig. 6) by 18-OH-DOC, in line with the findings obtained on rats[16,24].

Synergism between Glucocorticoids and 18-OH-DOC

Circulating levels of administered steroid have so far been measured by us only in dogs implanted with DOCA and with aldosterone. The levels of DOC and aldosterone fell precipitously within a few days after implantation and thus did not correlate with the hypertensive response (Figs. 7a and 7b). One interpretation for this might be that the hypertensive response is evoked by a metabolite of the administered steroid, present in the circulation or at a target site. Circulating cortisol levels (Figs. 7–8), however, rose markedly after steroid implantation and

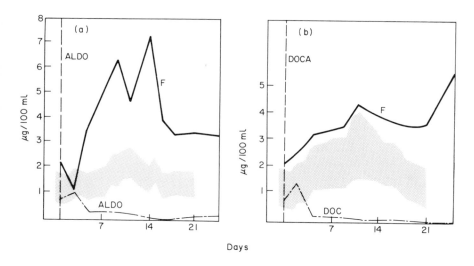

Days

Fig. 7.   Serum aldosterone (a), DOC (b) and cortisol levels, and blood pressures after implantation of aldosterone (4 mg/kg body wt.) and DOCA (3.2 mg/kg body wt.) in intact dogs maintained on saline (Exp. 2). Cortisol was measured by protein binding, aldosterone and DOC by radioimmunoassay, on two to three samples per week. Aldosterone and DOC concentrations fell from maximal values, on day 2, of 1.11 and 1.37 μg/100 ml respectively, to 0.30 and 0.18 μg on day 4. During the second week after implantation aldosterone values averaged 0.26 ± 0.03, and DOC 0.13 ± 0.05 μg/100 ml; during the third week, 0.047 ± 0.010 and 0.066 ± 0.040 μg/100 ml; and during the fourth week, 0.10 ± 0.05 and 0.013 ± 0.006 μg/100 ml. The b.p. values are taken from Figure 2.

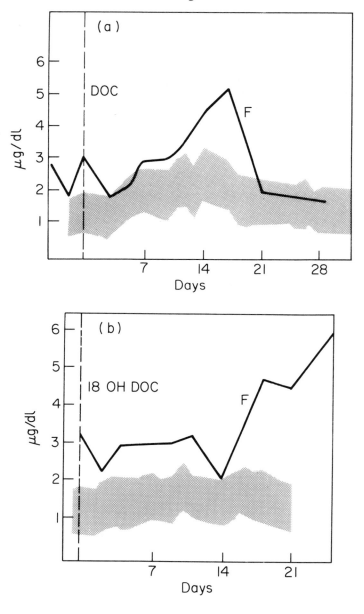

Fig. 8.   Serum cortisol levels and blood pressures (a) after implantation of unacetylated DOC (75 mg, 3.9 mg/kg body wt.) in an intact dog maintained on saline (Exp. 3), and serum cortisol levels and blood pressures (b) after implantation of 18-OH-DOC (75 mg; 7.5 mg/kg body wt.) in an intact dog maintained on saline (Exp. 2). Blood pressure in Fig. 8a were as follows: Day 1, 138/88; Day 14, 198/31; Day 21, 155/103. Blood pressures for 8b are taken from Fig. 2.

in some dogs were strikingly correlated with the increase in blood pressure, which suggests that a common denominator such as ACTH release, is responsible for these two responses. The possibility of a synergistic action between endogenous glucocorticoid and administered mineralocorticoid might also be entertained. This would accord with our earlier findings in rats processed for the induction of adrenal regeneration hypertension, in which thymus involution correlated significantly with blood pressure[27] and a positive correlation was apparent between the ratio of corticosterone to 18-OH-DOC in adrenal vein blood and the hypertensive response (Fig. 9). Synergistic effects are also indicated by the results

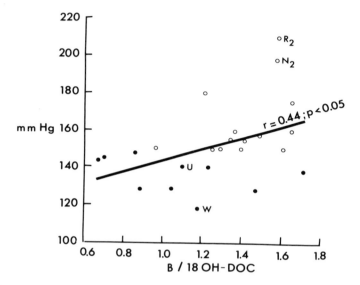

Fig. 9.   Positive correlation of blood pressure with corticosterone to 18-OH-DOC ratios in adrenal vein blood of unilaterally adrenonephrectomized rats bearing a regenerating adrenal gland. (Plot of data tabulated in 27). DOC secretion decreased with increasing blood pressure and was highest in rat W in which it approached the secretion of corticosterone.

of Fan *et al.* who induced a significant elevation in blood pressure and heart rate in sheep subjected to an infusion of 18-OH-DOC in combination with other steroids[25] and by the recent observations of Adam *et al.*[28], who found that the ring A-reduced derivative of cortisol, 5 α-dihydrocortisol, in itself does not influence sodium and potassium secretion in the rat but greatly potentiates the response to aldosterone.

The Effect of 18-OH-DOC on Mineral Metabolism

The effects of 18-OH-DOC on electrolyte balance have been studied in the rat with variable results[5,16,29]. The early assays, conducted by Giroud on the as yet unidentified material, yielded changes in Na^+/K^+ ratios ranging from near equal to one-tenth the activity of 18-OH-DOC[5]. In the assay performed by

Rochefort with crystalline 18-OH-DOC the sodium-retaining effect of 18-OH-DOC equalled that of DOC at a dose level of 10 μg[16]. The effect on sodium retention in the 18-OH-DOC-treated rats was, furthermore, not accompanied by a concomitant effect on potassium secretion, but by a disproportionate retention of water in relation to the sodium retained[16,43], an observation that would caution against a definition of mineralocorticoid activity and the implied hypertensive potential solely in terms of a balance between sodium retained and potassium excreted. A clear distinction between the control of these two ion movements has also been documented for aldosterone by Morris and Davis, who have reviewed the subject extensively[30]. Here amphibian membranes offer an ideal tool for comparing the capacity of agents on sodium transport, since this can be gauged from changes in short-circuit current across the membrane, which are mediated solely by the movement of sodium ions. Porter and Kimsey measured the effect of 18-OH-DOC by this technique in the toad bladder and found it to be active at a concentration of 0.7 μM [31]. Recent measurements conducted in the laboratory of Professor Jean Crabbé on the ventral skin of the toad have now demonstrated that in this tissue 18-OH-DOC may be as potent as aldosterone when both are compared at a concentration of 50 nM [32]. Further, 18-hydroxy-corticosterone (18-OH-B), which differs from 18-OH-DOC by the presence of an hydroxyl group at C-11, was active as well, whereas corticosterone and DOC caused only minor and statistically insignificant changes. This points to a physiological role also for 18-OH-B, a subject recently reviewed by Fraser and Lantos[33]. 18-OH-B is formed predominantly and perhaps exclusively in the zona glomerulosa of higher vertebrates and in the amphibian adrenal it is a major adrenocortical product. In amphibians, moreover, ACTH evokes a significant increase in the production of both aldosterone and 18-OH-B *in vitro*, exceeding that of corticosterone[34,35]. 18-OH-B is also a quantitatively important secretory product of the human adrenal where it is usually formed in higher quantity than aldosterone[36,37], and both angiotensin and ACTH have been found by Mason *et al.* to raise the plasma levels of this hormone[10].

Further, Damasco *et al.* have noted a specific effect of this steroid on H$^+$ ion secretion in the rat[28], which was not correlated with sodium transport, a property also documented for aldosterone by Al-Awqati *et al.* in the isolated toad bladder[39]. C-18 oxygenated steroids thus appear to feature not only in the control of sodium and potassium transport, but also in the regulation of pH and they may do this by distinct unrelated mechanisms.

18-OH-DOC Uptake in the Brain

Although steroid-mediated hypertension is primarily viewed in terms of affinities for receptor sites in the kidney or the vascular system, radiochemical and radioautographical studies implicate the central nervous system as an additional significant target site for adrenocortical steroids, which could be pertinent to their anaesthetic, feedback, and possibly their hypertensive activities as well. Nuclear localization within the central nervous system has now been established by radioautographic techniques not only for corticosterone but also for aldosterone[40,41], and conspicuous sites at which nuclear aggregations occur are the reticular formation of the lower brain stem, motor as opposed to sensory components of the cranial nerves, and the hippocampal formation, and here aldosterone in contrast to corticosterone appears to concentrate more intensely in its primitive remnants, the indusium griseum and hippocampus anterior. Significant nuclear localization also is found in the arachnoid, the olfactory nuclei, the septum and the piriform cortex, but no nuclear localization within the hypothalamus, an established target site for oestrogens and androgens, has as yet been noted by radioautographic techniques. The pattern of nuclear localization of one of the representatives of 18-oxygenated adrenocortical steroids in the central nervous system thus appears in some aspects distinct from the distribution of sex hormones and perhaps also from glucocorticoids. It should be noted, however, that in the rat, aldosterone is far more potent than corticosterone in suppressing the rise in circulating corticosterone measured 5 min after exposure to mild stress[42,43], a property usually associated with glucocorticoids, and DOC is also effective[44]. DOC is converted with high efficiency to ring A-reduced derivatives in brain tissue. These exceed in amount the unchanged material recovered after injection of the radioactive compound[45], pointing again to a role for hormonal conversion products in mediating biological effects, applicable not only to androgens but also to adrenocortical steroids. However, to what extent material localized by radioautography in specific cells of the central nervous system represents adrenocortical hormone or some derivative remains to be ascertained, as does the precise bearing of assorted visualized target sites to feedback and hypertensive action.

18-OH-DOC does not suppress plasma corticosterone levels in rats under conditions in which aldosterone, corticosterone and DOC are effective, but raises them, as has been shown by independent investigations from two laboratories[44,46]. In consideration of a possible involvement of the central nervous system also in the biological effects of 18-OH-DOC, evidence for its presence in the brain might be pertinent. Radioautographic evidence for nuclear localization of 18-OH-DOC has so far not been obtained in rat brain, although after injection of ^{3}H-labelled 18-OH-DOC diffusely distributed radioactive material is detected in both rat and frog brain by this technique (unpublished observations). However, endogenous 18-OH-DOC is readily detected in rat brain, as shown by Bartova, who noted regional differences, indicating preferential localization in the septum, and fluctuating levels depending on the activity of the pituitary–adrenal axis[47]. Further, she found that 18-OH-DOC administered *in vivo* was associated with a macromolecular complex in rat brain cytosol in amounts similar to those she obtained after injection of aldosterone.

CONCLUSION

In conclusion, 18-oxygenated adrenocortical steroids exhibit a variety of biological characteristics that could implicate them in hypertensive disease. Among these are the ability to alter ion transport; the sensitivity to ACTH, angiotensin and possibly neurohypophysial peptides; the localization in selected target sites, including the central nervous system; and the hypertensive potential established

210 M. K. Birmingham et al.

by direct evidence for some members of this group. 18-OH-DOC might be singled out because it is the member most responsive to ACTH, and appears to be sensitive to changes in ionic environment as well. 18-OH-DOC may therefore be an aetiological agent in inducing hypertension in those diseases in which there is excessive release of ACTH (e.g. Cushing's disease), and it may possibly have a role in inducing hypertension in response to psychological and possibly environmental stress.

ACKNOWLEDGEMENTS

This work was supported in part by the Medical Research Council of Canada and the Quebec Heart Foundation. We thank Mrs. H. Traikov for skilful technical assistance.

REFERENCES

1. Simpson, S. A. and Tait, J. F. (1953). *Mem. Soc. Endocrinol.* **2**, 9.
2. Birmingham, M. K. and Ward, P. J. (1961). *J. Biol. Chem.* **236**, 1661.
3. Péron, F. G. (1961). *Endocrinology* **69**, 39.
4. Birmingham, M. K. and Kurlents, E. (1959). *Can. J. Biochem. Physiol.* **37**, 510.
5. Ward, P. J. and Birmingham, M. K. (1960). *Biochem. J.* **76**, 269.
6. De Nicola, A. F. and Birmingham, M. K. (1968). *J. Clin. Endocrinol. Metab.* **28**, 1380.
7. Melby, J. C. *et al.* (1971). *Circ. Res.* **28**, Suppl. II, 143.
8. Williams, G. H. *et al.* (1976). *J. Clin. Invest.* **58**, 221.
9. Chandler, D. W. *et al.* (1976). *Steroids* **27**, 235.
10. Mason, P. A. *et al.* (1979). *J. Steroid Biochem.* **10**, 235.
11. Henry, J. P. and Cassel, J. C. (1969). *Amer. J. Epid.* **90**, 171.
12. Sheppard, H. *et al.* (1963). *Endocrinology* **73**, 819.
13. Bankiewicz, S. *et al.* (1968). *In* "Functions of the Adrenal Cortex", Vol. I (McKerns, K. W. ed.), p. 153, Appleton-Century-Crofts, New York.
14. Moore, T. J. *et al.* (1978). *Endocrinology* **103**, 152.
15. Dale, S. L. *et al.* (1976). *J. Clin. Endocrinol. Metab.* **43**, 803.
16. Birmingham, M. K. *et al.* (1968). *In* "Function of the Adrenal Cortex", Vol. II (McKerns, K. W. ed.), p. 647, Appleton-Century-Crofts, New York.
17. Melby, J. C. *et al.* (1972). *Recent Prog. Horm. Res.* **28**, 287.
18. Genest, J. *et al.* (1976). *Recent Prog. Horm. Res.* **32**, 377.
19. Vinson, G. P. *et al.* (1978). *J. Steroid Biochem.* **9**, 657.
20. De Nicola, A. F. *et al.* (1973). *J. Steroid Biochem.* **4**, 205.
21. Birmingham, M. K. (1971). 12th Annual Braun-Menéndez Lecture, Compania Impresaria, Buenos Aires.
22. Oliver, J. T. *et al.* (1973). *Science* **182**, 1249.
23. Rapp, J. P. *et al.* (1973). *Circ. Res.* **32**, Suppl. I, 139.
24. Hall, C. E. *et al.* (1978). *Endocrinology* **103**, 133.
25. Fan, J. S. K. *et al.* (1975). *Am. J. Physiol.* **228**, 1695.
26. Hepp, R. *et al.* (1974). *Acta. Endocrinol.* **75**, 539.
27. Birmingham, M. K. *et al.* (1973). *Endocrinology* **93**, 297.
28. Adam, W. R. *et al.* (1978). *Endocrinology* **103**, 465.

29.   Kagawa, C. M. and Pappo, R. (1962). *Proc. Soc. Exp. Biol. Med.* **109**, 982.
30.   Morris, D. J. and Davis, R. P. (1974). *Metabolism* **23**, 473.
31.   Porter, G. A. and Kimsey, J. (1971). *Endocrinology* **89**, 357.
32.   Beauwens, R. *et al. In preparation.*
33.   Fraser, R. and Lantos, C. P. (1978). *J. Steroid Biochem.* **9**, 273.
34.   Carstensens, H. *et al.* (1961). *Gen. Comp. Endocrinol.* **1**, 37.
35.   Kraulis, I. and Birmingham, M. K. (1964). *Acta. Endocrinol.* **47**, 76.
36.   De Nicola, A. F. *et al.* (1970). *J. Clin. Endocrinol. Metab.* **30**, 402.
37.   Marusik, E. T. and Murlow, P. J. (1969). *Proc. Soc. Exp. Biol. Med.* **131**, 778.
38.   Damasco, M. C. *et al.* (1976). *Gen. Comp. Endocrinol. Abstract 124.*
39.   Al-Awqati, Q. *et al.* (1976). *J. Clin. Invest.* **58**, 351.
40.   Ermisch, A. and Rühle, H. -J. (1978). *Brain Research* **147**, 154.
41.   Stumpf, W. E., Birmingham, M. F. *et al.* (1979). *Experientia* **35**. *In press.*
42.   Birmingham, M. K. *et al.* (1974). *In* "Oral Contraceptives and High Blood Pressure", (Fregly, M. J. and Fregly, M. S. eds.), p. 315, Dolphin Press, Gainesville.
43.   Birmingham, M. K. *et al.* (1974). *J. Steroid Biochem.* **5**, 789.
44.   Kraulis, I. *et al.* (1973). *J. Steroid Biochem.* **4**, 129.
45.   Kraulis, I. *et al.* (1975). *Brain Res.* **88**, 1.
46.   Jones, M. T. and Tiptaft, E. M. (1977). *Br. J. Pharmac.* **59**, 35.
47.   Bartova, A., *this volume.*

20

ENDOGENOUS LEVELS OF 18-OH-DOC AND RELATED STEROIDS IN THE BRAIN

A. Bartova

Allan Memorial Institute of Psychiatry, McGill University, Montreal, Canada

INTRODUCTION

There is now a good deal of evidence that many actions of steroid hormones are mediated by their interaction with specific receptor molecules located in the cytoplasm and nuclei of target tissues and that this initiates the hormonal effect[1,2]. The tissue uptake of the steroid hormone is affected by various factors including binding to plasma proteins, specificity of tissue receptors and saturation of the receptor sites. Studies on brain have demonstrated that this tissue retains the corticosteroids corticosterone, cortisol and aldosterone with selective affinity in limbic structures[3–7]. No information has hitherto been available regarding the uptake and retention of 18-hydroxy-11-deoxycorticosterone (18-OH-DOC) in the brain. This steroid possesses unique biochemical properties: 18-OH-DOC has high susceptibility to various inter- and intra-molecular reactions[9–11], has an extremely low affinity for plasma corticosteroid-binding globulin and exerts no feedback control on corticotropin (ACTH) secretion[12]. No specific receptors for this steroid have been detected in kidney, liver and heart[12,13], for the action of the hormone in these target organs was demonstrated to be through the receptors for other mineralocorticoids[12]. Previous experiments from this laboratory showed that endogenous levels of 18-OH-DOC in the rat brain are 30% of the plasma concentration and fluctuate with the physiological state[14]. In the present study, the distribution of the endogenous 18-OH-DOC in the rat brain is examined as is the uptake of the radioactive steroid into that tissue.

ENDOGENOUS AND EXOGENOUS (RADIOACTIVE) 18-OH-DOC
IN RAT BRAIN

Intact Sprague–Dawley male rats (160 g) were anaesthetized, blood was taken from the heart and the animals were perfused with dextran–saline. Brains were dissected as described by Glowinski and Inversen[15] and the brain regions were combined, extracted by homogenization in methylene chloride and analysed for 18-OH-DOC (by radioimmunoassay[16]) and B[17]. Results of six experiments are shown in Fig. 1. The highest concentration of 18-OH-DOC (8.2 ± 1.97 ng/g of tissue) was present in the septum, the lowest (2.3 ± 0.73 ng/g of tissue) in the hypothalamus. The remainder contained about equal amounts — cortex 4.3 ± 1.32, medulla 4.6 ± 2.36 and amygdala 3.4 ± 1.59 ng/g of tissue — of the hormone. A similar distribution was found for corticosterone, with the highest level in the septum and the lowest in the hypothalamus with intermediate levels in the rest of the tissue.

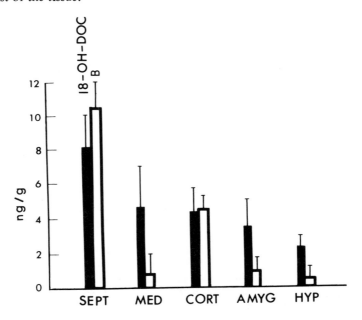

Fig. 1. Endogenous levels of 18-OH-DOC and corticosterone (B) in rat brain regions. Pooled brain sections of 20 intact rats were analysed for 18-OH-DOC and B. Closed bars represent 18-OH-DOC, open bars corticosterone. Vertical lines denote S.E. (n = 6).

For the determination of its uptake ^{3}H-labelled 18-OH-DOC (80 μCi) was injected intraperitoneally into rats adrenalectomized 4–7 days previously and 1 h later the animals were killed and the radioactivity in the brain regions was determined. The highest (2049 ± 111 d.p.m./g of tissue) and the lowest (1006 ± 125 d.p.m./g of tissue) concentrations of radioactivity were found in the septum and hypothalamus respectively. The medulla, amygdala and cortex contained intermediate amounts of radioactivity (Table I).

Table I. Distribution of the endogenous and radioactive 18-OH-DOC in the rat brain. A. Endogenous levels of the hormone were determined in the pooled brain sections of 20 animals. B. The uptake of the radioactive hormone was determined 1 h after the i.p. injection of ^{3}H-labelled 18-OH-DOC (80 μCi) into three adrenalectomized rats. The values represent mean of three to six determinations ± S.E.

Brain region	A 18-OH-DOC (ng/g of tissue)	B ^{3}H-18-OH-DOC (d.p.m./g of tissue)
1. Septum	8.20 ± 1.97	2049 ± 111
2. Medulla	4.6 ± 2.36	1881 ± 290
3. Cortex	4.3 ± 1.32	1386 ± 106
4. Amygdala	3.4 ± 1.59	1660 ± 102
5. Hypothalamus	2.3 ± 0.73	1006 ± 125

EFFECT OF ADRENALECTOMY OR TREATMENT WITH DEXAMETHASONE OR ACTH ON 18-OH-DOC IN RAT BRAIN

Concentrations of 18-OH-DOC were determined in the plasma and brains of four groups of rats: (a) in controls; (b) in adrenalectomized rats; (c) rats treated with dexamethasone for 5 days (2 mg/kg, twice daily administered intraperitoneally (i.p.)) and killed 2 h after the last injection; and (d) in rats treated with ACTH (4 U/kg in one i.p. dose) and killed 15 min after the injection. Results are shown in Table II. Control levels of 18-OH-DOC in the plasma were 7.88 ± 1.68 ng/ml and in the brain 2.22 ± 0.7 ng/g. Adrenalectomy and dexamethasone caused both plasma and brain levels of the hormone to decrease almost to undetectable values, 0.15 ± 0.03 and 0.52 ± 0.06 ng/ml, or 0.03 ± 0.01 and 0.06 ± 0.01 ng/g respectively, and ACTH caused a 10-fold increase in plasma as well as brain levels of 18-OH-DOC. When injected into humans, ACTH produced similar effects on plasma 18-OH-DOC levels (Fig. 2B). In this experiment, peripheral blood was taken before ACTH injection, then 25 U of ACTH (0.25 mg of Cortrosyn) was injected i.v. and the blood collection was continued for four

Table II. Effects of pharmacological and surgical manipulations on the plasma and brain levels of 18-OH-DOC. Rats were adrenalectomized 4–7 days before being killed, dexamethasone (2 mg/kg) was administered twice daily for 5 days and and animals were killed 2 h after the last injection. ACTH (4 U/kg) was injected in one i.p. dose and the rats were killed 15 min later. Controls were injected with saline. Values represent mean of four to six determinations ± S.E.

Treatment	18-OH-DOC (ng/ml plasma)	(ng/g brain)
1. Controls	7.88 ± 1.68	2.22 ± 0.73
2. Adrenalectomy	0.15 ± 0.03	0.03 ± 0.01
3. Dexamethasone	0.52 ± 0.06	0.06 ± 0.01
4. ACTH	78.62 ± 5.90	22.92 ± 8.71

A. *Bartova*

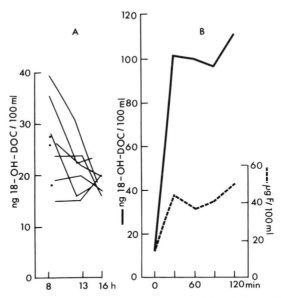

Fig. 2. (A) Diurnal variation of 18-OH-DOC in human peripheral plasma. Blood of seven volunteers (four men and three women) was drawn at 08.00–09.00 h, at 12.00–13.00 h and at 15.00–16.00 h and plasma analysed for 18-OH-DOC and cortisol F. (B) Effects of ACTH on plasma 18-OH-DOC and F. Peripheral blood was taken at 13.00 h, then 25 U of ACTH (0.25 mg Cortrosyn, Organon) was injected i.v. and the blood collection continued 30, 60, 90 and 120 min after the ACTH.

30 min intervals. At 30 min after ACTH administration, plasma levels of 18-OH-DOC increased about 10-fold, from 12.2 to 102 ng/100 ml. Cortisol determined simultaneously increased from 14.3 μg in the control to 46 μg/100 ml after the ACTH.

Diurnal fluctuations of plasma levels of 18-OH-DOC in seven volunteers (four men, three women) were determined at 08.00 h, 13.00 h and at 16.00 h (Fig. 2A). During the time interval between 08.00 and 13.00 h the concentration of the hormone decreased in four and remained practically unchanged in three persons. Similar fluctuations were seen between 13.00 and 16.00 h, declining in four and increasing in three persons.

To define further the uptake mechanism for 18-OH-DOC by the brain tissue, macromolecular binding of the radioactive hormone was assessed *in vivo*.

MACROMOLECULES CAPABLE OF BINDING 18-OH-DOC FROM RAT BRAIN NUCLEI AND CYTOSOL

Cell fractionation was performed by the method of McEwen *et al.*[18,19], preparations of cytosol from brains of adrenalectomized rats killed 1 h after i.p. injection of ^{3}H-labelled 18-OH-DOC were subjected to gel filtration on

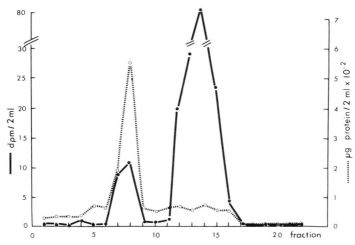

Fig. 3.   Elution pattern from Sephadex G-25 of protein (o) and radioactivity (o) in rat brain cytosol labelled *in vivo* with ³H-labelled 18-OH-DOC.

Sephadex G-25[19] and eluted with buffer containing 0.4 M NaCl. A representative elution pattern is shown in Fig. 3. One peak of radioactivity was eluted with the protein and represents ³H-labelled 18-OH-DOC bound to macromolecules. The second peak of radioactivity was eluted as free steroid in the effluent which contained no protein. The bound fraction represented 0.17 ± 0.06 fmol of ³H-labelled 18-OH-DOC/mg of protein (Table III). The radioactivity of the nuclear fraction was extracted with a buffer containing 0.4 M NaCl and the extract was filtered through a Sephadex G-200 column prepared and eluted with 0.4 M NaCl buffer[19]. A representative elution pattern is depicted in Fig. 4. One of the peaks of radioactivity was eluted with a protein peak representing the macromolecular bound ³H-labelled 18-OH-DOC and the second peak of the radioactivity was eluted at the low-molecular-weight region of the column with

Table III.   ³H-labelled 18-OH-DOC, [³H] aldosterone (³H-aldo) and [³H] corticosterone (³H-B) bound to macromolecules in brain cytosol, to nuclei or to high speed pellet (HSP). Macromolecular-bound steroids were determined in the protein fractions from the Sephadex G-25 and G-200 effluents of cytosol and of the 0.4 M NaCl extract of nuclei, respectively. The radioactivity of the high speed pellet was determined without further fractionation. Values represent mean ± S.E.

Cell fraction	Macromolecules bound (fmol/mg of protein)		
	³H-18-OH-DOC	³H-aldo	³H-B
Cytosol	0.17 ± 0.04	0.16 ± 0.02	4.93 ± 0.8
Nuclei	4.45 ± 0.03	10.82 ± 1.1	20.08 ± 1.6
HSP	0.05 ± 0.03	0.03 ± 0.01	4.54 ± 0.4

no protein present in the effluent. The bound fraction constituted 25 ± 4% of the total radioactivity, recovered from the column and 4.45 ± 0.5 fmol of ³H-labelled 18-OH-DOC were bound per mg of protein (Table III). The presence of the free steroid in the nuclear effluent is probably the result of the high salt concentration, which causes dissociation of the steroid–macromolecular complex. The high-speed pellet (containing synaptosomes, mitrochondria and plasma membranes, HSP) was analysed without further separation procedure and contained 0.05 ± 0.01 fmol of ³H-labelled 18-OH-DOC/mg of protein (Table III).

Parallel experiments with [³H] aldosterone injected into adrenalectomized rats in an equal amount (80 µCi/rat) gave results comparable with those obtained with ³H-labelled 18-OH-DOC (Table III). Higher values in all parameters were obtained with [³H] B. In the cytosol 4.93 ± 0.8 fmol of [³H] B were bound per mg of protein, in nuclei 20.08 ± 1.6 fmol/mg of protein and in the high-speed pellet, 4.54 ± 0.4 fmol/mg of protein (Table III).

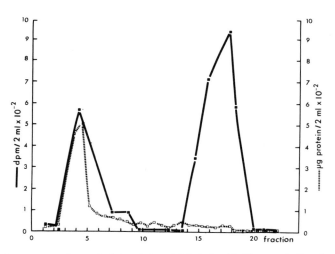

Fig. 4.   Elution pattern of protein (□) and dpm (■) in 0.4 M NaCl extract of rat brain and nuclei labelled *in vivo* with ³H-labelled 18-OH-DOC from a Sephadex G-200 column.

SEDIMENTATION PATTERN OF THE 18-OH-DOC BINDER FROM THE CYTOSOL

Sucrose gradient centrifugation[18,20] of brain cytosols labelled *in vivo* with ³H-labelled 18-OH-DOC (Fig. 5) indicates that in the presence of 0.4 M NaCl the radioactivity migrates prevalently in the top third of the gradient. This fraction represents 28% of the total radioactivity applied to the gradient. The second peak, occurring at the bottom third, contained 6% of the total radioactivity. According to the cytochrome *c* marker the prevalent ³H-labelled 18-OH-DOC binding material has an apparent *s* value of 3 and the minor peak one of 7.

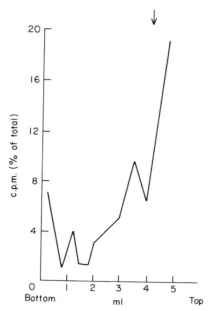

Fig. 5.   Separation of ³H-labelled 18-OH-DOC, bound to rat brain cytosolic macromolecules *in vivo*, by sucrose gradient centrifugation on 5–20% sucrose gradient containing 0.4 M NaCl. Arrow indicates the peak of cytochrome *c* marker.

CONCLUSION

These results demonstrate that the brain tissue retains considerable amounts of 18-OH-DOC, that the retained hormone fluctuates in response to pharmacological and surgical manipulations and that the uptake in the brain shows some gross regional differentiation. Cell-fractionation studies indicate some association of the 18-OH-DOC molecule with the brain cytosol and nuclear macromolecules with a preference for nuclear binding. Endocrine studies indicate that the brain is a target tissue for corticosteroids[21–23], thus glucocorticoids are implicated in neuronal processes underlying behaviour and regulation of ACTH secretion and aldosterone in electrolyte distribution in, or mediated through the central nervous system. The prevalent unbound 18-OH-DOC in the circulation and high (30%) retention by brain would facilitate a relatively large fraction of 18-OH-DOC available for the eventual brain target tissue binding. The precise role of 18-OH-DOC in the brain is unknown: its presence in the CNS points to a possible direct effect of the hormone on brain metabolism but the mechanism of this action has to be elucidated.

ACKNOWLEDGEMENT

The work of the author is supported by the Medical Research Council of Canada.

REFERENCES

1. Szego, C. (1957). *In* "Physiological Triggers", (Bulock, T. K. ed.), p. 152. American Physiological Society, Washington.
2. O'Malley, B. W. and Means, A. R. (1971). *Science* **183**, 610.
3. McEwen, B. S. *et al.* (1970). *Brain Res.* **17**, 471.
4. McEwen, B. S. and Wallach, G. (1973). *Brain Res.* **57**, 373.
5. Grosser, B. I. *et al.* (1973). *Brain Res.* **57**, 387.
6. Gerlach, J. L. and McEwen, B. S. (1972). *Science* **175**, 1133.
7. Carroll, B. J. *et al.* (1975). *Endocrinology* **98**, 676.
8. Anderson, III, N. and Fanestil, D. D. (1976). *Endocrinology* **98**, 676.
9. Birmingham, M. K. and Ward, J. P. (1961). *J. Biol. Chem.* **236**, 1661.
10. Domingues, O. V. (1965). *Steroids (Suppl. II)* **6**, 29.
11. Roy, A. K. *et al.* (1976). *J. Steroid. Biochem.* **7**, 81.
12. Fuller, P. J. and Funder, J. W. (1976). *J. Steroid. Biochem.* **7**, 673.
13. Feldman, D. and Funder, J. W. (1973). *Endocrinology* **92**, 1389.
14. Bartova, A. *et al.* (1977). Program of the 59th Annual Meeting of the Endocrine Society, Chicago, 280.
15. Glowinski, J. and Iversen, L. L. (1966). *J. Neurochem.* **13**, 655.
16. Bartova, A. *et al.* (1976). Abstracts of Short Communications and Poster Presentations of the Fifth International Congress of Endocrinology, Hamburg, 297.
17. Murphy, B. E. P. (1975). *J. Clin. Endocrinol. Metab.* **41**, 1050.
18. McEwen, B. S. *et al.* (1972). *Endocrinology* **80**, 217.
19. McEwen, B. S. and Plapinger, L. (1970). *Nature (London)* **226**, 265.
20. Martin, R. G. and Ames, B. N. (1961). *J. Biol. Chem.* **236**, 1372.
21. De Kloet, R. *et al.* (1975). *Endocrinology* **96**, 598.
22. McEwen, B. S. *et al.* (1972). *In* "Structure and Function of Nervous Tissue". (Bourne, G. D. ed.), Vol. 5, p. 205, Academic Press, New York.
23. McEwen, B. S. and Pfaff, D. W. (1973). *In* "Frontiers of Neuroendocrinology", (Ganong, W. F. and Martini, L. eds.), Vol. 3, p. 267, Oxford University Press, New York.

21

THE DIURNAL RHYTHMICITY OF BRAIN, PITUITARY AND ADRENOCORTICAL HORMONES

Janet Sadow

Department of Physiology, Medical Sciences, University of Leicester, U.K.

INTRODUCTION

The activity of the adrenal cortex has been known since 1943 to exhibit circadian periodicity[1]. For some years it was thought that the whole system (brain–pituitary–adrenal; BPA) together and separately followed this pattern with peak values of cortisol occurring in plasma between 06.00 h and 08.00 h in man[2] and peak values of corticosterone occurring between 16.00 and 20.00 h in the rat[3]. More recently it has become clear that circadian rhythmicity in the BPA is not a simple phenomenon of gradually increasing and then decreasing activity. Previous investigators had taken the mean value of blood corticosteroid levels derived from many rats or humans, or from a single subject at long sampling intervals[4]. From the work from several laboratories, it became evident that the circadian cycle of cortisol levels in man when analysed at short time intervals[5-8] is not a smooth curve. It was eventually demonstrated[9] that cortisol is secreted episodically in man, and that approximately half of the daily cortisol production is achieved during sleep in the early morning hours. From these studies, it has been deduced that the human adrenal is quiescent for at least 18 h of the day and secretes cortisol during a total of at most 6 h in the day[9].

RHYTHMS IN CIRCULATING ACTH AND CORTICOSTEROID LEVELS

When measured simultaneously at frequent intervals, increases in cortisol levels have usually been accompanied or immediately preceded by elevations in corticotropin (ACTH) levels in plasma[6]. However, the adrenal appears to

Janet Sadow

"ignore" some rises in ACTH, and cortisol levels occasionally increase in the absence of detected increases in ACTH[7]. The human adrenal gland has been shown to be least sensitive to injections of ACTH at the nadir of its activity cycle, and most sensitive during the peak of the cycle[10]. Similarly in the rat, adrenal responsiveness to ACTH has been estimated to increase by a factor of 12.5 between the morning trough and evening peak of the cycle[11].

In addition to circadian changes in ACTH and corticosteroid secretion, plasma corticosteroid levels are determined by daily changes in distribution volume, binding and metabolism of both ACTH and corticosteroids. There is little information available on the possible changes in these parameters for ACTH in the circulation. However, both in man[9] and rats[12] it appears that the half time for disappearance of corticosteroids from blood is longer at the time of the circadian maximum.

Episodic secretion of ACTH and corticosteroids are clearly under the entrainment of higher centres. It can be seen from the pre-dusk rise to peak of rat plasma corticosterone[3] and the marked increase in plasma cortisol concentrations that occur before activity in man[7,9] that the light–dark or activity cycle is important in the synchronization of the B–P–A axis. In addition to demonstrated rhythms in spontaneous activity of the B–P–A system, rhythms in responsiveness to exogenous stimuli that acutely activate the system have been demonstrated. In man, Takebe *et al.*[13] have shown that the plasma ACTH and adrenal responses to pyrogen are greater at 23.00 h (the time of minimum spontaneous activity) than at 09.00 h (the time of maximum spontaneous activity). Similarly, Engeland *et al.*[14] have shown that maximal ACTH responses to several stimuli occur in rats at lights-on (the time of minimum spontaneous activity) and minimum responses occur at lights-off (the time of maximal spontaneous activity).

However, there are other synchronizers in addition to the light–dark (activity) cycle. In rats allowed restricted access to food and/or water, the rhythm in plasma and adrenal corticosterone shifts to reach a peak just before the time of feeding (watering) independent of the light cycle[15,16]. Under such artificial conditions adrenal responsiveness to ACTH is maximal immediately before feeding in the absence of a demonstrable rhythm in ACTH[17]. However, in those studies there remained a minor effect of the light cycle on adrenal responsiveness to ACTH[17]. It has been demonstrated recently[18] that rats exposed to constant dim light, with free access to food, exhibit aperiodic feeding behaviour, plasma corticosterone concentrations and body temperature levels. Imposition of a restricted period of food access under the same lighting conditions is associated with the appearance of a circadian periodicity of both plasma corticosterone levels and body temperature levels, demonstrating food entrainment. Krieger and Hauser[18] linked this work with previous lesion work in the same laboratory to implicate the suprachiasmatic nucleus in some capacity of control.

RHYTHMS IN CORTICOLIBERIN (CRF) SECRETION

The activity of the 'CRF neuron'[19] is believed to be the humoral link between central nervous system and anterior pituitary secretion of ACTH. Almost exclusively applied in rats, the methodology for investigation and measurement of the biological activity of CRF has varied. Numerous assays have been developed[20-24]. CRF secretion *in vitro* may be obtained by measurement of CRF in the medium of incubates of isolated rat hypothalami[24-26]. This technique gives more information about the rate of release of CRF than can be gained from measuring hypothalamic CRF content by extraction techniques.

Circadian periodicity of hypothalamic CRF content has been thoroughly investigated by extraction techniques. Although there are discrepancies between laboratories, in general, it appears that the *content* of CRF in the hypothalamus does show rhythmicity. In some studies, the peak of CRF content occurred late in the afternoon[27-30,32] whereas a morning peak in CRF content was found by other workers[33-35]. CRF content did not alter significantly throughout the day in some studies[36,37]. Some reports described only a small fluctuation in CRF content[30,34,35], whereas other experiments showed significant changes[28,32,33]. Studies that did not find a rhythm in CRF content[36,37], also did not show marked changes after various treatments, suggesting that some aspect in the experimental procedure masked changes in CRF content. However, more recently, Dallman *et al.*[38], using an incubation technique, have shown a difference in CRF production from hypothalami removed from adrenalectomized rats (lights on and lights off) at 08.00 h and 20.00 h, thereby reflecting diurnal changes in CRF secretion in the absence of corticosteroid feedback at the time of removal.

In our own laboratory[39] we have demonstrated that when the isolated hypothalamus is incubated *in vitro*, the output of CRF is shown not to be a single steady process (Fig. 1). There is an initial rapid release during the first 15 min (phase 1) and another augmented release during the next 15 min (phase 2) falling to a slower steady output for at least the next 90 min. It is possible that the different phases in the release of CRF in our system correspond to different events in the synthesis, storage and exocytosis of CRF. The preparation has been shown by others to be viable over this period of time[40-42].

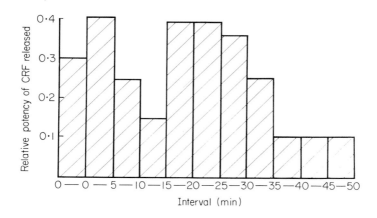

Fig. 1. The relative potency of CRF incubate produced in a series of 5 min intervals over 50 min. Relative potency is a measure of the potency of the incubate compared to an incubate obtained at 13.00 h having a potency of unity.

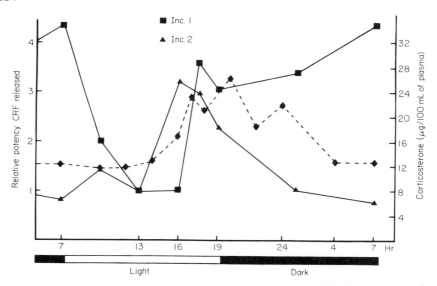

Fig. 2. The relative potency of CRF released during two successive 15 min incubations of the hypothalamus, Incubations 1 and 2, at different times in the day. Relative potency is a measure of the potency of the incubate compared with an incubate obtained at 13.00 h having a potency of unity. S.E.M. values have been omitted from this aggregate diagram for clarity. *n* is 15–21 for CRF estimates and 6 for blood corticosterone estimates.

It was decided therefore to investigate these two incubation periods 0–15 min (phase 1) and 15–30 min (phase 2) of a single isolated hypothalamus from rats at different times round the full 24 h cycle. The animals were kept two per cage in a quiet room before experiment, one being killed immediately before incubation at the time designated[26]. The results are plotted in full (Fig. 2) and compared with estimates of plasma corticosterone levels in other rats kept under identical conditions.

The circadian pattern in CRF release in Incubation 2 is quite different from that in Incubation 1. The afternoon rise in CRF secretion in Incubation 2 has occurred by 16.00 h, in advance of the rise in plasma corticosterone, whereas CRF secretion in Incubation 1, is still at its lowest at this time. Further, following the afternoon rise in CRF secretion during Incubation 2, production falls off during the night; in contrast, CRF secretion in Incubation 1 remains elevated during the dark period. Overall, the pattern of CRF secretion during Incubation 2 correlates better with the pattern expected of a system that would drive the diurnal rhythmicity of the B-P-A axis than the pattern in Incubation 1. It may be suggested that Incubation 1 represents a readily available pool, or content, which *follows* the pattern of plasma corticosterone rhythmicity rather than *causing* it, whereas Incubation 2 represents synthesis of CRF *de novo*, occurring in advance of circadian patterns of plasma corticosterone.

The phasic nature of the release of CRF, observed during a single incubation over 120 min at one particular time in the 24 h cycle, and the way in which the output of CRF during Incubations 1 and 2 vary independently over the 24 h cycle, together suggest that CRF output from the isolated hypothalamus incubated *in vitro* represents at least two events in the synthesis, storage and release of CRF from the CRF neurone. The significance of this is unclear, but it would indicate that the hypothalamus isolated and incubated *in vitro* provides a means of studying more complex phenomena in the dynamics of synthesis and release of CRF associated with the CRF neuron than may the simple measurement of "content", using extraction techniques to obtain the CRF sample at one single instant.

NEURAL REGULATORS OF CRF SECRETION

The neurons and their transmitter substances, which may influence the release of CRF, have recently been fully reviewed[42] and to complete this chapter, it is necessary to consider briefly how circadian periodicity within the CRF neuron is brought about in the intact system. Clues have already been cited in the work by Krieger and her colleagues[18], and it may be that circadian rhythms are programmed in the suprachiasmatic nucleus of the hypothalamus[43–47]. Various neurotransmitters have been implicated in the B–P–A axis causing an effect on CRF and ACTH release[42], serotonin(5-HT)[48–51], noradrenaline[52–54], acetylcholine[55–57], GABA[58] and prostaglandins[59]. Studies by Krieger and Krieger[60] have shown that chronic administration of reserpine or chlorpromazine in man does not affect circadian rhythmicity of plasma corticoids. Work done in our laboratory[61] has demonstrated that reserpine given to rats in a dose that has been shown to affect certain stress responses, does not interfere with circadian rhythmicity. Atropine was shown to block the circadian rhythm in cats[62].

In summary therefore it is possible that the rhythmicity of the CRF neuron is regulated by acetylcholine as the 'normal' transmitter with the possibility of noradrenaline as general suppressor of the B–P–A axis[52–54] with GABA as the specific inhibitory-neuron transmitter, with 5-HT periodically controlling disinhibitions programmed in at critical times[63].

Although the circadian rhythmicity of B–P–A axis has been discussed at length there are areas left uncovered, the questions left unanswered, such as the effects of the rhythmicity of corticosteroids and ACTH, on the feedback mechanisms they influence? Further, what are the controlling events of 'feedback' when there is a virtual absence of circulating cortisol in man, in the absence of an episode of secretion from the adrenal gland[9]?

Finally, it might be considered that corticosteroid feedback during normal circadian rhythms is far from important and that all that is needed of the various parts of the system is fast oscillatory phenomena that can be "entrained" and "damped" as necessary by the synchronizer or clock.

REFERENCES

1. Pincus, G. (1943). *J. Clin. Endocrinol. Metab.* **3**, 195.
2. Mills, J. N. (1966). *Physiol. Rev.* **46**, 128.
3. Guillemin, R. *et al.* (1959). *Proc. Soc. Exp. Biol. Med.* **101**, 394.
4. Krieger, D. *et al.* (1970). *J. Clin. Endocrinol. Metab.* **32**, 266.
5. Orth, D. N. *et al.* (1967). *J. Clin. Endocrinol. Metab.* **27**, 549.
6. Berson, S. A. and Yalow, R. S. (1968). *J. Clin. Invest.* **47** 2725.
7. Krieger, D. T. and Allen, W. (1975). *J. Clin. Endocrinol. Metab.* **10**, 675.
8. Orth, D. N. and Island, D. P. (1969). *J. Clin. Endocrinol. Metab.* **29**, 479.
9. Weitzman *et al.* (1971). *J. Clin. Endocrinol. Metab.* **33**, 14.
10. Forsham, P. H. *et al.* (1955). Ciba Colloquim on Endocrinology, Vol. 8, (Wolstenholme G. E. W. and Cameron, M. P. eds.), Little Brown and Co., Boston.
11. Dallman, M. F. *et al.* (1978). *Am. J. Physiol.* **235**, 210R.
12. Gibbs, F. (1970). *Am. J. Physiol.* **219**, 288.
13. Takebe, K. C. *et al.* (1966). *J. Clin. Endocrinol. Metab.* **26**, 437.
14. Engeland *et al.* (1977). *Endocrinology* **100**, 138.
15. Johnson, J. T. and Levine, S. (1973). *Neuroendocrinol.* **11**, 268.
16. Gray, G. D. *et al.* (1978). *Neuroendocrinol.* **25**, 236.
17. Wilkinson, C. W. *et al.* (1979). *Endocrinology (in press).*
18. Krieger, D. and Hauser, H. (1978). *Proc. Natl. Acad. Sci. USA.* **75**, 1577.
19. Saffran, M. and Schally, A. V. (1955). *Endocrinology* **56**, 523.
20. Mulder, G. H. *et al.* (1976). *Neurosci. Lett.* **2**, 73.
21. Portanova, R. and Sayers, G. (1973). *Neuroendocrinol.* **12**, 236.
22. Buckingham, J. C. and Hodges, J. R. (1977). *J. Endocrinol.* **73**, 30P.
23. De Wied, D. *et al.* (1969). *Endocrinology* **85**, 561.
24. Thomas, P. and Sadow, J. (1974). *J. Endocrinol.* **64**, 59P.
25. Bradbury, M. W. B. *et al.* (1974). *J. Physiol.* **239**, 269.
26. Sadow, J. and Thomas, P. (1976). *J. Physiol.* **258**, 9P.
27. David-Nelson, M. A. and Brodish, A. (1969). *Endocrinology* **85**, 861.
28. Hiroshige, T. *et al.* (1969). *Jap. J. Physiol.* **19**, 866.
29. Hiroshige, T. and Sato, T. (1970). *Endocrinol. Jap.* **17**, 1.
30. Retiene, K. and Schulz, F. (1970). *Horm. Metab. Res.* **2**, 221.
31. Takebe, K. and Sakakura, M. (1972). *Endocrinol. Jap.* **19**, 567.
32. Ixart, G. *et al.* (1977). *J. Endocrinol.* **72**, 113.
33. Chiefetz, P. N. *et al.* (1969). *Endocrinology* **81**, 1117.
34. Seiden, G. and Brodish, A. (1972). *Endocrinology* **90**, 1401.
35. Chiappa, S. A. and Fink, G. (1977). *J. Endocrinol.* **72**, 195.
36. Sirett, N. E. and Purves, H. D. (1973). *In* "Brain–Pituitary–Adrenal Interelationships", (Brodish, A. and Redgate, E. S. eds.), pp. 79–98, Karger, Basel.
37. Yasuda, N. and Greer, M. A. (1976). *Neuroendocrinol.* **22**, 48.
38. Dallman, M. *et al.* (1977). *J. Physiol.* **266**, 84.
39. Kamstra, G. S. *et al.* (1978). *J. Physiol. (in press).*
40. Hillhouse, E. W. and Jones, M. T. (1976). *J. Endocrinol.* **71**, 21.
41. Bradbury, M. W. B. *et al.* (1974). *J. Physiol.* **239**, 269.
42. Carpetner, W. T. and Gruen, P. H. (1978). Handbook of Psychopharmacology No. 13. (Iverson, L. *et al.* eds.), Plenum, N.Y. and London.
43. Krieger, D. T. (1975). *J. Steroid Biochem.* **6**, 785.
44. Krieger, D. T. (1976). Brain and Endocrine System Symposium., Longbeach Calif.

45.   Liddle, G. W. (1974). *In* "Textbook of Endocrinology", (Williams, R. H., ed.), pp. 233–283, Saunders, Philadelphia.
46.   Moore, R. Y. (1974). The Neurosciences-Third Study Programme, pp. 537–542, MIT Press, Cambridge, Mass.
47.   Rusak, B. and Zucker, I. (1975). *Ann. Rev. Physiol.* **26**, 137.
48.   Chambers, J. W. and Brown, G. M. (1976). *Endocrinology* **98**, 420.
49.   Naumenko, E. V. (1968). *Brain Res.* **11**, 1.
50.   Telegdy, G. and Vermes, L. (1973). *In* "Brain–Pituitary–Adrenal Interelationships", (Brodish, A. and Redgate, E. S. eds.), pp. 332–33, Karger, Basel.
51.   Scapagnini, U. *et al.* (1971). *Neuroendocrinol.* **7**, 90.
52.   Ganong, W. F. (1972). *In* "Brain–Endocrine Interaction: Median Eminence", (Knigge, K. M. *et al.* eds.), pp. 254–266, Karger, Basel.
53.   Nakai, Y. *et al.* (1973). *Acta. Endocrinol.* **74**, 263.
54.   Van Loon, G. R. (1973). *In* "Frontiers in Neuroendocrinology", (Ganong, W. F. and Martini, L. eds.), pp. 209–247, O.U.P., New York.
55.   Hedge, G. A. and Smelik, P. G. (1968). *Science* **159**, 890.
56.   Krieger, D. T. and Krieger, H. P. (1970). *Am. J. Physiol.* **218**, 1632.
57.   Hedge, G. A. and De Wied, D. (1971). *Endocrinology* **88**, 257.
58.   Jones, M. T. *et al.* (1976). *In* "Frontiers in Neuroendocrinology", Vol. 4, (Martini, L. and Ganong, W. F. eds.), pp. 195–226, Raven Press, New York.
59.   Labrie, F. *et al.* (1976). *In* "Frontiers in Neuroendocrinology", Vol. 4, (Martini, L. and Ganong, W. F. eds.), pp. 63–93, Raven Press, New York.
60.   Krieger, D. T. and Krieger, H. P. (1967). *Neuroendocrinol.* **2**, 232.
61.   Thomas, P. and Sadow, J. (1975). *Acta. Endocrinol. (kbh) Supp.* **199**, 209.
62.   Krieger, D. T. and Krieger, H. P. (1967). *Science* **155**, 1421.
63.   Krieger, D. T. *et al.* (1971). *J. Clin. Endocrinol. Metab.* **32**, 266.

22

POSSIBLE ROLES FOR ADRENAL LYSOSOMES IN CONTROLLING THE RESPONSE TO CORTICOTROPIN (ACTH)

Vineeta Prasad and Sukumar Chattopadhyay

*Hormone Research Unit, Department of Physiology,
Institute of Medical Sciences, Banaras Hindu University, Varanasi, India.*

INTRODUCTION

The demonstration by Hechter[1] that perfusion of corticotropin (ACTH) into bovine adrenal glands causes a rapid release of corticosteroids opened up an era in which evidence has accumulated on possible mechanisms involved in this response. Thus, since adrenal cortices store only small quantities of steroid[2], it follows that synthesis *de novo* must precede any sustained secretion. In turn this observation suggested that a rate-limiting step in corticosteroid biosynthesis should exist and at this point ACTH might act to allow the generation of the quanta of steroid required in response to stress.

The knowledge that an early committed stage in any biosynthetic pathway is the most likely point at which regulatory influences may be exerted, caused close scrutiny of the release of cholesterol from lipid storage droplets, its passage into the mitochondrion and its subsequent conversion into pregnenolone in that organelle. Observations were made that provided some support for regulation at each of these points.

In the bovine adrenal cortex, ACTH was observed to cause the activation of phosphorylase, a key glycogenolytic enzyme, and if the resulting glucose 1-phosphate (and hence glucose 6-phosphate) were channelled into the pentose phosphate pathway the resulting NADPH might stimulate side-chain cleavage of cholesterol. However, the cellular concentration of NADPH showed no direct relation to the rate of corticosteroidogenesis, nor was it clear how NADPH generated in the cytosol could act as a substrate in the mitochondrion.

The elucidation of the spatial arrangement of the enzymes involved in steroidogenesis within the cells of the adrenal cortex suggested another possible means of control of the early stages of the pathway. Thus pregnenolone is formed in the mitochondria and the next stage in the sequence (the formation of progesterone) occurs in association with the smooth endoplasmic reticulum. Therefore, since pregnenolone as a product of the side-chain cleavage reaction exerts product inhibition it might be expected that accelerated removal of pregnenolone from the mitochondrial milieu might in turn accelerate corticoidogenesis.

More evidence on a possible influence of ACTH at an early stage of steroidogenesis come from the demonstration that protein synthesis inhibitors block the effect of the peptide. It is suggested that part of the effect of ACTH is mediated *via* a labile protein, possibly a cholesterol carrier protein, more likely, in view of recent work[3], a protein that enhances the binding of cholesterol to the adrenal mitochondrial cytochrome P-450 responsible for the removal of the side-chain.

In summary, the present view seems to be that increased activity of the adrenal cortex in response to ACTH may involve (i) enhanced passage of intermediates such as cholesterol or pregnenolone across mitochondrial membrances, (ii) increased availability of NADPH within the mitochondrion or (iii) induction of specific proteins responsible for the binding of cholesterol. These various data suggest that the search for a single mechanism to explain the action of ACTH is naive and the interaction of the above and other metabolic events might best explain adrenal activation.

POSSIBLE ROLES FOR ADRENAL LYSOSOMES

A.   Lysosomes and the Promotion of Corticosteroidogenesis

Despite the fact that several potentially rate-limiting steps in corticosteroid formation seem to involve hydrolytic cleavage reactions, scant attention has been paid to the possible roles of those organelles that are rich in hydrolases, namely the lysosomes. Thus the mobilization of cholesteryl esters[4] and the rapid turnover of the protein that is involved in the binding of cholesterol to cytochrome P-450 must derive from the hydrolysis of ester and peptide bonds respectively.

The existence of lysosomes as a distinct class of cytoplasmic granules emerged from the characterization of acid phosphatase[5]. Differential centrifugation of the intracellular organelles indicated that acid hydrolases (enzymes with an acid pH optimum) were present in latent form in the lysosomes and were released on treatment with solubilizers. De Duve[5] visualized the lysosomes as an organelle containing acid hydrolases bounded by a continuous membrane.

A possible role for lysosomes comes from the work of Szego[6,7]. He showed that in the preputial gland or the uterus, vacuoles containing target-specific hormones can be formed, which fuse with primary lysosomes and can be transported by them to the nucleus. Thus lysosomes might have a role in the function of some hormones.

An early study of the involvement of lysosomes in the *zona fasciculata* of the rat adrenal cortex was that of Szabo *et al.* [8]. They found that after treatment of intact rats with ACTH the lysosomes in this zone increased in size and number and that lysosome–lipid conglomerates are formed. Hypophysectomy leads to a time-dependent decline in the size and number of lysosomes. When ACTH is given to such animals 2 to 4 weeks after the operation, the lysosomes appear conspicuously large around lipid droplets, which frequently coalesce with them. These results suggest a role for a lysosomal interaction with lipid stores, possibly involving the mobilization of cholesterol, although whether these changes are sufficiently rapid is not clear. Lysosomes in the adrenal cortex also contain active arylsulphatase B[9,10] and it may be that sulphation–de-sulphation reactions are of importance in the synthesis and secretion of corticosteroids.

All of the observations on lysosomes suggest roles for the organelles and their enzyme complements when the latter are firmly retained within the former. It may be that in certain circumstances the escape of the enzymes from lysosomes is of functional significance.

B.   Lysosomes and the Limiting of Corticosteroidogenesis

The structure-linked latency of lysosomal acid hydrolases led De Duve and his associates[11] to examine the effects of various lipids on the solubilization of these enzymes. The rate of release of acid phosphatase from lysosome-rich fractions of rat liver showed an increase in the presence of digitonin and vitamin A and was decreased by cholesterol, cortisone and hydrocortisone. The rate of release of acid phosphatase was reduced by steroids of known antiinflammatory activity whereas other steroids had no effect[12]. This was followed by a large number of observations indicating that corticosteroids may retard the release of acid hydrolases from lysosomes damaged by hypervitaminosis A, ultraviolet irradiation or trauma in systems that ranged from isolated organelles to whole animals[13].

The activation of the adrenal cortex in response to a severe injury to an organism and the consequent release of glucocorticoids has been assumed necessary for the defence of that organism against stress. However, the signs of stress develop in parallel with the increased activity of the adrenal cortex. The progressive tissue injury, in spite of adrenal activation and its arrest by the administration of supraphysiological amounts of glucocorticoids, led to the suggestion that such activation of the adrenal cortex as occurs in stress is inadequate to provide circulating levels of glucocorticoids sufficient to stabilize lysosomal membranes in damaged tissues. It might appear therefore somewhat surprising that in such conditions maximal steroidogenesis does not occur and may be further stimulated by ACTH. This implies the existence of a factor(s) that limits adrenal steroidogenesis in stress. This may involve the further supply of ACTH or it may be an inherent property of the adrenal itself.

One hypothesis to explain adrenal self-limitation would be that stimulation of the gland by its trophic hormone ACTH, leads to the release of lysosomal enzymes as a concomitant of the response. The work of Szego[6] on preputial lysosomes suggests that the trophic hormone for this gland (oestradiol-17-β)

can cause the intracellular release of acid hydrolases (this finding is complicated by the trophic hormone also being a steroid that is taken up into secondary lysosomes). However, in the case of the adrenal cortex the response would also go hand-in-hand with the intracellular accumulation of corticosterone or cortisol and this might serve to limit responsivity of the tissue by stabilizing lysosomal membranes.

It seemed to us therefore that the possibility that increased availability of glucocorticoids in the cellular milieu of the adrenal cortex leads to lysosomal stabilization, which could in turn be reflected in an inhibition of necessary metabolic functions, required investigation. In designing the experiments, we were aware of the possibility that if there is a cellular mechanism that limits activation of the gland, it may be altered when the organism is exposed repeatedly to the same stimulus owing to an adjustment of intracellular controls. Therefore quantitation of adrenal function was carried out after multiple as well as single exposures to the same stressor, namely gridshock.

It was observed that the concentration of the lysosomal marker enzymes acid phosphatase and β-glucuronidase free in the cytosol decreased at 1 h and increased at 24 h (relative to controls) after exposure of rats to gridshock for 15 min (controlled input of 70 V/1.2 mamp, 75 times/min). When the exposures were repeated once a day for 7 days and the determinations were again made 1 h and 24 h after the last gridshock, it was found that at both times the concentrations of the free enzymes was elevated (Fig. 1). In addition, it was found that in intact rats pre-treated with triamcinolone the concentrations of the enzymes in the adrenal cytosol were increased. Since the two enzymes determined may well derive from distinct lysosomal populations, perhaps a truer indication of

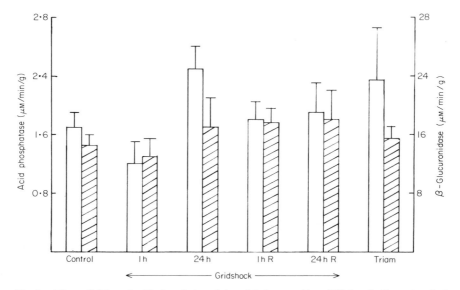

Fig. 1. The activities of acid phosphatase (□) and β-glucuronidase (▨) free in the cytosol of rat adrenal cortical cells 1 and 24 h after gridshock or gridshock repeated daily for 7 days (R) or after triamcinolone (triam).

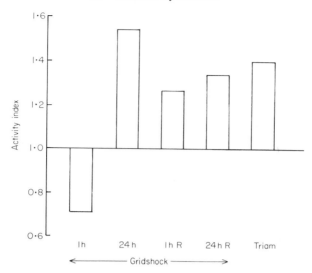

Fig. 2. An activity index for acid phosphatase and β-glucuronidase found free in the cytosol of rat adrenal cortical cells 1 and 24 h after gridshock or gridshock repeated daily for 7 days (R) or after triamcinolone (triam).

stability–lability may be obtained by expressing the product of the two activities as an activity index relative to the control values set at unity (Fig. 2).

From these data we may conclude that 1 h after the first gridshock there is evidence that lysosomes are stabilized such that their enzymic contents are not released. This contrasts with an apparent labilization 24 h and also at both 1 and 24 h after the last of seven daily treatments. In the experiment with triamcinolone, in which endogenous ACTH and hence adrenal corticosterone would be expected to be reduced, more lysosomal enzymes were present in the cytosol. Therefore in the adrenals of rats subjected to stress there is at 1 h an effect consistent with lysosomal stabilization due to corticosterone, and in animals with expected low adrenal corticosterone the results fit with a postulated increased labilization of the organelle.

CONCLUSION

Activation of the adrenal cortex seems to involve a whole constellation of metabolic changes. Some of these are rapid and are probably concerned with the immediate secretory response of the tissue to stress. Others seem to take more time to be fully established and these may reflect more long-term modulations of adrenal function.

ACKNOWLEDGEMENT

The work of the authors was supported by a grant from C.S.I.R., India.

REFERENCES

1. Hechter, O. (1949). *Fed. Proc.* **8**, 70.
2. Vernikos-Danellis, J. *et al.* (1966). *Endocrinol.* **79**, 624.
3. Simpson, E. R. *et al.* (1978). *J. Biol. Chem.* **253**, 3135.
4. Beckett, G. J. and Boyd, G. S. (1977). *Eur. J. Biochem.* **72**, 223.
5. De Duve, C. *et al.* (1951). *Nature (London).* **167**, 389.
6. Szego, C. H. (1974). *Rec. Prog. Horm. Res.* **30**, 171.
7. Szego, C. H. (1975). *In* "Lysosomes in Biology and Pathology", Vol. 4, (Dingle, J. T. and Dean, R. T. eds.), North Holland, Amsterdam.
8. Szabo, D. *et al.* (1967). *Hisotchemie* **10**, 321.
9. Rappay, Gy. *et al.* (1973). *Histochemie* **34**, 271.
10. Bascy, E. and Rappay, Gy. (1973). *In* "Electron Microscopy and Cytochemistry" (Wisse, E. *et al.* eds.), North Holland, Amsterdam.
11. De Duve, C. *et al.* (1962). *Biochem. Pharmacol.* **9**, 97.
12. Beaufay, H. and de Duve, C. (1957). *Arch. Int. Physiol. Biochem.* **65**, 156.
13. Weissman, G. (1967). *Ann. Rev. Med.* **18**, 97.

23

STUDIES OF THE HUMAN FETAL PITUITARY–
ADRENAL AXIS IN TISSUE CULTURE

†C. J. P. Giroud, C. Goodyer, G. Hall and C. Branchaud

*Endocrine Research Unit, Montreal Children's Hospital
Research Institute, Montreal, Canada.*

Explanatory note:

The work I am about to present is not my own but that of the late Claude Giroud who was killed in a tragic automobile accident in January last year. For the past 5 years he and his colleagues Charlotte Branchaud, Cindy Goodyer and George Hall have been investigating the interplay between the human fetal pituitary, adrenal and placenta in tissue culture.   B. E. P. MURPHY.

INTRODUCTION

Some aspects of fetal adrenal function are well known — the human fetal adrenal is an active androgen-secreting organ, producing large amounts of the C_{19}-steroid dehydroepiandrosterone sulfate (DHA-S), which is then utilized by the placenta to make estrogens. *In vivo*, the DHA-S is predominantly hydroxylated by the fetal liver before its transformation within the placenta to estriol. A second pathway involves the utilization of DHA-S itself by the placenta with the resultant formation of estrone and estradiol. Although a great deal of information is available regarding steroid biosynthesis and metabolism in the fetoplacental unit, relatively little is known about the regulatory mechanisms controlling the various phases of hormonogenesis. This has been the focus of these investigations[1–4].

Not only is the human fetal adrenal very large relative to body size during fetal life, but its structure is quite different from that found in the adult. There are two clearly defined zones, an outer narrow rim of cells just below the capsule, which is called the definitive or neo-cortex, and an inner mass of cells, comprising roughly 80% of the gland, called the fetal zone. Not only is there a marked difference in the size of the two zones, but the cell types are also quite different; the definitive zone is comprised of small cells with densely staining nuclei whereas the fetal zone consists of much larger cells with more lightly stained nuclei.

FETAL ADRENAL TISSUE IN CULTURE

The major contribution of the fetal adrenal during fetal life is its production of DHA-S and this has been found to come mainly from the fetal cortex. The neo-cortex, under culture conditions at least, produces a small amount of cortisol as well. It was of interest to study the biosynthetic pathways in both of these zones using as an endpoint the production of DHA-S and cortisol.

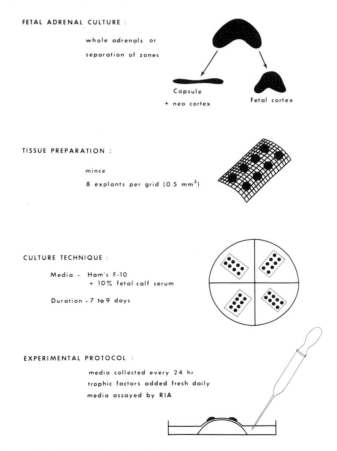

Fig. 1.   Preparation of fetal adrenal explants.

In all cases the tissues studied were obtained at the time of therapeutic abortion by hysterotomy. The gestational age of the fetuses ranged between 10 and 18 weeks. Definitive zone explants were found to be relatively free of fetal zone cells. By contrast, the fetal zone explants showed about 5% contamination by definitive zone cells.

The tissues were minced and then eight pieces were placed on stainless-steel grids and maintained for 7–9 days in Ham's F-10 culture medium supplemented with 10% fetal calf serum and antibiotics (Fig. 1). Since the long-term effects of exposure to the various corticotropic factors were of interest, the media were collected every 24 h during the week-long culture, fresh hormones being added with each medium change. The media samples were then extracted and subsequently assayed for both DHA-S and cortisol by radioimmunoassay. Morphological studies of the fetal adrenal under culture conditions showed that the tissue could be well maintained for at least 1 week *in vitro* but only if corticotropin (ACTH) or another corticotropic factor was present in the medium.

Effect of ACTH and Related Peptides

When the media from these cultures were assayed for steroids, both DHA-S and cortisol were found, with the DHA-S concentration being much higher than that of cortisol (Fig. 2). There is very good agreement with the morphological data in that control cultures maintained with medium alone stopped producing the two hormones within a few days. On the other hand, ACTH, either in the form of Duracton (the $ACTH_{1-39}$ extracted from porcine pituitaries) or as Cortrosyn (synthetic $ACTH_{1-24}$), maintained and even stimulated hormone production.

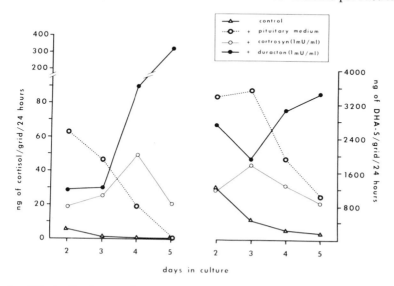

Fig. 2. Effects of various corticotropins and of homologous pituitary medium on the biosynthesis of DHA-S and cortisol by whole human fetal adrenal explants. △, Control; --○--, + pituitary medium; —○—, + Cortrosyn (ImU/mL); ●, + Duracton (ImU/mL).

Also, it was found that media taken from homologous human fetal pituitary cultures and added to the fetal adrenal cultures stimulated the production of both DHA-S and cortisol (Fig. 2 and 3).

In addition to explants of whole adrenals, results were obtained from cultures of the separated zones (Fig. 4). DHA-S was produced predominantly by the fetal zone, and cortisol by the definitive zone — results that correlate well with the data of others who have studied the distribution of enzymes necessary for the production of these hormones[5]. Human ACTH was able to stimulate DHA-S production in both zones. Cortisol production was also stimulated by human ACTH in both zones but predominantly in the neocortex. That in the fetal cortex may have been due to contamination by definitive zone cells as mentioned above.

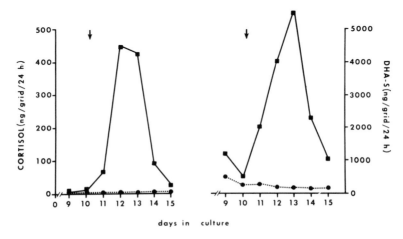

days in culture

Fig. 3. Re-stimulation of steroid production of fetal adrenal mixed zone explants by heterologous pituitary medium. Arrows indicate the first of daily additions of the pituitary medium. This demonstrates that the transient stimulatory effect of pituitary medium seen in both Figs. 2 and 3 is due to the fact that the pituitary ceases to produce its corticotropic factor after a few days in culture rather than to a loss in the responsiveness of the adrenal tissue. Gestation was 13 weeks. •, Control; ▪, human fetal pituitary culture medium.

Although it is possible that the pituitary corticotropic factor is simply ACTH, studies by other laboratories have suggested that one or more other pituitary hormones may also be involved, such as melanotropin (αMSH) or corticotropin-like intermediate lobe peptide (CLIP). A gradual transition in the ratio of these latter two peptides to ACTH have been found from fetal life through to the adult[6]. During fetal life the small peptides predominated, with the reverse being the case in the adult pituitary. In these tissue culture studies CLIP (not shown) had no effect, whereas αMSH stimulated production of DHA-S in both zones (Fig. 5). However, the concentration of αMSH required was 1 μM compared to 1 nM for human ACTH. Cortisol was also stimulated. When both CLIP and αMSH were added at the same time, there was no greater effect than that observed with αMSH alone. Thus in these studies ACTH was the most effective corticotropic factor. Other pituitary hormones implicated in fetal growth and development, i.e. growth hormone and prolactin, were also tested but had no effect.

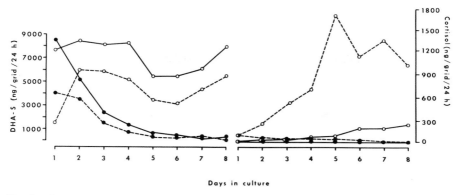

Fig. 4.   Steroid production by separated adrenal zones without (●, control) and with (○) human ACTH (22 nM); ——, fetal cortex; - - - -, neocortex.

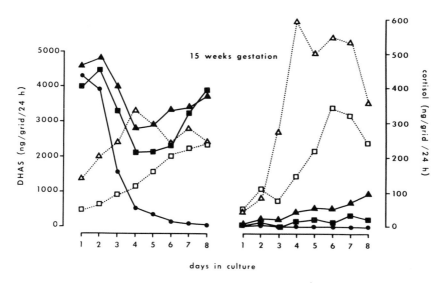

Fig. 5.   Stimulation of steroid production of separated adrenal zones by ACTH and αMSH. Fetal zone: ●, control; ▲, human ACTH; ■, αMSH. Neocortex: △, human ACTH; □, αMSH.

Effect of Placental Hormones

Similarly, possible placental involvement was examined and the effects of the placental peptide hormones human choriogonadotropin (HCG) and human placental lactogen (HPL) were tested. Preliminary results again showed no effect either on DHA-S or cortisol production by the fetal adrenal cultures.

FETAL PITUITARY IN CULTURE

One might wonder why, if ACTH is so effective, one should go on looking for a fetal corticotropic factor. There are several reasons: for instance we know that the human fetal adrenal develops normally for the first half of gestation whether or not a fetal pituitary is present, but after 20 weeks in an anencephalic the fetal zone atrophies. Also it is well known that immediately following birth, despite normal pituitary function in the newborn, the fetal zone atrophies, leaving the definitive zone cells to proliferate and form an adult-type cortex. Thus there would appear to be some specifically fetal corticotropic factor(s), other than ACTH, which is involved in the development and maintenance of the fetal zone of the fetal adrenal.

In considering the pituitary, it was desirable to define several aspects of fetal pituitary function. First, the ability of the gland to secrete its hormones under culture conditions; secondly, the relationship of fetal pituitary function to gestational age; and thirdly, the age of onset of fetal pituitary responsiveness to hypothalamic factors, such as luliberin (LRF), thyroliberin (TRF) and somatostatin.

Both explant and monolayer culture techniques were used successfully. Explant cultures were prepared in a fashion similar to that for the adrenal. For the monolayer preparation, the glands were minced and the tissue was exposed to 0.25% trypsin for dispersion. The cells were harvested, resuspended in medium (again Ham's F-10 supplemented with 10% fetal calf serum and antibiotics) and planted in tissue-culture flasks. These cultures were maintained for 2 to 4 weeks during which time the media were collected daily in order to analyze pituitary activity as a function of time in culture as well as gestational age.

Effect of Hypothalamic Releasing and Inhibiting Hormones

Every 2 to 3 days, a short-term test with hypothalamic factors was undertaken. This consisted of a 4 h control incubation followed, after two rinses, with a 4 h incubation in the presence of either LRH, TRH or somatostatin. The media were subsequently assayed for their content of growth hormone, lutropin (LH), follitropin (FSH), thyrotropin (TSH) and prolactin by radioimmunoassay and, on several occasions, for corticotropic activity by bioassay.

Light and electron microscopic investigations showed that the tissue did well under conditions of culture, and that under either explant or monolayer culture four different types of epithelial cells could be distinguished based on their granule cell population.

When the media were analyzed for pituitary trophic hormones, there was a general trend of secretion with time in culture. The data shown in Fig. 6 are from a culture of a fetal pituitary (19 weeks gestation) but they are representative of all those examined. Secretion of growth hormone, LH and FSH declined during the the first few days in culture, then stabilized for at least 2 weeks. TSH secretion dropped off rapidly and was lost within the first 2 weeks. The production of prolactin, unlike that of all the other trophic hormones, after the initial decline increased and this increase continued for several weeks.

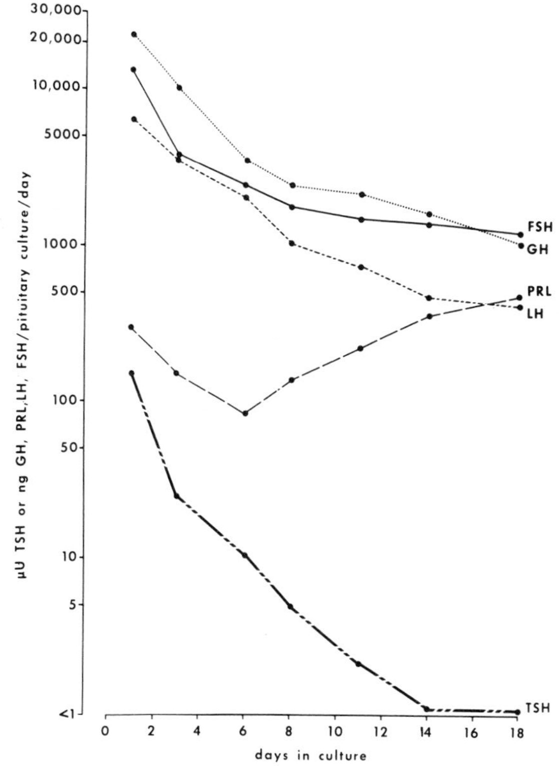

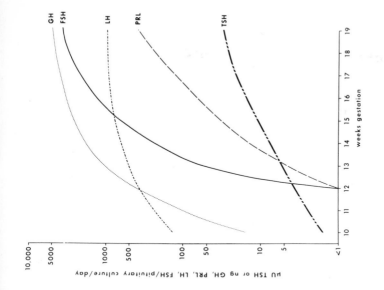

Fig. 7. Pituitary hormone production as a function of gestational age.

Fig. 6. Trophic hormone production by a fetal (19 weeks gestation) pituitary.

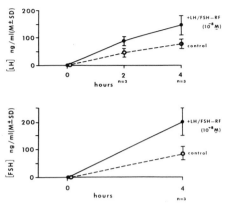

Fig. 8.　　Effect of LRH on LH and FSH secretion by fetal pituitary. ●, LH or FSH in presence of 10 nM gonadoliberin (LRH); ○, control.

When the secretion data were analyzed as a function of gestational age, it was found that the older the fetus the greater the secretion and the longer the hormones were secreted *in vitro* (Fig. 7). Growth hormone, LH and TSH secretion were evident by 10 weeks, ACTH (i.e. corticotropic activity) as early as 11 weeks, and FSH and prolactin after 12 weeks of fetal life.

When the cultures were tested with LRH, it was able to stimulate both LH and FSH secretion 2–4-fold (Fig. 8) as early as 13 weeks gestation. TRH, as early as 10 weeks of gestation, was able to stimulate TSH secretion 2–5-fold (Fig. 9); and somatostatin at 10 weeks of gestation was able to inhibit GH release from 14 to 78% (Fig. 10).

Thus the human fetal pituitary is capable of synthesizing, storing and secreting its trophic hormones by the third month of gestation; and beginning at 10 to 13 weeks, the fetal pituitary cells can respond to three hypothalamic peptides, LRH, TRH and somatostatin. Thus the hypothalamus could begin to influence pituitary function by the end of the third month of gestation.

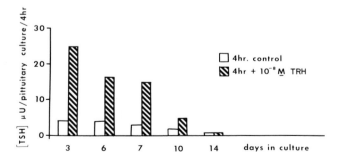

Fig. 9.　　Effect of TRH on TSH secretion by fetal pituitary. □, 4 h control; ■, 4 h + 10 nM TRH.

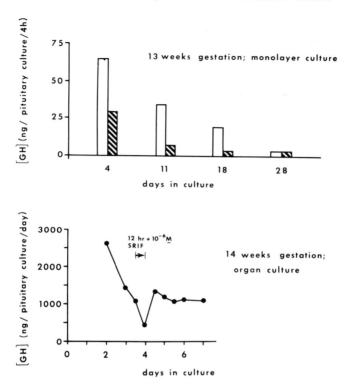

Fig. 10. Effect of somatostatin (10 nM) on growth hormone (GH) release by fetal pituitary. ▫, 4 h control; ▨, 4 h + 10 nM somatostatin.

PLACENTAL TISSUE IN CULTURE

We now come to the placenta — its production of steroid hormones: progesterone, estrone and estradiol — and the interrelationship of the placenta and the fetal adrenal. Both mid-term and term placenta were studied in monolayer culture, as for the pituitary. The media were collected every 24 h and trophic factors or precursors were added fresh daily; the media were assayed for estrone, estradiol and progesterone after extraction of the media, and for HCG and HPL.

Mid-term placental monolayer cultures produced both estradiol and estrone, with estradiol predominating. There was significant incorporation of tracer ^{14}C-DHA-S into both estrogens. Term placental cultures yielded similar results. The amount of estradiol and estrone produced was shown to be related to the amount of precursors used. That is, in the presence of tracer amounts of precursors, production was low. Addition of adrenal medium to the placental cultures also increased estrogen production (Fig. 11), presumably due to the presence of DHA-S in the adrenal medium.

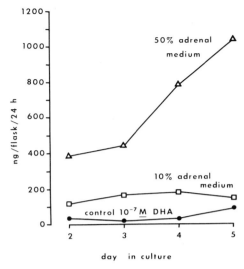

Fig. 11. Effect of adrenal medium on estradiol production by mid-term placental monolayer cultures.

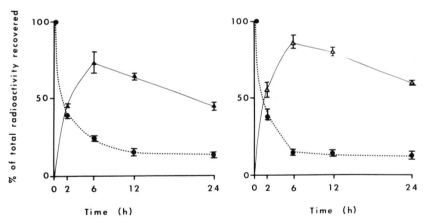

Fig. 12. Incorporation of [³H] pregnenolone into progesterone by mid-term and term placental monolayer cultures. •, Labelled substrate; ▲, mid-term production; △, term production.

The fact that the placental monolayers are able to incorporate DHA-S into estrone and estradiol demonstrates the presence of 3β-hydroxysteroid dehydrogenase isomerase. Not only is this a key enzyme in the estrogen biosynthetic process, but it is also responsible for the conversion of pregnenolone into progesterone in steroid-producing tissues. Fig. 12 shows the progressive disappearance of [³H-] pregnenolone and the rapid incorporation of the radioactivity into

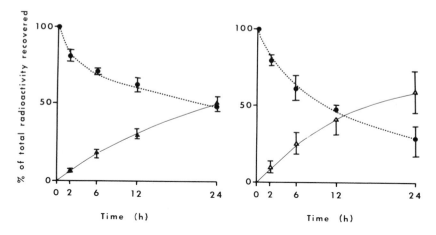

Fig. 13.   Formation of cortisone from [¹⁴C] cortisol by placental monolayer cultures.
Symbols as in Fig. 12.

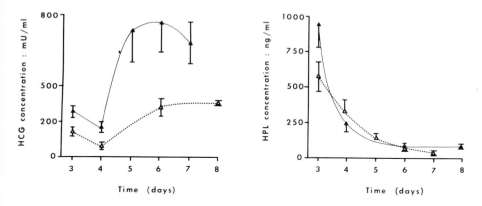

Fig. 14.   Production of HCG and HPL by mid-term and term placental cultures. Symbols
as in Fig. 12.

progesterone over a 24 h period in both mid-term and term placental cultures.
The presence of 11β-hydroxysteroid dehydrogenase in placental cultures was
demonstrated by the progressive incorporation of [¹⁴C-] cortisol into cortisone
over a 24 h period of observation, again in both mid-term and term placental
cultures (Fig. 13). There was a progressive increase in HCG production as a
function of time in culture and rapid decrease in HPL production by both mid-
term and term cultures (Fig. 14).

CONCLUSION

It has been shown that in culture, the fetal zone and the neocortex of the human fetal adrenal, the fetal pituitary and the mid-term and term placenta produce the respective hormones attributed to these tissues *in vivo*. The fetal adrenal responds to the tropic effect of human fetal pituitary medium as well as to ACTH and related peptides. The fetal pituitary is capable of synthesizing, storing and secreting trophic hormones and by 10 to 13 weeks of gestation is responsive to hypothalamic releasing and inhibiting factors as well. The placenta produces estrogens, progesterone, HCG and HPL and greatly augments its estrogen production when provided with DHA-S or adrenal medium. It is proposed that this tissue culture model is suited for the study of factors affecting hormonogenesis in the human feto-placental unit.

ACKNOWLEDGEMENTS

The authors are grateful to the editors of *Steroids* and *The Journal of Clinical Endocrinology and Metabolism* for permission to reprint the following: Figure 3 from *Steroids* (1977) **29**: 407; Figure 4 from *Steroids* (1978) **31**: 557; Figures 6, 8 and 9 from *The Journal of Clinical Endocrinology and Metabolism* (1977) **45**: 73, and Figures 12, 13 and 14 from *Steroids* (1977) **30**: 569.

REFERENCES

1. Goodyer, C. G. *et al.* (1977). *Steroids* **29**, 407.
2. Hall, C. St. G. *et al.* (1977). *Steroids* **30**, 569.
3. Goodyer, C. G. *et al.* (1977). *J. Clin. Endocrinol. Metab.* **45**, 73.
4. Branchaud, C. T. *et al.* (1978). *Steroids* **31**, 557.
5. Goldman, A. S. *et al.* (1966). *J. Clin. Endocrinol. Metab.* **26**, 14.
6. Silman, R. E. *et al.* (1976). *Nature (London)* **260**, 716.

24

A ROLE FOR CORTISONE IN HUMAN FETAL DEVELOPMENT

Beverley E. Pearson Murphy

Reproductive Physiology Unit, Montreal General Hospital, Montreal, Canada.

INTRODUCTION

Although cortisone (E) has long been known to be a more prominent steroid than cortisol (F) in human placenta and fetal serum, little attention has been paid to its possible significance in fetal life. It was observed as long ago as 1952 that E levels were high in human placenta[1]. In 1960 Baird and Bush[2] showed that amniotic fluid at term contained F/E in the ratio 1/2 and in the same year Osinski[3] demonstrated that with addition of cofactors, F and E were inter-converted in the placenta. These observations were ignored, however, when in 1961 Migeon *et al.*[4] provided evidence that F crossed the placenta "freely" i.e. unchanged. However, it was recognized in 1962 by Bro-Rasmussen *et al.*[5] that in cord serum at term F/E was only 0.5.

THE MEASUREMENT OF CORTISOL IN HUMAN FETAL FLUIDS AND TISSUES

Before embarking on the major topic of this chapter — the interconversion of cortisol-cortisone — a word of caution is in order about measurements of cortisol in human fetal fluids and tissues. There have been many articles published recently using radioimmunoassay methods validated for adult serum. That these are entirely inadequate is demonstrated in Table I where two of these methods (Lab 1,2) using antibodies to the same hapten conjugate (at C21) gave entirely different results although both claimed high specificity for cortisol. Both gave

247

Table I.   Cortisol in amniotic fluid. RTA, Radiotransinassay; RIA, radioimmuno-assay; BSA, bovine serum albumin.

	Lab. 1	Lab. 2	Lab. 3
No. of samples	43	114	98
Entity measured	"Total cortisol"	Cortisol	Cortisol
Method	RIA	RIA	RTA
Binding protein	-antibody to cortisol-21-hemisuccinate-BSA	same as	horse transcortin
Mean cortisol (ng/ml)			
at 20–34 wk	32	139	10
at 35–40 wk gestation	72	170	27
Reference	20	21	22

values that were very much higher than the true values for cortisol determined by a similar assay, i.e. without extraction or chromatography, employing horse transcortin as the binding protein (Lab 3). This radiotransinassay, which was developed in our own laboratory[19], was shown to give – for amniotic fluid though not for fetal serum – values almost identical with those obtained after chromatography on Sephadex LH-20 and by double-isotope derivative assay. These results emphasize the point that all radioimmunoassays for steroids in fetal material should be validated by chromatography since we are still far from knowing the identity of all the steroids present in the feto-placental unit.

CONVERSION OF CORTISOL INTO CORTISONE

In our own laboratory, when we repeated Migeon's experiment of injecting radioactive F into women at midpregnancy and examining the radioactivity of the fetal blood and placenta 20 min later, we found that most of the radioactivity was in the form of E rather than F[6].

Other important evidence as to the importance of E in the human fetus was provided in 1970 by Pasqualini *et al.*[7] who showed that when tracer E and F were infused *in vivo* into the umbilical vein 20 min before therapeutic abortion at about 18 weeks gestation, much of the F had been converted into E but little E was converted into F except in the placenta. On the other hand, in 1973 Smith *et al.*[8] found that in tissue cultures of fetal lung, E was converted into F but not the reverse. By this time, Beitins *et al.*[9] had concluded that the bulk of fetal E was mainly maternal in origin.

Our own studies were extended by simply surveying the concentrations of F and E in various tissues in early and late pregnancy (Table II). At 10 to 20 weeks, maternal serum contained mainly F (F/E = 7.5) and this ratio remained essentially unchanged throughout pregnancy. Placenta contained mainly E throughout pregnancy. In cord arterial serum, the F/E ratio in early pregnancy was about 0.4 rising to 0.6 in late pregnancy (i.e. delivery by Caesarean section) and to 1.1

Table II.   Concentrations of cortisol (F) and cortisone (E) in various tissues. Values are means ± S.E.

Gestational age (weeks)	Tissue	n	Steroid (ng/ml)		F/E Ratio
			Cortisol	Cortisone	
11–16	Amniotic fluid	11	3.0 ± 0.6	9.2 ± 1.6	0.33 ± 0.04
11–22	Cord arterial serum	8	8.9 ± 3.0	20.2 ± 5.0	0.44 ± 0.14
11–22	Cord venous serum	9	4.0 ± 2.2	28.9 ± 9.5	0.14 ± 0.03
11–22	Fetal adrenal	6	207.0 ± 54.0	116.0 ± 25.0	1.80 ± 0.60
11–22	Placenta	5	2.2 ± 0.5	103.0 ± 32.0	0.02 ± 0.01
17–22	Amniotic fluid	11	4.7 ± 0.9	6.7 ± 1.0	0.66 ± 0.07
17–22	Maternal serum	6	150.0 ± 10.0	20.0 ± 4.0	7.50 ± 1.70
36–40 (no labour)	Amniotic fluid	7	18.0 ± 3.0	10.6 ± 2.6	1.80 ± 1.80
(no labour)	Cord arterial serum	5	36.0 ± 7.1	62.0 ± 6.9	0.57 ± 0.11
(no labour)	Cord venous serum	5	20.5 ± 5.6	70.0 ± 3.6	0.29 ± 0.08
(no labour)	Placenta	6	11.0 ± 4.1	256.0 ± 10.0	0.04 ± 0.02
(no labour)	Maternal serum	6	300.0 ± 48.0	40.0 ± 7.0	7.50 ± 2.50
36–40 (spontaneous onset labour)	Amniotic fluid	5	28.5 ± 8.3	18.9 ± 7.1	1.50 ± 1.00
	Cord arterial serum	6	120.0 ± 25.0	108.0 ± 15.0	1.20 ± 0.40
	Cord venous serum	6	98.0 ± 27.0	143.0 ± 17.0	0.76 ± 0.11

at delivery (i.e. vaginal delivery of spontaneous onset). In cord venous serum the low ratio of 0.1 at 10–20 weeks rose to 0.3 in late pregnancy and to 0.7 at spontaneous vaginal delivery. In amniotic fluid there appeared to be an earlier rise at about 18 weeks gestation with a ratio of F/E in excess of 1 thereafter.

We were puzzled as to why the F/E ratio should be so much higher in amniotic fluid than in fetal serum since it is generally believed that most of the amniotic fluid steroids are derived from fetal urine. We studied fetal kidney and skin[10] to see if they might be responsible, but in vain, and we finally looked at the fetal membranes.

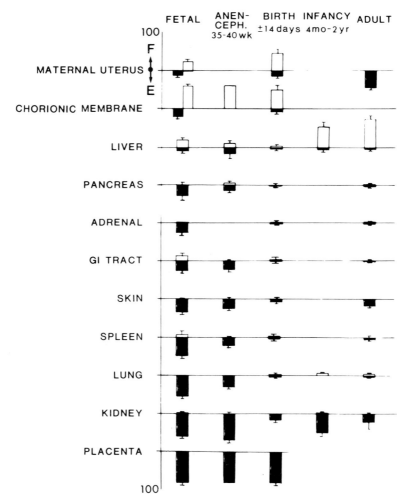

Fig. 1. Conversion of F–E in fetal tissues and maternal uterus. Downward solid bars indicate conversion of F into E, upward open bars the conversion of E into F, as %. 100% represents the distance between horizontal lines.

CONVERSION OF CORTISONE INTO CORTISOL BY THE MEMBRANES

The fetal membranes (the inner amnion and the outer chorion laeve) which form the sac containing the amniotic fluid bathing the fetus, are fetal tissues, the chorion laeve being continuous with the placenta proper (chorion frondosum). Traditionally they have been ignored; however, it is now being recognized that they are rich sources of enzymes and are probably very important in determining the onset of parturition. Much to our surprise, on adding tracers to membranes at various gestational ages we found that after 18 weeks or so the membranes began to convert E into F and this was continued to term with a variable drop at the time of delivery[10]. Thus in the latter half of pregnancy the activity in the absence of added cofactors is opposite in the placenta and the contiguous membranes. This appeared to explain Pasqualini's finding of activity in both directions since he had not bothered to remove the membranes from his "Placentas"[7].

These observations led us to an examination of the behaviour of individual fetal tissues and of the maternal uterus (Fig. 1). The uterus was found to behave in much the same way as the fetal chorion laeve i.e. reversal of activity from oxidative to reductive occurred at mid-pregnancy. Fetal tissues were almost all reductive in early pregnancy but showed little or no activity at or shortly after birth (autopsy material). After birth, activity varied with the tissue, uterus, kidney and skin being oxidative, whereas the liver became strongly reductive over the first few years. The overall pattern of activity is summarized in Fig. 2.

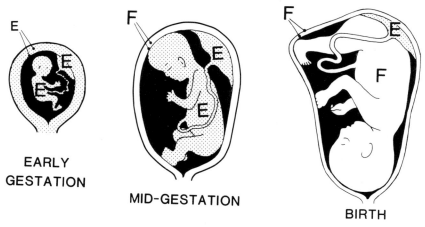

EARLY GESTATION

MID-GESTATION

BIRTH

Fig. 2.   Summary of E–F interconversion. The predominant steroid at each site is indicated.

FACTORS THAT INFLUENCE INTERCONVERSION

Why is there so little activity in fetal tissues at birth? What factors control oxidoreduction in these tissues? Using the placenta as a test system, the effects on conversion of F into E and E into F of maternal and fetal serum were studied (Fig. 3). Both types of serum greatly inhibited the reaction F into E, but the

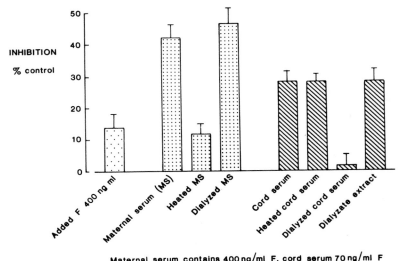

Maternal serum contains 400 ng/ml F, cord serum 70 ng/ml F

Fig. 3. Inhibition of placental conversion of F into E. Standard errors are indicated.

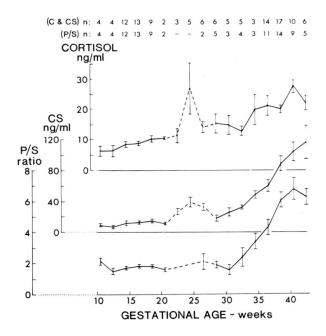

Fig. 4. Levels of cortisol and glucocorticoid conjugates (CS) and the palmitic/stearic ratio (P/S) in amniotic fluid throughout pregnancy. Means ± S.E. are shown. Reproduced from ref. 15.

nature of the inhibition appeared to be quite different, that in maternal serum being heat-labile and undialyzable (suggesting it to be due to transcortin) whereas that in fetal serum at delivery was heat-stable, dialyzable and extractable into organic solvents. We are currently trying to make a positive identification of these factors.

Another question we wanted to answer was: when does this change in F metabolism occur in the fetus? Amniotic fluid is the only fetal fluid obtainable in the human at all gestational ages but owing to the membrane contribution of F, the amniotic fluid F level cannot be used as a reliable indicator of fetal F production. We therefore looked at conjugated F in amniotic fluid (Fig. 4), which is known to be present mainly as the sulfate — an entity which is believed to be secreted either entirely or in large part by the fetal adrenal cortex itself[11]. This material was less variable than F and showed a steady rise from about 33 weeks onward, a rise that closely parallelled that of the palmitic/stearic (P/S) ratio, a reliable indicator of fetal lung maturation[12].

The correlation of the conjugated material (CS) with P/S was 0.80 compared with a value of 0.55 for amniotic fluid F vs P/S.

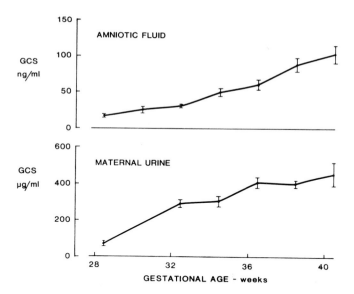

Fig. 5. Levels of glucocorticoid conjugates (GCS) in amniotic fluid and maternal urine compared in two different groups of patients. Means ± S.E. are shown.

Since the amniotic fluid F conjugate appears to reflect fetal lung maturation might this relationship hold true for maternal F conjugate? Our preliminary data, shown in Fig. 5, suggest that it might, but it will require much more work to establish any clinical validity of such a test.

THE SIGNIFICANCE OF CORTISOL–CORTISONE INTERCONVERSION

What is the biological significance of the changing F–E interconversion during fetal life, at birth and subsequently? It is known that high F levels in early fetal life may, in many species, have deleterious effects on fetal development — cleft lip in mice being a well-known example[13,14]. It thus seems possible that 11β-hydroxysteroid dehydrogenase, by converting F into its inactive analogue E, can maintain a low F level in fetal tissues without decreasing fetal adrenocortical production of a steroid that is vital for survival after birth. Oxidation of the bulk

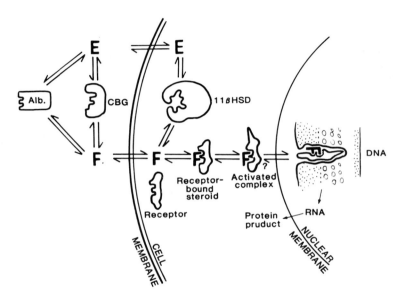

Fig. 6.   Mechanism of cortisol action. The current concept is modified to include diversion of F from glucorticoid receptors by enzymic conversion into E, and the reverse.

of the cortisol coming across the placenta from the mother achieves the same purpose and permits the fetus to exert some degree of autonomy over its cortisol production *via* the feedback mechanism. Presumably in fetal tissues F is diverted away from the glucocorticoid receptors (known to be present from the early weeks of pregnancy) in the manner depicted in Fig. 6 because of the large amount of enzyme present. The presence of an enzyme inhibitor at about the time of birth would allow a greater amount of F to bind to cytosol receptors thereby effecting the maturational processes known to occur in various species at this time[15]. Thus a rise in F could be brought about by a decrease in metabolism rather than an increase in production. The F production from E by the membranes may act to decrease the immune response of the mother toward the fetal allograft. Thus cortisone would appear to have an important role to play in the development of the human fetus. That it may play a similar role in some animal species is suggested by the work of Burton *et al.*[16] in rats and that of Pasqualini *et al.*[17] in guinea pigs.

We have also shown that the currently used drugs betamethasone and dexa-methasone are not metabolized in this manner by the placenta and presumably not by other fetal tissues[18]. Prednisone, on the other hand, is converted by the maternal liver into prednisolone and by the placenta back into prednisone. Thus if administered to the mother for the prevention of the respiratory distress syndrome, dexamethasone and betamethasone are much more potent than cortisol or prednisone. On the other hand, we know very little about their handling by fetal tissues, a fact that should make us cautious in their use. It would seem more logical to administer the natural glucocorticoid cortisol *via* the amniotic fluid since available studies suggest that amniotic fluid is swallowed in large quantities by the fetus. Even if some F is converted into E by the fetal gut a considerable amount could be absorbed into the circulation. Since a much smaller dose would be required intra-amniotically than if injected into the mother this would be a particularly desirable mode of administration in the diabetic mother where gluco-corticoid administration will alter insulin requirements.

CONCLUSION

Our studies, based on determinations of tissue concentrations of cortisol and cortisone and of their interconversion in fetal tissues and maternal uterus, suggest that conversion of cortisol into cortisone in virtually all fetal tissues (except the fetal membranes) and particularly in the placenta (chorion frondosum) protects the fetus until late pregnancy from concentrations of cortisol derived from the mother and from its own adrenals which would otherwise inhibit growth. On the other hand, production of cortisol from cortisone in the chorion laeve and uterine wall throughout the latter half of pregnancy may help to prevent rejection of the fetal allograft. At the time of birth, interconversion appears to be inhibited by a dialyzable, extractable, heat-stable factor in fetal serum.

REFERENCES

1. DeCourcy, C. *et al.* (1952). *Nature (London)* **170**, 494.
2. Baird, C. W. and Bush, I. E. (1960). *Acta. Endocrinol.* **34**, 97..
3. Osinski, P. A. (1960). *Nature (London)* **187**, 777.
4. Migeon, C. A. *et al.* (1961). *Rec. Progr. Horm. Res.* **17**, 207.
5. Bro-Rasmussen, F. *et al.* (1962). *Acta. Endocrinol.* **40**, 579.
6. Murphy, B. E. P. *et al.* (1974). *Am. J. Obstet. Gynecol.* **118**, 538.
7. Pasqualini, J. R. *et al.* (1970). *J. Steroid Biochem.* 1, **209**.
8. Smith, B. T. *et al.* (1973). *Steroids* 22, 515.
9. Beitins, I. Z. *et al.* (1973). *Ped. Res.* 7, 509.
10. Murphy, B. E. P. *et al.* (1977). *Nature (London)* **266**, 179.
11. Giroud, C. J. P. (1971). *Clin. Obstet. Gynecol.* **14**, 745.
12. Murphy, B. E. P. (1978). *J. Clin. Endocrinol. Metab.* **17**, 212.
13. Hall, B. K. and Kalliecharan, R. (1976). *Teratology* **12**, 111.
14. Chen, T. L. *et al.* (1977). *Endocrinology* **100**, 619.
15. Liggins, G. C. (1976). *Am. J. Obstet. Gynecol.* **126**, 931.
16. Burton, A. F. *et al.* (1970). *Can. J. Biochem.* **48**, 178.
17. Pasqualini, J. R. *et al.* (1970). *J. Steroid Biochem.* 1, 341.

18. Blanford, A. T. and Murphy, B. E. P. (1977). *Am. J. Obstet. Gynecol.* **127**, 264.
19. Murphy, B. E. P. (1975). *J. Clin. Endocrinol. Metab.* **41**, 1050.
20. Fencl, M. deM. and Tulchinsky, D. (1975). *New Eng. J. Med.* **292**, 133.
21. Sivakumaran, T. *et al.* (1975). *Am. J. Obstet. Gynecol.* **122**, 291.
22. Sharp-Cageorge, S. M. *et al.* (1977). *New Eng. J. Med.* **296**, 89.

25

PITUITARY-DEPENDENT CUSHING'S DISEASE

Lesley H. Rees

*Department of Chemical Endocrinology, St. Bartholomew's Hospital,
London EC1A 7BE, U.K.*

INTRODUCTION

Cushing's syndrome is the result of prolonged raised circulating levels of free corticosteroid in the plasma. Although the clinical diagnosis may be relatively easily made when the disease is florid, difficulties may frequently arise due to an atypical presentation or a mild or intermittent illness. Thus the diagnosis of Cushing's syndrome is not based solely on the clinical findings but must be based on the biochemical evidence of elevated corticosteroid secretion. Because corticosteroid secretion may be increased in other disorders such as obesity, depression and under conditions of 'stress', a variety of complicated investigative procedures may be required to arrive at the correct diagnosis. There is no single test alone which will make the diagnosis of Cushing's syndrome in the first instance and further elucidation of the underlying aetiology of the syndrome is even more complex.

Table I.   Causes of Cushing's Syndrome.

1.	Pituitary-dependent Cushing's disease.
2.	Adrenocortical tumours — adenoma or carcinoma.
3.	Ectopic ACTH syndrome.
4.	Iatrogenic: (a) Corticosteroid administration
	(b) ACTH administration
	(c) Alcohol[a]

[a]References 34 and 35.

There are three main causes of Cushing's syndrome (Table I) although a similar clinical picture indistinguishable from Cushing's syndrome may be caused by the iatrogenic administration of exogenous corticosteroids, corticotropin (ACTH) or alcohol. Although pituitary-dependent Cushing's disease is stated to be the commonest cause of Cushing's syndrome and in conjunction with adrenal tumours is normally regarded as accounting for two-thirds of all cases, it is probable that both ectopic ACTH production and alcohol-induced Cushing's syndrome are under-diagnosed[1].

CUSHING'S SYNDROME

Clinical Features

The clinical features of Cushing's syndrome are easily recognized and include weight gain with fat being distributed mainly in the trunk, head and neck. Facial plethora is associated with mooning of the face the overall central adiposity contrasting with loss of proximal muscle mass in the arms and legs. Most patients have clinically demonstrable myopathy, and histological changes similar to those seen in patients treated long-term with exogenous glucocorticoids[2]. Generalized symptoms include tiredness, weakness, ankle oedema, loss of libido, amenorrhoea, hirsuties and acne. Easy bruisibility of the skin with purple striae on the abdomen or upper arms may be present and pigmentation, most marked over the knuckles, in the palmar creases, in the buccal mucosa and in recent surgical scars or areas exposed to sunlight. Other symptoms may be due to diabetes mellitus, osteoporosis with or without pathological fractures and a host of psychiatric disorders. Thus in a review of 500 patients with Cushing's syndrome, psychiatric symptoms were a major feature in 40%[3]; depression is most commonly seen and can be alleviated by reduction of plasma corticosteroid levels to normal either by medical or surgical adrenalectomy[4].

Biochemical Diagnosis of Cushing's Syndrome

In the first instance the correct diagnosis of Cushing's syndrome must be established before the differential diagnosis of pituitary-dependent Cushing's disease can be made.

1. Loss of circadian rhythm of plasma corticosteroids and urinary corticosteroid excretion

The demonstration of the loss of circadian rhythmicity of plasma corticosteroids[5,6] is the cornerstone of initial diagnosis. Thus although plasma cortisol levels may remain within the normal range at 09.00 h, they are almost always raised at 24.00 h. However, raised corticosteroid levels may be associated with 'stress' so that the midnight blood should only be taken after the patient has been 'settled' in hospital for 48 h. Corticosteroid measurements on a single 09.00 h blood sample is of no value in the diagnosis of Cushing's syndrome.

Demonstration of a raised excretion of urinary corticosteroids or their metabolites may be of value, although in a series of 60 patients with Cushing's syndrome 23% showed levels of 17-oxogenic corticosteroids (17-OGS) within the normal range[7]. Measurement of urinary 'free' cortisol is of more value; this can be done either by a modification of the Mattingly fluorogenic corticosteroid method, competitive protein binding or radioimmunoassay[8]. This measurement has the major advantage that it reflects 'free' plasma cortisol levels and is elevated in the majority of patients with Cushing's syndrome[9].

2.   Dexamethasone-suppression test

The low-dose dexamethasone-suppression test is the test most used in the initial diagnosis of Cushing's syndrome. Although a variety of different test procedures have been designed, that first described by Liddle and colleagues[10] is still widely used. Thus after 48 h treatment with 0.5 mg of dexamethasone 6 hourly, the urinary excretion of urinary 17-hydroxycorticosteroids (17-OHCS) falls below 8.5 μmol/day (25 mg/day) and the plasma fluorogenic corticosteroids at 09.00 h should fall below 200 nmol/l (6 μg/100 ml). Although this protocol has stood the test of time, nonetheless it may occasionally be unreliable since some patients with pituitary-dependent Cushing's disease may demonstrate suppression and patients with depressive illness may show resistance to suppression[11]. In this latter group other clinical features suggestive of Cushing's syndrome may be present present such as obesity etc., which may cause diagnostic confusion.

3.   Insulin tolerance test

During the induction of hypoglycaemia by exogenous insulin administration in normal subjects, a rise in plasma corticosteroids occurs; thus levels in normals either rise in excess of 100% of basal value of > 580 nmol/l (21 μg/100 ml) whereas in patients with Cushing's syndrome no rise occurs. This test is invaluable in the establishment of the diagnosis of Cushing's syndrome, since responsiveness is preserved in the diagnostically confusing groups of patients with depression or in those who are 'stressed'.

4.   Plasma ACTH/LPH

Since plasma immunoreactive ACTH levels lie within the normal range at 09.00 h in about 50% of patients with pituitary-dependent Cushing's disease, its measurement is of little value in the initial diagnosis of Cushing's syndrome but is only of value in establishing the differential diagnosis. More recently, with the use of an N-terminal radioimmunoassay for lipotropin (LPH) we have shown that basal LPH levels are virtually always raised in patients with Cushing's disease and also in those with the ectopic ACTH syndrome[12]. It is possible therefore that the measurement of N-terminal LPH may help to distinguish patients with ACTH-dependent Cushing's syndrome from normals.

Differential Diagnosis of Cushing's Syndrome

Since the availability of plasma ACTH radioimmunoassays, the diagnosis of corticosteroid-secreting adrenal tumours as a cause of Cushing's syndrome has been simplified, since ACTH/LPH is suppressed due to negative feedback. Thus the main problem lies in distinguishing pituitary-dependent Cushing's disease from the ectopic ACTH syndrome. It is unusual for patients with Cushing's disease to exhibit any degree of hypokalaemia, whereas this is an almost invariable accompaniment of ectopic ACTH secretion. A number of dynamic test procedures are used, most of which are based on the observation that in most patients with pituitary-dependent Cushing's disease it is possible to demonstrate some maintenance of the normal corticosteroid feedback mechanisms, whereas patients with the ectopic ACTH syndrome do not.

Although some degree of negative feedback is present in Cushing's disease, the threshold is higher than normal and administration of larger doses of exogenous steroid are required to suppress plasma and urinary corticosteroids. Thus 98% of patients with Cushing's disease will show at least a 40% suppression of plasma and urinary corticosteroids after treatment with 8 mg of dexamethasone/day for 48 h. Only a small number (5%) of patients with ectopic ACTH secretion show an equivalent degree of suppression.

Patients with Cushing's disease are also capable of responding to a fall in plasma cortisol induced by the administration of oral metyrapone (2-methyl-1, 2-bis-(3-pyridyl)-1-propanone). Thus the falling level of circulating cortisol, induced by administration of this inhibitor of adrenal 11-β-hydroxylase to such patients leads, to a rise in plasma ACTH and an increased secretion of the 11-deoxy precursors of cortisol which can be measured in the urine as a rise in urinary 17-OHCS. In contrast, patients with Cushing's syndrome caused by either an adrenal tumour or the ectopic ACTH syndrome do not show such a rise. Since the adrenal glands in Cushing's disease are hyperplastic the increase in urinary 17-OHCS is exaggerated. The standard test consists of the administration of oral metyrapone (750 mg 4 hourly) and measurement of plasma cortisol at zero, 1, 2, 3, 4 and 24 h and the measurement of 17-OHCS for 2 days before, the day of and the day after metyrapone treatment. Urinary 17-OHCS usually rise to greater than twice basal levels, either on the day of or the day after metyrapone. Plasma cortisol in patients on metyrapone must always be measured by a fluorimetric technique since most competitive-binding assays will measure 11-deoxycortisol, levels of which become greatly elevated in the presence of a 11-β-hydroxylase block.

Patients with Cushing's disease usually have lower cortisol/ACTH/LPH levels than patients with the ectopic ACTH syndrome. However the differential diagnosis is difficult and simultaneous ACTH/LPH measurements may be helpful. Thus, a retrospective comparison of simultaneously measured ACTH/LPH levels in patients with Cushing's disease and the ectopic ACTH syndrome has shown that the ratio of ACTH/LPH is higher in patients with Cushing's disease[13].

The Aetiology of Cushing's Disease

Only a small number (< 10%) of patients with pituitary-dependent Cushing's disease have an abnormality demonstrable on plain X-ray of the pituitary fossa and large tumours are exceedingly rare. Thus a review of 22 patients with Cushing's disease presenting at a hospital between 1968 and 1978 revealed only two with suprasella extension of the tumour and resultant visual-field defect. Similarly, a recent radiological review of the skull X-ray of 86 patients with Cushing's disease showed normal pituitary fossa appearances in 66[14], although this low incidence does not correlate with the high incidence of pituitary microadenomas found either at pituitary surgery or during postmortem examination.

It is of especial interest that Cushing (1932) found pituitary adenomas in seven of nine patients with Cushing's disease who came to autopsy. Interestingly, one of his patients described in the classic review was subsequently shown to have a basophil adenoma at autopsy. More recently, a review of microsurgery under-taken in 20 consecutive patients with Cushing's disease demonstrated pituitary adenomas in 18 which were subsequently confirmed in 15. All the plain pituitary skull X-rays were considered normal[14].

There has been much debate over the years as to whether Cushing's disease is a primary hypothalamic or pituitary disorder. It was usually regarded to be a disorder resulting from increased secretion of hypothalamic corticotropin-releasing factor (corticoliberin, CRF) activity[15]. Since some of the mechanisms controlling normal ACTH secretion are 'normal' such as ACTH secretion in response to lowering of plasma cortisol and suppression after high-dose dexa-methasone, it was held that this suggested that pituitary function was not autonomous and that the disorder was primarily hypothalamic. Although such theories remain purely speculative, Liddle has listed the criteria necessary to test this hypothesis[16]. Thus in order to prove that the disorder is hypothalamic in origin, it is necessary to show that (i) the disorder is cured by disruption of hypothalamic–pituitary connections, (ii) demonstration of whether removal of pituitary adenoma cures Cushing's disease without impairment of other anterior pituitary function, (iii) demonstration of high CRF levels in Cushing's disease and (iv) clear evidence that the pharmacological inhibitors of CRF secretion will ameliorate or cure the disorder. Much evidence exists to suggest that in Cushing's disease the pituitary corticotrophs act independently of the hypothalamus. Thus in the patient originally described by Liddle[16], stalk section had no effect on her disease, although it rendered the patient deficient in thyrotropin (TSH) and gonadotropin secretion. Similar data have been obtained by Hardy and colleagues[17] who have treated Cushing's disease by selective removal of pituitary microadenomata, which while leaving the remainder of anterior pituitary function intact, resulted in 'cure' of Cushing's disease. Similarly, in a series of 20 patients undergoing transphenoidal hypophysectomy, Tyrrell and colleagues[18] reported the resolution of hypercortisolaemia in 17 of 18 patients in whom adenomectomy was feasible, although of 12 patients followed by Carmalt for 11 years[19] after transphenoidal hypophysectomy, none regained full pituitary function. It is also clear that it is *not* possible to show that pituitary microadenomas do not result from prolonged hypothalamic hyperstimulation and that they will not recur after adenomectomy.

Since the nature of CRF remains unknown and since its pharmacological control is ill-understood, the role of hypothalamic CRF in the aetiology of Cushing's disease remains obscure. A large amount of confusing data exists impli-cating the involvement of both serotonin (5-HT)[20], L-DOPA and the catechola-mines[21] in its aetiology. The dopamine agonist bromocriptine has been used to control ACTH secretion in Cushing's disease and Nelson's syndrome[22], although the numbers of responsive patients is small. However, Krieger and her colleagues[23] report clinical responsiveness in approximately one-third of patients treated with the 5-HT antagonist cyproheptadine, although in the remainder increasing obesity, drowsiness and psychopathy may be exacerbated. It seems likely that several diseases of different aetiologies lie under the diagnostic umbrella of Cushing's disease, although they are all ultimately mediated by pituitary ACTH secretion.

The Treatment of Cushing's Disease

1. *Pituitary surgery and pituitary irradiation*

When a large pituitary tumour with a suprasella extension and a visual-field defect is present, transfrontal craniotomy should be performed to decompress the tumour before external irradiation. Although the latter treatment alone is effective therapy in children with Cushing's disease[24], the result of radiotherapy alone in adults is disappointing[15,25]. Thus pituitary irradiation alone will cure only 10–20% of adults, with many years elapsing between the treatment and clinical and biochemical remission. During this period adjuvant therapy will be required such as 'medical' or surgical adrenalectomy. Others recommend the use of pituitary implantation with radioactive gold or yttrium[26].

More recently, as discussed earlier, microsurgery directed at pituitary adenoma removal has become more fashionable and although a high cure rate is reported, the expertise is not sufficiently widespread nor has the follow-up been of sufficient length for full evaluation to be undertaken.

2. *Medical adrenalectomy*

The use of the drug metyrapone, which blocks 11-β-hydroxylase in the adrenal cortex, can be used both in the preparation of any patient with Cushing's syndrome before surgery or investigation, or in the long-term management of patients with Cushing's disease in conjunction with external pituitary irradiation[27]. Although it has been stated that it would not be possible to use this drug in Cushing's disease since plasma ACTH would rise and override the enzyme blockade[28] this has not been our experience[27]. Thus such breakthrough does *not* occur and plasma fluorogenic corticosteroid levels can be maintained between 300 and 400 nmol/l with doses of metyrapone of between 500 mg to 6 g/day. Repeated assessment of the plasma cortisol levels is required throughout the day since the accumulative effect of the drug means that the sensitivity varies requiring fine adjustment of the metyrapone dose.

Clinical improvement after the institution of metyrapone treatment is rapid; skin-flaking and improvement in myopathy occurring as rapidly as that seen after bilateral adrenalectomy.

Although metyrapone is not the only drug capable of inducing medical adrenalectomy, other drugs such as aminoglutethimide[29,30] and o,p^1-DDD (1,1-dichlora-2-(o-chloro)phenyl)-2-2(p-chlorophenyl)ethane) may be associated with a high incidence of often unacceptable side-effects.

3. *Surgical adrenalectomy*

Although this remains an effective treatment for Cushing's disease, this operation carries a high morbidity and mortality in an unprepared patient. Thus in a review of 29 consecutive patients treated by bilateral adrenalectomy published by Scott and colleagues[31] a high incidence of complications was recorded including wound infections, postoperative haemorrhage and pulmonary embolus in over one-third of the patients. Such problems are hardly surprising since most patients go to surgery with untreated hypertension, diabetes mellitus, bleeding diatheses and a predilection for poor wound healing. Preoperative preparation with metyrapone, rendering the patient eucorticoid before surgery, will reduce such complications to a minimum.

Unilateral or subtotal adrenalectomy is an ill-conceived form of treatment in Cushing's disease since continued ACTH drive merely results in hypertrophy of remaining adrenal tissue until the original hypercortisolaemia is achieved.

NELSON'S SYNDROME

In a proportion of patients with Cushing's disease treated by bilateral adrenalectomy alone, plasma ACTH levels rise in association with a pituitary tumour and skin pigmentation, a condition known as Nelson's syndrome[32]. Occasionally this may be associated with the presence of an aggressive locally invasive tumour which may prove difficult to control. This can usually be prevented by instituting external pituitary irradiation at the time of or soon after bilateral adrenalectomy[33].

REFERENCES

1. Rees, L. H. *et al.* (1977). *Ann. N. Y. Acad. Sci.* **297**, 603.
2. Djaldetti, M. *et al.* (1977). *Am. J. Med. Sci.* **273**, 273.
3. Mason, A. S. (1971). *Proc. Roy. Soc. Med.* **64**, 749.
4. Jeffcoate, W. J. *et al.* (1979). *Brit. Med. J. (in press).*
5. Doe, R. P. *et al.* (1960). *J. Clin. Endocrinol. Metab.* **20**, 253.
6. Ekman, H. *et al.* (1961). *J. Clin. Endocrinol. Metab.* **21**, 684.
7. Cope, C. L. and Pearson, J. (1963). *J. Clin. Path.* **18**, 82.
8. Beardwell, C. G. *et al.* (1968). *J. Endocrinol.* **42**, 79.
9. Mattingly, D. *et al.* (1964). *Lancet* **2**, 1046.
10. Liddle, G. W. (1960). *J. Clin. Endocrinol. Metab.* **20**, 1539.
11. Butler, P. W. P. and Besser, G. M. (1968). *Lancet* **1**, 1234.
12. Jeffcoate, W. J. *et al.* (1979). *J. Endocrinol.* **80**, 6P.
13. Gilkes, J. J. H. (1977). *Brit. Med. J.* **1**, 996.
14. MacErlean, D. P. and Doyle, T. H. (1976). *Br. J. Radiol.* **49**, 820.
15. Daughaday, W. M. (1978). *New Eng. J. Med.* **298**, 793.
16. Liddle, G. W. (1977). *Ann. N. Y. Acad. Sci.* **297**, 594.
17. Hardy, J. (1971). *J. Neurosurg.* **34**, 582.
18. Tyrrell, J. B. *et al.* (1978). *New Eng. J. Med.* **298**, 753.
19. Carmalt, M. H. B. *et al.* (1977). *Quart. J. Med.* **46**, 119.
20. Krieger, D. T. (1977). *Ann. N. Y. Acad. Sci.* **297**, 527.
21. Ganong, W. F. (1977). *Ann. N. Y. Acad. Sci.* **297**, 509.
22. Besser, G. M. *et al.* (1976). V Int. Congr. Endocrinol. Abstract No. 4941. Hamburg.

23. Krieger, D. T. *et al.* (1975). *New Eng. J. Med.* **293**, 893.
24. Jennings, A. S. *et al.* (1977). *New Eng. J. Med.* **297**, 957.
25. Orth, D. N. (1972). *In* "Cushing's Syndrome" (Binder, C. and Hall, P. E. eds.), pp. 148–160, Heinemann, London.
26. Burke, C. W. *et al.* (1973). *Quart. J. Med.* **42**, 693.
27. Jeffcoate, W. J. *et al.* (1977). *Brit. Med. J.* **2**, 215.
28. Orth, D. N. (1978). *Ann. Int. Med.* **89**, 128.
29. Fishman, L. M. *et al.* (1967). *J. Clin. Endocrinol. Metab.* **27**, 481.
30. Zachmann, M. *et al.* (1977). *Clin. Endocrinol.* **7**, 63.
31. Scott, H. W. *et al.* (1977). *Ann. Surg.* **185**, 524.
32. Nelson, D. H. *et al.* (1958). *New Eng. J. Med.* **259**, 161.
33. Orth, D. N. and Liddle, G. W. (1971). *New Eng. J. Med.* **285**, 243.
34. Smals, A. G. *et al.* (1976). *Brit. Med. J.* **2**, 1298.
35. Rees, L. H. *et al.* (1977). *Lancet* **1**, 726.

26

ADRENOCORTICAL FUNCTIONS IN PSYCHIATRIC DISORDERS

Sarada Subrahmanyam, R. Chandramouli, S. Sivakumar, and
V. S. Amanullah Baig

*Department of Physiology, P. G. Institute of Basic Medical Sciences,
University of Madras, Madras 600042, India*

INTRODUCTION

The secretion of cortisol from the adrenal cortex is under the control of corticotropin (ACTH) which in turn is regulated by the secretion of corticotropin-releasing factor (CRF; corticoliberin). The CRF cells are located within the hypothalamus which comes under the regulatory influences of the limbic system and the neocortex. There is therefore a hierarchy of neural influences, which may affect the secretion of cortisol. The main stimuli to CRF and ACTH secretion are stress and those environmental cues that entrain the intrinsic circadian rhythm. In man, the normal circadian rhythm in plasma cortisol shows a peak concentration in the early morning and a nadir in the evening[1].

Mason[1] has pointed out that psychological influences are the most potent neural stimuli that affect the pituitary–adrenocortical system. Psychological stresses represent a diverse group of stimuli producing emotional disequilibrium. Such stimuli include oral examination, appearing for an interview, quarrels, anxiety, anger etc.

The investigation of the hypothalamo–pituitary–adrenocortical activity in psychoses has been undertaken by several laboratories[2,3,4]. The data obtained have been interpreted in two basically different ways. Either they have been taken to indicate the level of emotional stress or turmoil or to reflect an abnormality of the hypothalamic regulatory system due to changes in neurotransmitter function which may be an integral part of the disease process.

265

Table I. Daily urinary steroid excretion (mg/24 h). Values are means ± S.D. ID, intense depression; DD, decreased depression.

Steroids	Groups					
	Manic depressive		Neurotic depressive		Neurotic and Manic depressive	
	ID	DD	ID	DD	ID	DD
17 KGS	40.6 ± 10.2	22.3 ± 1.4	30.2 ± 6.8	19.0 ± 5.3	39.0 ± 9.8	24.8 ± 8.4
Range	30.8 – 60.5	20.6 – 25.2	18.6 – 50.5	12.4 – 28.6	20.6 – 60.8	10.6 – 26.4
17 KS	15.6 ± 4.9	8.6 ± 2.8	8.4 ± 2.2	7.8 ± 2.2	10.2 ± 2.4	8.6 ± 2.4
Range	8.6 – 20.2	8.0 – 10.4	3.8 – 16.0	4.0 – 10.6	4.2 – 20.2	4.2 –11.2
17 OHCS	11.6 ± 3.6	8.2 ± 2.4	4.9 ± 2.1	3.3 ± 0.8	8.0 ± 2.8	4.6 ± 1.6
Range	4.8 – 19.8	5.2 – 10.6	2.0 – 7.2	1.6 – 6.0	2.6 – 16.2	2.0 – 10.8

In the current work we have investigated adrenocortical activity in schizophrenia and depressive illness. The cases were selected from the Government Hospital and the Institute of Neurology of the State of Madras. Patients suffering from depression were treated with imipramine, tranquilizers and ECT. Selected patients suffering from mania were given tranquilizers and lithium. In the case of schizophrenia, the patients were treated with antipsychotic drugs.

ADRENOCORTICAL FUNCTION IN DEPRESSION AND SCHIZOPHRENIA

Plasma cortisol was estimated by the method of Mattingly[5], urinary 17-OHCS (17-hydroxycorticosteroids) and 17-KS (17-oxosteroids) by the method of Glenn and Nelson[6], 17-KGS (17-oxogenic corticosteroids) by the method of Appleby[7] and CSF (cerebrospinal fluid) cortisol by a modification of the method of Murphy *et al.*[8]. The degree of depression was measured by the Hamilton rating scale.

Table I shows urinary excretion of 17-OHCS, 17-KGS and 17-KS in three types of depressed patients, namely manic depressives, neurotic depressives and a combination of both. The data were collected during both intense depression and during recovery. The values were highest in manic depressives at the height of the illness and declined in all groups on clinical improvement.

Plasma cortisol was next measured, at the same time of day, in eleven patients suffering from endogenous depression and eight patients suffering from reactive depression before and after treatment (Fig. 1).

Plasma cortisol concentration was elevated in patients suffering from both forms of the illness but declined to normal values only in the endogenous

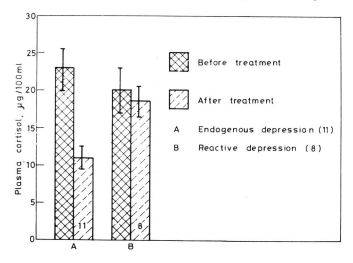

Fig. 1. Plasma cortisol concentration measured before and after treatment in eleven patients suffering from endogenous depression (A) and eight patients with reactive depression (B).

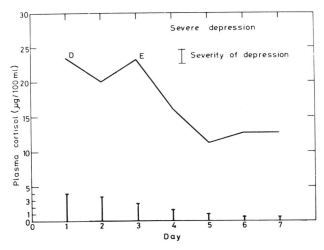

Fig. 2. The correlation between the severity of depression and plasma cortisol concentration in a single patient over a period of 1 week. This patient was treated with drugs and E.C.T.

depressives after treatment. Surprisingly no such decline was seen in the plasma cortisol concentration of patients suffering from reactive depression. This appears to be in conflict with the data presented in Table I. However, plasma values measure activity in the axis at only one point in time, whereas the urinary values reflect activity over the 24 h period. It is likely therefore that the urinary values are more reliable and that adrenocortical activity returns to normal values in both forms of depression with clinical improvement. The correlation between clinical

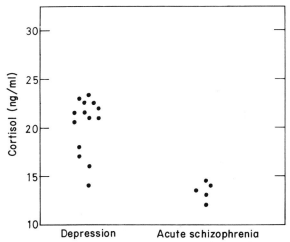

Fig. 3. Cortisol levels in cerebrospinal fluid of patients suffering from acute depression and acute schizophrenia.

status and plasma cortisol in a single case of endogenous depression is shown in
Fig. 2. This patient was successfully treated by drugs and ECT and the plasma
cortisol levels returned to normal within 1 week. Concurrently there was a considerable improvement in his mood.

The cortisol concentration in the CSF was measured at the same time of day
in 14 patients suffering from acute depressive illness and five suffering from acute
schizophrenia (Fig. 3). CSF cortisol levels were considerably higher in the depressed than in the schizophrenic patients — the levels in the latter group being close
to those we find in normal individuals.

Various terms have been used to describe the different stages of schizophrenia.
The acute phase (psychotic turmoil) may pass through the stage of organic
psychosis into anaclitic depression. Alternatively the psychotic turmoil may pass
to stage A (parasitic phase) and then to stage B (compliance phase) leading
eventually to recovery[2]. Urinary 17-OHCS excretion in the different recognized
stages is shown in Table II. In schizophrenia, during the acute psychotic turmoil,
the urinary 17-OHCS were roughly 250% higher than after recovery. The initial
values are all significantly ($p < 0.05$) higher than the subsequent values.

Table II.   17-OHCS excretion (mg/day)

	Psychotic turmoil	Organic psychosis		Depression
1.	16.9	6.2		9.4
2.	18.6	4.4		7.6
	Turmoil	Stage A	Stage B	Recovery
1.	15.2	12.8	10.4	6.5
2.	12.6	9.6	6.6	5.5
3.	14.4	10.6	8.4	4.8
4.	12.2	9.4	6.6	4.6

Interpretation of the changes in plasma cortisol concentrations in psychosis

The results of the present investigation in acute schizophrenics bear out the
speculation of Mann and Semrad[9] and confirm the findings of the earlier study
by Sachar *et al.*[2]. The state of acute psychotic turmoil in schizophrenics is
associated with hypersecretion of the adrenal cortex. Marked fall to normal in the
phase of organized psychosis indicates the return of endocrine functions to normal.
There is an increase in the corticosteroid excretion in the anaclitic depression phase
compared with the phase of organized psychosis.

In the alternative pathway to recovery from psychotic turmoil, gradual
diminution of corticosteroid excretion occurred during the "parasitic" and
"compliance" phase and reached normal values in the recovery stage. Thus
psychological factors probably explain the pattern of adrenocortical secretion in
schizophrenia.

Gibbons (1964) showed that patients suffering from depressive illness commonly had elevated plasma 11-OHCS and that this is associated with a raised cortisol secretion rate. In severely depressed patients, several investigators have compared plasma cortisol levels with normal controls. The first investigation was conducted in 1956 by Board *et al.*[11].

The increased adrenocortical activity in endogenous and manic depressives is presumably due to raised ACTH secretion which in turn is the result of neural activation of ACTH-releasing mechanism of the hypothalamus. Though depressive patients appear to be dull and moody, intense mental activity is going on in the brain. Thus a plausible explanation of increased adrenocortical activity in depression may be the result of emotional arousal. Studies on normal subjects undergoing prolonged psychological stress suggest that persistently increased adrenocortical activity occur only in a few, since most of them adjust to the situation[2]. In severe depressive illness, adjustment does not occur during the illness suggesting that there may be some primary hypothalamic dysfunction. It is most unlikely that anxiety, often a component of depression, can fully account for the activation of the adrenocortical axis since the levels are raised during sleep and the patients mood usually improves as the day progresses. Plasma cortisol, however, remains elevated. Recently Sachar[4] reported that there is a subgroup of melancholics, who respond very favourably to antidepressants, who have significant neuroendocrine dysfunction. The secretory pattern of cortisol in these patients (see Fig. 4) shows hypersecretion in the afternoon, evening and

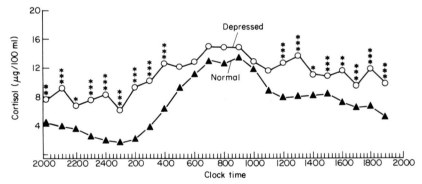

Fig. 4. Mean hourly cortisol concentration in the plasma of seven depressed and 54 normal individuals. * $p < 0.05$, ** $p < 0.01$, *** $p < 0.001$. Reproduced by permission from Sachar[4].

early morning hours. The differences, compared with controls, were greatest in the evening and early morning when cortisol secretion is normally at its nadir. In these patients cortisol had a normal half-life and so the cortisol levels probably reflect accurately the pattern in ACTH secretion. Sachar[4] had stated that such a secretory pattern is difficult to explain on the basis of a stress response (induced by the disease) since the pattern is seen during sleep, as well as during the waking hours. In addition, drugs that reduce the level of anxiety have no effect on cortisol secretion in these patients.

Can the changes seen in cortisol secretion be explained in terms of the presumed changes in neurotransmission, which may be part and parcel of endogenous depression? The answer is probably "yes". The drugs that are useful in treating endogenous depression, namely the monoamine uptake blockers and the mono-amino-oxidase inhibitors (MAO-inhibitors), will increase the amount of noradrenaline available at the postsynaptic site. There is good evidence to show that noradrenaline exerts an inhibitory effect on CRF secretion[12,13]. If there is a decrease in noradrenergic function in depressive illness, then a concomitant increase in hypothalamic–pituitary–adrenocortical function would be expected. In depression therefore the best assessment that can be made is that the increase in cortisol secretion is due to two factors — anxiety and impaired central neurotransmission, particularly noradrenergic function.

REFERENCES

1. Mason, J. (1968). *J. Psychosom. Med.* **30**, 563.
2. Sachar, E. *et al.* (1963). *J. Psychosom. Med.* **25**, 510.
3. Seligman, M. E. P. (1975). *In* "Helplessness in Depression, Development and Death", W. H. Freeman and Company, San Francisco.
4. Sachar, E. (1977). *Ann. N.Y. Acad. Sci.* **297**, 621.
5. Mattingly, D. (1962). *J. Clin. Path.* **15**, 374.
6. Glenn, E. M. and Nelson, D. H. (1953). *J. Clin. Endocrinol.* **13**, 911.
7. Appleby, J. I. *et al.* (1955). *Biochem. J.* **60**, 453.
8. Murphy, B. *et al.* (1963). *J. Clin. Endocrinol.* **23**, 293.
9. Mann, J. and Semrad, E. (1969). *In* "Conversion as process and conversion as symptoms in psychosis", International University Press, New York.
10. Gibbons, J. L. (1964). *Arch. Gen. Psychiat.* **10**, 572.
11. Board, F. *et al.* (1956). *J. Psychosom. Med.* **18**, 324.
12. Van Loon, G. R. (1973). *In* "Frontiers in Neuroendocrinology" (Ganong W.F. and Martini, L. eds.), p. 209, Oxford University Press.
13. Jones, M. T. *et al.* (1976). *In* "Frontiers in Neuroendocrinology" (Martini, L. and Ganong, W. F. eds.), p. 195, Raven Press, New York.

27

YOGA IN RELATION TO THE BRAIN-PITUITARY ADRENOCORTICAL AXIS

K. N. Udupa and R. H. Singh

Institute of Medical Sciences, Banaras Hindu University, Varanasi, India.

INTRODUCTION

In 1893 Swami Vivekananda, a noted exponent of yoga, suggested that yoga should be studied scientifically and not relegated to the realm of mysticism[1]. Few scientific investigations were conducted, however, until 1961 when Anand and Chinna[2] and Wenger et al.[3] reported on their studies on well-known practitioners of yoga. These yogis claimed to be able to stop both pulse and heart beat, but clinical observations showed that they were using the valsalva manoeuvre. The resulting increase in thoracic pressure reduced cardiac output (by reducing venous return) and this made the pulse barely perceptible. The skeletal muscular sounds masked the heart sounds but ECG recordings showed the heart had not stopped. One practitioner of yoga who only claimed he could slow his heart rate did succeed in doing so; he used a different muscular technique. His success in controlling the heart rate was via an increase in vagal tone consequent on his striated muscular efforts.

Subsequently Wallace and Benson[4] studied the effects of meditation and showed that it caused a fall in O_2 consumption, plasma lactate concentration and a decrease in cardiac output and blood pressure. They concluded that meditation was "a wakeful hypo-metabolic state". This relaxed state is, of course, the opposite of the "fight or flight" response of stress associated with its increased arousal and raised blood pressure and oxygen consumption. It seems natural to test whether techniques such as meditation and other yoga practices might be used to ameliorate the stresses of everyday life.

273

The profound muscular and mental relaxation produced by meditation and yoga exercises have been used to reduce blood pressure in hypertensive patients. Thus Datey et al.[5] found that "shavasan" exercises reduced the blood pressure in hypertensive patients. He postulated that this exercise influences the hypothalamus through the continuous feedback from slow rhythmic proprioceptive and enteroceptive impulses which re-set the blood pressure controller at a lower level. When meditation has been re-enforced with bio-feedback techniques a fall in blood pressure has also been achieved. In patients where continued drug treatment was necessary, a significant reduction in the dose of antihypertensive drugs was achieved with this combined treatment[6,7].

In the past decade we have conducted studies in healthy volunteers on the effect of various yoga practices[8-11]. We have investigated the effect of these practices on their sense of well being and some physiological parameters including adrenomedullary and adrenocortical function. In psychological studies, the memory quotient, performance quotient, level of neuroticism, mental fatigue and health complaint scores were assessed by standard testing methods as described previously[9]. Plasma cortisol concentration was measured by Mattingley's fluorimetric assay[12], the urinary 17-hydroxycorticosteroids (17-OHCS) as described by Appleby et al.[13], 17-keto(oxo) steroids (17-KS) were estimated as described by King and Wooton[14]. The plasma catecholamines, cholinesterase and erythrocyte acetylcholine concentrations were also measured as reported previously[8].

THE EFFECT OF YOGA POSTURES

Ten persons were asked to perform a set of 12 standard yoga postures for 1 h a day for a period of 6 months. They were assessed before, during and at the end of the course. The results are shown in Table I. The studies with psychological parameters clearly indicate that after 6 months practice of 12 yogic postures there was a statistically significant improvement in the performance, memory quotients and neuroticism levels. There was also a decrease in mental fatigue and also in the C.M.I. complaint score. In the same way, there was a statistically significant

Table I. Psychological changes induced by a 6 months practice of twelve postures of yoga. Values are mean ± S.D.

Observations	Initial	After 3rd month	After 6th month
1. Performance quotient	93.15 ± 12.50	102.00 ± 16.40	108.20 ± 14.70 $p < 0.02$
2. Memory quotient	89.75 ± 9.15	97.30 ± 13.20	100.80 ± 9.60 $p < 0.02$
3. Neuroticism	19.50 ± 9.95	11.40 ± 10.70	9.82 ± 8.40 $p < 0.05$
4. Mental fatigue index	1.59	0.40	1.20
5. Health index in C.M.I. complaint scores	192.00	114.00	94.00

Table II. Physiological changes induced by 6 months practice of twelve postures of yoga.

S.No.	Observations	Initial	After 3rd month	After 6th month
1	1. Urinary catechol-amines (mg of VMA/ 24 h)	3.14 ± 2.12	3.33 ± 2.38	4.37 ± 1.63 N.S.
2	2. Urinary 17-OHCS (mg/24 h)	3.65 ± 2.02	5.80 ± 3.01	10.30 ± 4.10 $p < 0.001$
3	3. Urinary 17-KS (mg/24 h)	11.46 ± 8.33	5.87 ± 4.04	7.30 ± 2.30 N.S.
4	4. Acetylcholine (μg/100 ml)	181.70 ± 149.30 —	101.10 ± 34.30 $p < 0.1$	58.70 ± 18.05 $p < 0.01$
5	5. Cholinesterase (pH units/h)	1.170 ± 0.309 —	0.894 ± 0.313 $p < 0.05$	0.950 ± 0.087 $p < 0.05$

reduction in the erythrocyte acetylcholine and cholinesterase content of the blood (Table II). However, on the examination of adrenocortical function, it was observed that there was a significant increase in the urinary excretion of 17-OHCS indicating an increase in the total activity of the adrenal cortex. Medullary activity was not significantly changed.

THE EFFECT OF BREATH CONTROL

Ten other volunteers were submitted to breath control practices for a similar 6 month period and were studied in the same way. The results of 6 months practice of breath control also showed a similar activation in the function of adrenal cortex. Thus there was a significant rise of plasma cortisol, urinary 17-OHCS and urinary 17-KS (Table III). However, urinary VMA (vanillylmandelic acid) rose indicating an overall increase in the function of the adrenal medulla, but the values did not reach statistical significance.

Table III. Physiological changes induced by 6 months practice of breath control. Values are mean ± S.D.

S. No.	Observations	Initial	After 3rd month	After 6th month
1	Plasma cortisol (μg/100 ml)	18.00 ± 7.07	24.36 ± 10.00	25.30 ± 1.39 $p < 0.001$
2	Urinary 17-OHCS (mg/24 h)	5.76 ± 1.04	7.26 ± 0.70	7.90 ± 0.70 $p < 0.001$
3	Urinary 17-KS (mg/24 h)	4.85 ± 1.11	5.54 ± 1.08	6.37 ± 1.47 $p < 0.02$
4	Urinary VMA (mg/24 h)	3.66 ± 1.22	3.66 ± 1.93	4.40 ± 1.40 N.S.

THE EFFECT OF MEDITATION

The third group of 10 volunteers underwent an intensive course of meditation (vipasana) for 10 days. The results of 10 days intensive meditation showed a statistically significant increase in the acetylcholine and cholinesterase with a significant decrease in the plasma catecholamine level (Table IV). The studies on adrenocortical function after meditation showed no significant change and neither was there a significant change in the VMA excretion.

Table IV. Physiological changes induced by a 10-day course of meditation. Values are mean ± S.E.M.

S.No.	Observations	Before the course	After the course	Comparison
1	Plasma cortisol (μg/100 ml)	9.12 ± 0.85	8.50 ± 1.22	$p < 0.50$
2	Urinary 17-OHCS (mg/g creatinine)	7.27 ± 0.99	5.88 ± 1.24	$p < 0.30$
3	Urinary 17-KS (mg/g creatinine)	3.42 ± 0.28	4.93 ± 0.65	$p < 0.10$
4	Urinary VMA (mg/g creatinine)	1.62 ± 0.27	2.14 ± 0.29	$p < 0.10$
5	Plasma catechol-amine (μg/ml)	21.90 ± 0.76	18.36 ± 1.06	$p < 0.05$
6	Erythrocyte ACh (μg/ml)	0.301 ± 0.100	0.349 ± 0.120	$p < 0.01$
7	Erythrocyte ChE L(P.U./ml)	112.25 ± 3.22	161.19 ± 2.55	$p < 0.05$

Table V. Physiological changes induced by combined practice of yoga postures, breath control and meditation. Values are mean with number of observations in parentheses.

S.No.	Observations	Before the course	After the course	Comparison
1	Plasma cortisol (μg/100 g)	19.04 (5)	32.00 (5)	$p < 0.05$
2	Urinary 17-OHCS (mg/g creatinine)	6.72 (5)	7.30 (5)	$p < 0.05$
3	Urinary 17-KS (mg/g creatinine)	3.86 (5)	8.03 (5)	$p < 0.05$
4	Urinary VMA (mg/g creatinine)	2.480 (5)	1.614	$p < 0.05$
5	Plasma catechol-amines (μg/100 g)	42.60 (5)	32.30 (5)	$p < 0.001$
6	Erythrocyte ACh (μg/ml)	1.006 (5)	0.462 (5)	$p < 0.001$
7	Erythrocyte ChE (P.U./ml)	101.0	72.00	$p < 0.001$

COMBINED YOGA PRACTICES

When all three methods of yogic practices were combined in a group of five volunteers there was a decrease in the erythrocyte acetylcholine and plasma cholinesterase, as well as in the level of plasma catecholamines (Table V). However, there was activation of adrenocortical function as shown by an increase in the level of plasma cortisol, urinary 17-OHCS and 17-KS excretion. As would be expected from the catecholamine levels the urinary VMA was decreased at the end of 3 months.

CONCLUSIONS

Although the various yogic practices are known to produce beneficial results, very few scientific studies had so far been conducted to test their utility for the average man. Therefore in this study, the utility of all the three types of yogic practices separately and jointly was investigated. As already observed the practice of 12 yogic postures produced a tranquilizing effect. The practice of breath control also showed almost similar results. Intensive practice of meditation showed a significant decrease in the activity of the adrenal medulla. When all the three methods of yogic practices were combined, one could clearly observe a tranquilizing effect of yoga as shown by a decrease in the catecholamine levels in the blood. Surprisingly, this was associated with simultaneous increase in the adrenocortical function.

An increase in adrenocortical activity usually represents a response to a stressful situation. Yet the data from both the psychological tests and adrenomedullary function demonstrate that yoga is not stressful; indeed it has a tranquilizing effect. The assumption that an increase in adrenocortical activity represents a stress response is obviously not always a valid conclusion.

From these studies one can say that to derive full benefit from yoga all the three yoga methods should be practiced together. This was also suggested by the Sage Patanjali about 2500 years ago. However, they will have to be individualized and adapted to meet the health needs of each person for the maintenance of good health in the treatment of stress disorders.

REFERENCES

1. Vivekananda, Swami (1970). Raja Yoga, Calcutta, Advaita Ashram.
2. Anand, B. K. and Chinna, B. S. (1961). *Ind. Jour. Med. Research* **49**, 82.
3. Wenger, M. A. *et al.* (1961). *Circulation* **24**, 1319.
4. Wallace, R. K. and Benson, H. (1972). *Scientific American* **226**, 84.
5. Datey, K. K. *et al.* (1969). *Angiology* **20**, 325.
6. Patel, C. H. (1973). *Lancet* **2**, 1053.
7. Patel, C. H. (1975). *Lancet* **1**, 62.
8. Udupa, K. N. and Singh, R. H. (1972). *J.A.M.A.* **220**, 1365.
9. Udupa, K. N. *et al.* (1973). *Ind. J. Med. Res.* **61**, 237.
10. Udupa, K. N. (1976). A manual of Science and Philosophy of Yoga, Varanasi, *Journal of Research in Indian Medicine.*

11.   Udupa, K. N. (1978). Disorders of Stress and their management by Yoga, Varanasi, B.H.U. Press.
12.   Mattingly, D. J. (1964). *Clin. Path.* **15**, 374.
13.   Appleby, *et al.* (1965). *Biochem. J.* **60**, 460.
14.   King, E. A. and Wooton, I. P. D. (1964). *In* "Medical Biochemistry", 4th Edition. J. A. Churchill Ltd., London.

AN OVERALL VIEW OF THE HYPOTHALAMO-
PITUITARY–ADRENOCORTICAL AXIS

L. Martini and M. T. Jones

Istituto di Endocrinologia, Universita di Milano and
*Sherrington School of Physiology, St. Thomas's Hospital Medical School,
London, U.K.*

The interrelationships between the brain, the anterior pituitary and the adrenal cortex have been the subject of a large number of investigations in past decades. Probably, this is the area of neuroendocrinology that has been most extensively explored. But even so, there are still many gaps in our knowledge of this complicated system.

The Organizing Committee of the 5th International Congress on Hormonal Steroids was very pleased to be able to list the Varanasi Meeting as a Satellite Symposium of the Steroid Congress in New Delhi. The Committee felt that the time was ripe for reviewing this field, and for analyzing the most provocative data collected in the last few years.

The first chapter deals with the corticotropin (ACTH)- and lipotropin (LPH)-related peptides found in the anterior and intermediate lobes of the pituitary gland. Lowry *et al.* provide evidence in favour of ACTH and LPH existing in a precursor form in the same granules of "corticotroph" cells. It is clear that a family of peptides are found in vertebrate pituitary glands which are basically divisible into two groups, those related to ACTH and those related to LPH. α-MSH (melanotropin) and CLIP (corticotropin-like intermediate-lobe peptide) eminate from ACTH, whereas β-MSH, α-, β- and γ-endorphins and N-terminal fragments are all post-translational fragments of LPH. The common cell (the "corticotroph") manufactures both ACTH and LPH but its anatomical location (whether in the anterior or intermediate lobe) dictates the type of peptide secreted. ACTH and LPH are released into the circulation from the anterior lobe, with the possible breakdown of the LPH to give β-endorphin. All the small peptides including the endorphins are released from the pars intermedia.

279

The pattern of ACTH- and LPH-related peptides is by no means consistent across species. In primates the smaller pars intermedia is only present at the foetal stage but decreases or disappears after birth. Lowry and his co-workers suggest that many peptides may act centrally (as suggested by Dr. Bohus) rather than peripherally but they also make the intriguing suggestion that these peptides may play a lesser role in learning and behaviour in primates with their highly developed neocortex.

Bohus shows the bewildering (and often contradictory) effects of the various neuropeptides. He demonstrates that the behavioural effects of the endorphins involve both opiate and non-opiate receptors. There is an interaction between ACTH fragments and opiate receptors since ACTH fragments can antagonize morphine-induced analgesia. ACTH- and LPH-related peptides are present in the brain and persist after hypophysectomy. However, hypophysectomized animals show behavioural deficits that can only be corrected by replacement therapy with ACTH and the endorphins. So the pituitary is an important source of these peptides in modulating behaviour. The role of ACTH and the endorphins (and enkephalins) within the central nervous system as neurotransmitters or modulators of neurotransmitters has yet to be determined.

The secretion of ACTH and α-MSH from the intermediate lobe is under inhibitory control of dopaminergic secretomotor innervation, but CLIP is only influenced by humoral factors of hypothalamic origin. This suggests that if CLIP and α-MSH are derived from the same prohormone (ACTH) the mechanisms of release are different. It will be interesting to determine how this differential release is brought about at the cellular level.

A matter of great potential interest is Dr. Edwardson's observations on the role of CLIP in the control of insulin secretion. Obviously this work is in its early stages, but already it is clear that the circulating level of CLIP is influenced by metabolic substrates, particularly glucose. Diet also plays a role, for normal animals made obese (by being placed on a very high-fat diet) have a large increase in the amount of CLIP in their intermediate lobe. It will be important to know whether CLIP circulates in man and whether it has an effect in obese patients. If it is found in man, then we will have to re-think our current concepts on its source, since the intermediate lobe is not found in man except at the foetal stage of development.

Corticotropin-releasing factor (CRF; corticoliberin) was the first postulated hypothalamic neurohormone, but it appears it will be among the last to be identified. This must lead us to ask why this should be so. It is possible that vasopressin is the true CRF and that we have been searching for a non-existant hormone. This appears too simplistic an explanation as Dr. Gillies' elegant experiments suggest that vasopressin does require some "potentiating factors" of hypothalamic origin to enable it to exert its full ACTH-releasing propensity. Dr. Gillham and co-workers have posed the question whether there are one or two (or even more) CRFs in addition to vasopressin. Dr. Mialhe's laboratory comes to quite different conclusions from Dr. Gillies on the relative importance of vasopressin and other CRF material in hypothalamic extracts. There are significant methodological differences in assays and it is tempting to suggest that progress would be faster if these could be resolved.

It may be that different releasing factors are secreted in response to different stimuli. Both Drs. Smelik and Mialhe refer to the deficit in the corticotrophic response to neurogenic stress in animals deprived of both the posterior and inter-mediate lobes. It is unlikely that the intermediate lobe plays a major part since, as indicated by both Dr. Smelik and Dr. Edwardson, little ACTH is present in the intermediate lobe. Moreover, transplanted intermediate lobes in hypophysec-tomized rats are incapable of maintaining corticotrophic function although α-MSH levels are normal. This implies a role for the posterior pituitary gland in ACTH secretion. ADH may not be the only CRF material in the posterior lobe because Dr. Makara shows the presence of CRF in the posterior lobe (his assay system cannot detect even large amounts of vasopressin). It should not be too surprising if CRF is found in the posterior pituitary since it is a down-growth from the hypothalamus and posterior lobe extracts were the original source used in the earliest attempts to isolate CRF.

A theme that repeatedly occurs in the present volume is the importance of the paraventricular nucleus (PVN) as a nucleus involved in ACTH control. Dr. Gillies makes the point that vasopressin release from the zona interna and zona externa could be separately controlled and thus allow independent regula-tion of the stress response and antidiuresis. Dr. Gann shows that stimulation of the PVN releases ACTH but stimulation of the supraoptic nucleus (SON) did not. Yet both stimulators elevate peripheral vasopressin levels. Clearly, the PVN does release CRF material (via the median eminence) which activates ACTH release. Some of the projections from the PVN terminate in the median eminence and contain in their nerve endings material that appears to be vasopressin. Dr. Makara's data would suggest that CRF also has its origin in this nucleus and not from nuclei within the median basal hypothalamus. Was Dr. Gann stimulating a CRF in addition to vasopressin? These speculations will doubtlessly be resolved in the not too distant future.

Neurotransmitter control of ACTH secretion is extensively reviewed. Professor Hodges reports on the excitatory effects of acetylcholine and serotonin on the release and synthesis of CRF. Acetylcholine acts principally through nicotinic cholinoceptive receptors. The inhibitory effect of noradrenaline (via an α-adrenoceptive mechanism) and γ-aminobutyric acid (GABA) are also referred to. The role of GABA is further reviewed by Dr. Makara. A problem that has previously proved difficult is resolved by Professor Scapagnini who shows that it is possible to reconcile the inhibitory role of noradrenaline in CRF secretion with the observation that prolonged depletion of noradrenaline in experimental animals results in little disturbance in ACTH release. In his chapter, Professor Scapagnini refers to the various compensatory mechanisms whereby the improved noradrenergic system may restore the situation to the *status quo ante*. These mechanisms include increased turnover of noradrenaline in the nerve fibres and the development of "end organ" super-sensitivity. An intriguing observation is that super-sensitivity occurs in corticosteroid receptors in the hippocampus following adrenalectomy. The development of the gross super-sensitivity seen *in extremis* in response to neuronal destruction or adrenalectomy may reflect the more subtle ways in which a plastic nervous system sets about compensating for deficits in neuronal function.

Dr. Palkovits reports on the changes induced in brain neurotransmitters under stress conditions and the difficulties in determining the cause–effect relationship.

The problem is particularly acute here since the secretion of several hormones occur in response to stress. In addition, he gives a comprehensive account of the changes that occur in both nerve terminals as well as cell bodies.

The work of mapping out pathways involved in a particular stimulus to ACTH secretion is a painstaking but fundamental approach and is represented by only one chapter, that of Dr. Gann. He focuses on the identification of central neurons that are responsive to haemodynamic changes and tested the effect on ACTH secretion of electrical stimulation of these neurons. In this way he has demonstrated physiological and anatomical connections of areas implicated in the control of ACTH. This work has demonstrated the presence of several connected areas, from the medulla to the hypothalamus, implicated in the control of ACTH. This work shows the elegant results obtained when a neurophysiological approach is combined with the measurement of endocrinological correlates.

Another major topic covered is the role of corticosteroid negative-feedback mechanisms. Evidence from experiments both *in vivo* and *in vitro* are reported. First, there are two separate mechanisms, fast and delayed feedback, which appear to represent facets of an integrated control mechanism. Further, the role of neuronal inputs from the adrenal glands has a bearing on feedback control as is emphasized by Dr. Dallman. In addition, there are steroid-resistant as well as steroid-sensitive stimuli. Dr. Dallman's work also suggests the exciting possibility that an endocrine homunculus may exist in the hypothalamus.

The sites of corticosteroid feedback include the hypothalamus, anterior pituitary and, in all probability, the neural inputs to the hypothalamus. Doubtlessly the relative importance of these sites depends on the particular stimulus to CRF or ACTH secretion. Stimuli reaching the pituitary *via* the systemic circulation by-pass the higher feedback sites but stimuli acting *via* the central nervous system may be subject to feedback at multiple sites.

Studies using the hypothalamus *in vitro* have demonstrated that corticosteroids inhibit CRF secretion. However, these observations are difficult to reconcile with Dr. Stumpf's failure to demonstrate nuclear labelling within the hypothalamus. Other studies have, however, demonstrated corticosteroid binding sites in the hypothalamus, though the degree of binding is considerably lower than in the pituitary but is on par with that in the hippocampus. Dr. Stumpf's demonstration that aldosterone may be concentrated in several brain structures is certainly of importance. These data may provide a link between the adrenal cortex on the one hand and isorenin on the other hand. He illustrated that glucocorticoids are taken up in various brain regions, and these may form the neural substrate for the behavioural effects of corticosteroids referred to by Dr. Bohus.

There are two chapters that deal with the problems of corticoid feedback in man. Professor Daly studies the effect of infusing physiological doses of cortisol on the episodic secretion of ACTH. He demonstrates that small rises in plasma cortisol result in an immediate decline in plasma ACTH concentration. Much of his data is compatible with the fast (rate-sensitive) feedback hypothesis as it appears that a rise in cortisol level (and not the actual level itself) is the signal that inhibits ACTH secretion. The feedback mechanism is sufficiently sensitive to function as a servo-mechanism but further research will be needed to determine whether a rate-sensitive mechanism is the best explanation of the experimental observations. An interesting but puzzling finding reported by Daly is that episodes of ACTH secretion were not always followed by a corresponding secretion of cortisol. It is obvious that the coupling of ACTH–cortisol secretion may not be as tight as was originally assumed.

Professor Brooks and his colleagues study the effects of intermediates in the cortisol synthetic pathway on feedback control in man, since experiments in the rat showed that 11-deoxycortisol and 17 α-OH progesterone blocked the feedback effect of cortisol. They therefore tested the hypothesis that the breakthrough from the suppressive effect of dexamethasone in patients suffering from adreno-genital syndrome is due to the interference of 17 α-OH progesterone on the feedback mechanism. They found no evidence that 17 α-OH progesterone had any influence on the feedback mechanism. They also investigated the effect of metyrapone (an 11 β-hydroxylase inhibitor) and found a compensatory increase in adrenocortical activity sufficient to restore cortisol levels to within normal values. Although these results provided an elegant example of feedback control, the results show that the precursor 11-deoxycortisol does not interfere with the fast-feedback effect of cortisol. It is obvious that there are differences in the corticosteroid receptors in the rat and man. This is a cautionary tale since most of the work in the development of synthetic corticosteroids is carried out in the rat.

Professor Rees gives a comprehensive account of Cushing's syndrome including its clinical features and various causes. Professor Rees emphasizes that two forms of the disease remain underdiagnozed — the ectopic ACTH syndrome and alcohol-induced Cushing's syndrome; the recognition of the latter condition has only recently been reported. She reviews the biochemical tests that can distinguish pituitary-dependent Cushing's disease and the ectopic ACTH syndrome. Recently the use of an N-terminal radioimmunoassay for LPH has assisted in distinguishing patients with ACTH-dependent Cushing's disease from the normal. In addition, simultaneous determination of ACTH and LPH allows a differential diagnosis between patients afflicted with Cushing's disease and those affected by the ectopic ACTH syndrome to be made. What is known of the aetiology of Cushing's disease is reviewed and it is suggested that what appears as a single clinical entity is a collection of several diseases of separate origin, either in the hypothalamus or in the pituitary. The burden of the evidence favours a primary dysfunction at the pituitary level in most cases.

Professor Rees makes a plea for the pretreatment of patients with metyrapone (which blocks the 11 β-hydroxylase in the adrenal cortex) before surgery to reduce the high mortality rate. She also advocates its use in conjunction with external pituitary irradiation in the treatment of Cushing's disease. The metabolic effects of 11-deoxycortisol are very weak, in comparison with cortisol, and the clinical improvement after institution of the treatment is rapid. This contrasts with Professor Brooks' observation that in normal individuals given metyrapone the adrenal seems capable of compensating by adjustments in total steroid synthesis to make good the potential cortisol deficit.

Dr. Subrahmanyam reports on pituitary–adrenocortical activity in patients suffering from depressive illness and schizophrenia. She comes to the conclusion, on the basis of her own work and that of others, that the raised levels of cortisol found in some phases of schizophrenia reflect the state of psychological turmoil. In depressive illness the situation is different because the level of cortisol in the plasma is raised even when the patient is asleep and unaffected by tranquilizers. There may be a subgroup of depressive patients in whom the high levels of cortisol are best ascribed to impaired noradrenergic function in the brain. Such an explanation would agree with several observations, including the fact that most anti-depressants influence noradrenergic function and noradrenaline is an inhibitory neurotransmitter to CRF secretion. If a deficit in central noradrenergic function is at the root of some forms of depressive illness then it would not be surprising if these patients had elevated plasma cortisol. The particular high cortisol secretion in depressive illness may result in the condition and Cushing's syndrome being confused. This problem is referred to by Professor Rees who also points out that on the other side of the coin psychiatric disturbance may be a presenting symptom in Cushing's syndrome.

Dr. Udupa studies the role of various yoga practices on psychological status and on adrenocortical and medullary function. It is noteworthy that not all the practices have similar effects on adrenal function. Thus meditation reduced the level of circulating catecholamines but breath control and yoga postures had no such effect. On the other hand, the practice of breath control and yoga postures both increased adrenocortical activity. We are used to the concept of adreno-cortical function reflecting the level of arousal or stress but here we have a clear example of raised cortisol levels in tranquil and unstressed individuals. The tranquil state of subjects carrying out a combination of all three yoga practices is attested to by both psychological tests and lowered adrenomedullary activity. The important lesson that should be learned from Dr. Udupa's study is that although it is true that stress will cause the release of cortisol, we must not jump to the conclusion that a raised cortisol level necessarily indicates a state of stress.

Dr. Sadow deals with the assessment of the levels of activity in the component parts of the brain–pituitary–adrenocortical system operating in the circadian rhythm in plasma ACTH and cortisol concentrations. She reviews what is known about the changes in sensitivity of the component parts at the peak and nadir of the rhythm and the factors that influence the clearance of corticosteroids. Her own work shows the important role that the hypothalamus plays in initiating the rhythm. Her review includes the role thought to be played by various neuro-transmitters in initiating these changes in CRF secretion and how maturation of various neurotransmitter pathways is believed to be a necessary prerequisite for the development of the rhythm.

Two chapters deal with the developmental changes that occur in adrenocortical function during intra-uterine life – one by Dr. Giroud and the other by Dr. Murphy. The late Dr. Giroud showed that the foetal zone and the neocortex of the human foetal adrenal respond to ACTH to release dehydroepiandrosterone sulphate and cortisol respectively. He showed that the foetal pituitary is capable of synthesizing and releasing trophic hormones by the third month of intra-uterine life. Though α-MSH is present in high amounts in the foetal pituitary and is capable of stimulating both adrenal zones, its potency is only about one-thousandth that of ACTH. Therefore it is unlikely that it is the most important peptide for adrenocortical activation during foetal development.

Dr. Murphy, in her chapter, deals with the conversion of the cortisol into the metabolically inactive cortisone. This occurs, until late pregnancy, in all foetal tissue and in the placenta and so protects the foetus from the metabolic effects of cortisol derived from its own adrenals or the mother. The converse (i.e. conversion of cortisone into cortisol) occurs in the chorion and uterine wall during the latter half of pregnancy; this may help prevent rejection of the foetal allograft.

Drs. Prasad and Chattopadhyay deal with the activation of adrenal cortex and point out the whole constellation of metabolic changes that must occur. Some of these are rapid whereas others require more time and reflect long-term modulations of adrenal function and this may involve changes in lysosomal activity.

It is now almost 20 years since Birmingham and Ward isolated 18-OH-DOC, the most prominent 18-oxygenated steroid in the rat and which is also secreted in man. In the rat it is sometimes the most prevalent adrenocortical hormone; it is secreted by the zona fasciculata and the reticularis, and is under the control of ACTH. In the human, plasma levels of 18-OH-DOC can increase ten-fold in response to ACTH.

Considerable interest in this steroid has arisen recently because of the suggestion that it may be involved in the genesis of hypertension, since 18-OH-DOC is controlled by ACTH it might be implicated in some forms of hypertension induced by chronic stress. It has been thought for some time that disturbance in arteriolar cation contents (or ratios) may induce increased vascular responsiveness to sympathetic tone and circulating angiotensin II. Dr. Birmingham has shown that 18-OH-DOC has both mineralocorticoid and glucocorticoid activity and is a hypertensive agent. However, the sodium retention caused by 18-OH-DOC is not accompanied by a concomitant excretion of potassium and there is a disproportionate retention of water in relation to the sodium retained.

Dr. Bartova shows that brain tissue retains 18-OH-DOC and cell-fractionation studies indicate some association with brain cytosol and nuclear macromolecules and nuclear binding. The highest concentrations are found in the septum, but considerable amounts are found in the amygdala, cortex and medulla. The precise role of 18-OH-DOC in the brain is unknown and its possible behavioural effects deserve investigation. It is also possible that the medullary uptake might be related to the hypertensive effects of 18-OH-DOC since the vasomotor centre is located in this region.

Thus the effects of 18-OH-DOC still remains, to some extent, an enigma. Are its (as yet) uninvestigated effects on behaviour important or is it an important hypertensive agent in low or normal renin hypertension? This, like other problems raised in the current publication, remains to be clarified in the future.

SUBJECT INDEX

Acetylcholine
  effect on CRF secretion, 116, 166–169
  effect of meditation on, 276
ACTH *see* adrenocorticotropic hormone
Addison's disease, 183
Adenohypophysis *see* Anterior pituitary
Adrenal cortex,
  action on ACTH on, 229, 230
  cholesterol in, 229, 230
  self limitation, 231
  stimulation in stress, 231
Adrenal, fetal
  cortisol secretion from, 235–9
  DHA-S secretion from, 235–9
  effect of ACTH on, 237
  effect of CLIP on, 237–8
  effect of HCG on, 239
  effect of HPL on, 239
  effect of α-MSH on, 237–8
  tissue culture of, 236–239
Adrenalectomy
  effect on ACTH secretion, 163
  effect on brain peptides, 11
  effect on feedback *in vivo*, 157–158
  stress response after, 163
Adrenal sensitivity in circadian rhythm, 222
Adrenocortical function
  in depression, 265–271
  in schizophrenia, 265–271
Adrenocorticotropic hormone (ACTH)
  on behaviour, 8–11, 14

Adrenocorticotropic hormone (ACTH) *cont.*
  of brain origin, 11
  chronic treatment with, 150–151
  circadian rhythm of, 221–222
  effect on 18-OH-DOC, 197, 215–6
  effect on fetal adrenal, 237–8
  factors releasing, 41, 66
  "hunting mechanism", 1
  as insulin secretagogue, 20
  interrelationship with LPH, 4, 5, 6
  in intermediate lobe, 17, 21, 29–37
  in obese mice, 17–21, 26, 27
  in posterior lobe, 30
  in rat, 3, 4
  release
    effect of adrenalectomy on, 163
    effect of arginine vasopressin antiserum on, 415
    antero-lateral nucleus intercalatus, involvement in, 76, 77
    effect of catecholamines, 87–94 127–136
    to electrical stimulation, 76–83
    with haemodynamic changes, 75–83
    inhibitory and facilitatory areas of brain in, 76, 77, 82, 83
    neural pathways in control of, 75–85
    vasopressin stimulation of, 66
  retrograde transport of, 10
  effect of steroids on, 163–180
  in sheep, 213
  in stress, 231

Adrenocorticotropic hormone
(ACTH) *cont.*
  secretion *see* release
  synthesis, 158
ACTH, of intermediate lobe
  control of secretion of, 31–37
  function, 31
  effect of K^+ on, 34
  measurement of, 29, 30
  effect of neurotransmitters on, 34–37
  as precursor, 30
  structure, 29
Adrenocorticotropic hormone/
      lipotropin related peptides
  anterior pituitary cell column,
      secretion of, 4, 5
  in behaviour, 8–14
  in intermediate lobe, 30, 31
  in monkey, 3
  in sheep, 2, 3
  in rat, 3, 4, 6
α-Adrenoreceptors involved in control
    of CRF secretion, 116–118
Aldosterone
  effects of, 197, 201
  regions of uptake in brain, 137–146
γ-Amino butyric acid, *see* GABA
Androgens
  in fetal adrenal, 235–9
  stimulation by ACTH, 237–8
  stimulation by CLIP, 237–8
  stimulation by α-MSH, 237–8
Angiotensin II, effect on 18-OH-DOC,
    198
Anterior-pituitary
  delayed feedback of steroids, 174–176
  fast feedback of steroids, 171–173
  transcortin-like binding protein in,
      150
  effect of steroids on, 153, 166, 171–180
Autoradiographic techniques, applica-
    tion of, 137–146

Behaviour,
  conditioned, involvement of
      pituitary gland, 8
  effect of corticosteroids on, 11–14
  effect of pituitary and hypothalamic
      peptides on, 7–15

Behaviour *cont.*
  receptor systems in 10
Betamethasone, in fetus, 255
Breath control, effect on adrenal
    corticosteroids, 275

Catecholamines
  effect of ACTH on, 93, 94
  humoral control, 91, 92
  effect of glucocorticoids on, 93
  effect of meditation on, 276
  neural control, 92
  in stress, 87, 88–94
Chemical stimulation of CRF, 100
p-Chlorophenylalanine, effect on HPA
    axis, 130–132
Cholesterol
  corticoidogenesis from, 229, 230
  release from lipid storage droplets,
      229
Cholinesterase, effect of meditation on,
    276
Cholinoceptors, type involved in con-
    trol of CRF secretion, 116
Circadian rhythm
  of ACTH, 221–222
  of corticosteroids, 221–222
  of CRF, 222–225
  in man, 183–187
  of neurotransmitters, 224–225
Circadian rhythms, 183–187, 221–226
Congenital adrenal hyperplasia,
    anomalous observations, 189
Corticoliberin *see* corticotropin-
    releasing factor (CRF)
Corticosteroid feedback
  adrenal factor, 149
  antagonism, 189–194
  GABA involvement, 168
  on humans, 183–5, 189–195
  interactions between fast and de-
      layed, 178–180
  of intermediates of cortisol synthesis,
      189–194
  norepinephrine involvement, 168
  physiological importance, 182
  receptors involved, 164
  site of action, 164–178
Corticosteroidogenesis
  ACTH in, 229, 230
  cholesterol in, 229, 230

Corticosteroidogenesis *cont.*
  role of lysosomes in, 230–233
  NADPH in, 229, 230
  pregnenolone in, 230
  in stress, 231
Corticosteroids
  in Addison's disease, 181
  in behaviour, 12–14
  brain uptake sites, 164
  chronic treatment, 150–151
  circadian periodicity of, 183–187,
    221–222
  effect on CRF, 118
  dissociation from ACTH release,
    183–185
  episodic secretion, 183–184
  feedback on ACTH secretion, 12,
    149–161, 163–171, 176–180
  effect on GABA synthesis, 124
  hippocampal uptake of, 12
  HPA axis, regulation of, 181–187
  effect on lysosomes, 230–233
  in obese mice, 20
  receptors, 164, 213
  treatment timecourse, 150–153
  uptake, 213
Corticosterone
  hippocampal receptors, 11, 12
  regions of uptake in brain, 137–146
Corticosterone uptake in hippocampus
    and septrum, 133
Corticotropin-like intermediate lobe
    peptide (CLIP)
  control of secretion, 22–26
  on fetal adrenal, 237–8
  effect of glucose on, 24, 25
  effect of hypothalamic extract on,
    23, 24
  as insulin secretagogue, 20, 21
  in intermediate lobe, 17, 21, 22, 29,
    30, 31
  in monkey, 3
  effect of neurotransmitters on, 23
  in obese mice, 17, 21, 27
  in rat, 3, 4
  in sheep, 2, 3
Corticotropin releasing factor (CRF)
  effect of acetylcholine on, 166–169
  in Brattleboro rats, 57, 58, 66, 72
  effect of Ca^{2+} on, 169
  cell body location, 97–112
  effect of cholinomimetics on, 100

Corticotropin releasing factor
(CRF) *cont.*
  chromatography of, 42, 43, 55–58
  circadian rhythm of, 223–225, 265,
    270, 271
  content, 157–158
  effect of corticosteroids on, 118
  effect of cylohexamide on, 48
  electrophoresis of, 43, 44
  effect of ether on, 105–108
  effect of GABA on, 121–125
  effect of GABA antagonists on, 100
  effect of 5-hydroxytryptamine on,
    100, 130–136
  in hypothalamic extract, 41, 52–58,
    63, 64
  from hypothalamus *in vitro*, 42, 43
  location, 85, 98, 99
  effect of MAO inhibitors on, 271
  effect of monoamine uptake blockers
    on, 271
  nature of, 51
  in neural lobe of pituitary, 108–112
  effect of norepinephrine on, 93, 94,
    127–129
  in obese mice, 19, 20
  paraventricular nuclei involvement,
    108–112
  in posterior lobe, 53, 55
  effect of potassium on, 169
  effect of psychological influences on,
    265, 270
  purification, 42–44
  receptor sites, 70
  relationship to other CRF's, 44
  regulation of, 48, 265, 270, 271
  effect of steroids on, 166–171
  stimulation of ACTH secretion, 97
  subcellular location, 70–72
  after surgical isolation of MBH,
    99–108, 111, 112
  synergistic factor, 55–57
  synthesis, 157–158
  vasopressin as, 46, 47
  with vasopressin antibody, 53, 64–68
Corticotrophin-releasing hormone
    (CRH) *see* corticotropin-releasing
    factor (CRF)
Cortisol
  binding in fetus, 254
  circadian periodicity, 183–7
  in CSF, 269

Cortisol *cont.*
  in depression, secretion of, 267–269
  dissociation from ACTH release, 183–5
  episodic secretions, 183–5
  feedback inhibition, 181–187
  interconversion with cortisone, 247–255
  measurement, 247–8
  in plasma, 267–8
  urinary, 267
Cortisone
  in development of fetus, 254
  F/E ratio in developing fetus, 248–250
  interconversion with cortisol, 247–255
  levels in placenta and fetus, 247–250
CRF *see* corticotropin releasing factor
Cushing's disease, 260–3
  aetiology, 260–1
  treatment, 262–3
Cushing's syndrome, 257–260
  biochemical diagnosis, 258–259
  clinical features, 258
  differential diagnosis, 259–260
Cyclohexamide, effect on CRF synthesis, 158

Dehydroepiandrosterone sulphate (DHA-S)
  adrenal zone for secretion of, 237
  effect of CLIP, 237–8
  in fetal adrenal, 235–9
  effect of α-MSH, 237–8
  in placenta, 235, 239
  stimulation by ACTH, 237–8
  in tissue culture, 236–9
Delayed feedback of corticosteroids, 149, 153–156
  site of action, 153–155
Deoxycorticosterone (DOC)
  effects on blood pressure, 200–201
  effect on Na^+ and K^+, 205
11-Deoxycortisol
  feedback, 192–194
  effect of metyraponeon, 192–194
Depressive illness
  effect on adrenocortical activity, 267–269

Depressive illness *cont.*
  circadian rhythm of ACTH in, 270
  hypothalamus in 270
  effect of monoamine oxidase inhibitors in, 271
  effect of monoamine uptake blockers in, 271
Dexamethasone
  in fetus, 255
  regions of uptake in brain, 137–146
  suppression test, 259
DHA-S, *see* dehydroepiandrosterone sulphate
5, 6-Dihydroxytryptamine, effect on HPA axis, 132
5, 7-Dihydroxytryptamine, effect on circadian rhythm, 135
Dopamine
  effect on ACTH secretion, 93, 94
  in stress, 87, 88–94
Dopamine-β-hydroxylase activity in stress, 91

Electrical stimulation, of CRF, 100–102
Endorphins
  in behaviour, 7–11, 14
  of brain origin, 9, 11
  in mental disorders, 7, 8
α-Endorphin, 1–6
β-Endorphin, 1–6
  in monkey, 3
  in rat, 3, 4
Endotoxin, effect on corticoid response, 150
Met-Enkephalin, in behaviour, 9
Epinephrine, in stress, 87, 88–94

Fast feedback of corticosteroid, 149, 156–157
  site of action, 157
Fetal development
  role of cortisone, 247–255
Fetal membranes
  in conversion of cortisone to cortisol, 251
  in parturition, 251
Fetal tissues, interconversion of cortisone and cortisol, 251
Fornix lesion, effect on circadian rhythm, 132–133

GABA
    in control of CRF secretion, 121–
        125
    distribution, 121
    on the hypothalamus *in vitro*, 122
    effect on isolated medial basal
        hypothalamus *in situ*, 122
Glial cell uptake of steroids, 145–146
Glutamic acid decarboxylase (GAD)
    distribution, 121
    inhibition, 122

Haemodynamic changes, effect on
    ACTH secretion, 75–83
Hippocampus,
    role in behaviour, 12
18-Hydroxy-DOC (18-OH-DOC)
    effect of ACTH on, 197, 215–6
    angiotensin II on, 198
    binding macromolecules, 216–8
    in Brattleboro rats, 199
    control of, 197–205
    diurnal fluctuations, 216
    in humans, 197
    in hypertension, 197–210
    effect on mineral metabolism,
        207–8
    originates from 198
    plasma concentrations, 213
    properties of, 197–205, 213
    synergism with glucocorticoids,
        205–7
    uptake in brain, 214–6
18-OH-DOC uptake effect of adrenal-
    ectomy on, 215–6
    effect of dexamethasone on, 215–6
6-Hydroxydopamine treatment,
    effect on HPA axis, 128, 129
17-Hydroxy progesterone
    administration, 190
    antagonism of feedback, 189–192
11β-Hydroxysteroid dehydrogenase,
    in fetus, 254
5-Hydroxytryptamine
    effect on ACTH secretion, 94
    in control of circadian rhythm, 130
    effect on CRF secretion, 116
    in stress, 87, 88–94, 130
Hypertension
    effect of 18-OH-DOC in, 197–8
    renin hypertension, 199

Hypophysectomy, effect on brain
    peptides, 8, 11
Hypothalamic islands, 99–108
    effect of ether on, 105–108
Hypothalamo-pituitary-adrenocortical
    axis
    effect of breath control on, 275
    effect of meditation on, 276
    effect of yoga on, 273–7
Hypothalamus
    effect of acetylcholine on, 100,
        168–171
    areas involved in ACTH control, 76–
        85
    effect of GABA on, 168
    effect on norepinephrine on, 168
    effect of steroids on, 166–171
Hypothalamus *in vitro*
    effect of acetylcholine on, 100
    release of CRF, 42–48
    effect of 5-hydroxytryptamine on,
        100

Insulin tolerance test, 259
Intermediate lobe peptides, in obesity,
    17–27
Intermediate lobe, *see* pars intermedia

Lateral retrochiasmatic area (RCAL),
    in stress response, 99
Lipotropin (LPH), 1–6, 11
    of brain origin, 11
    interrelationship with ACTH, 4, 5, 6
    stimulation of secretion, 4, 5, 6
β-Lipotropin
    in behaviour, 8–11, 14
    in intermediate lobe, 31
    effect of AVP antiserum on, 4, 5
    secretion, effect of AVP antiserum
        on, 4, 5
γ-Lipotropin, in monkey, 3
Lysosomes
    acid hydrolases, 232
    effect of ACTH on, 230
    role in corticosteroidogenesis, 230–
        233
    effect of hypophysectomy on, 231
    structure, 230

Medial basal hypothalamus
    chemical stimulation of isolated, 100

Medial basal hypothalamus *cont.*
    CRF cells location, 97–112
    electrical stimulation, 100–102
    surgical isolation, 99–108, 111, 112
Meditation
    effect on drug treatment, 274
    in hypertensive patients, 273–4
    effects on metabolism, 273–277
α-Melanocyte stimulating hormone (α-
    MSH)
    on behaviour, 8, 11
    on fetal adrenal, 237–8
    in intermediate lobe, 17, 21, 22, 29–
        37
    in monkey, 3
    in obese mice, 17–27
    in rat, 3, 4
    in sheep, 2, 3
β-Melanocyte stimulating hormone (β-
    MSH)
    in monkey, 3
    in rat, 3, 4
    in sheep, 2, 3
Mental disorders
    β-endorphin and fragments in, 7
    vasopressin in, 7
α-Methyl-*p*-tyrosine treatment, effect
    on HPA axis, 128
Metyrapone, 194, 195, 262
    effect on cortisol half life, 194
    treatment in Cushing's disease, 194–
        195
    effect in normal humans, 194–195

NADPH, in corticoidogenesis, 229,
    230
Nelson's syndrome, 263
N-Fragment, 2
Neural lobe
    CRF-like activity of, 108–112
    stimulation of, 109
Norepinephrine
    effect on CRF secretion, 116–118
    effect on the HPA system, 93, 94,
        127
    involvement of locus coeruleus, 89,
        93
    in stress, 87–94, 128
    synthesis and release of, 89, 90

Obese (ob/ob) mouse
    hypothalamo-pituitary-adreno-
        cortical system of, 19, 20
    physiological abnormalities of, 18
18-OH-DOC, *see* 18-hydroxy DOC

Pars intermedia, in human, 2
Pituitary cell culture, 240–242
Pituitary, fetal
    release of gonadotropins, 240–2
    release of growth hormone, 240–2
    release of prolactin on, 240–2
Pituitary insulin secretagogue, in obese
    mice, 20
Pituitary transplantation, 99
Placenta
    interconversion of E-F, 247–255
    utilization of DHA-S, 235
Placental tissue culture, 243–245
Prednisolone, in fetus, 255

Quipazine, effect on circadian rhythm,
    132

Rate-sensitive feedback of corticos-
    teroids, *see* fast feedback
Receptor supersensitivity, 128, 132,
    133, 136
Reserpine, effect on HPA axis, 127–
    128

Schizophrenia
    effect on adrenocortical activity,
        269, 270
    role of brain peptides in, 7, 8
    phases of, 269, 270
    psychosis, 269, 270
Septal lesions
    effect on circadian rhythm, 132–
        133
Serotonin, *see* 5-hydroxytryptamine
Stress, pathways involved in, 151, 155,
    158, 161
Synergistic factor, of CRF, 55–57

Triamcinolone, effect on lysosomes,
    232
Tryptophan hydroxylase activity,
    after PCPA treatment, 131, 132
    in stress, 88, 89
Tyrosine hydroxylase activity
    after norepinephrine depletion,
        128
    in stress, 88, 91

Vasopressin
    effect on ACTH secretion, 51, 52
    Brattleboro rats, effect of, 66
    chromatography of, 55–58
    as CRF, 46, 47, 63–73
    effect on CRF action, 68, 69

Vasopressin *cont.*
  electrophoresis of, comparison to
    CRF, 44
  immunological characterization, 52,
    53
  in mental disorders, 8
  portal blood concentrations, 52
  receptor sites, 65, 66, 70
  in stress, 72
  subcellular location, 70–72

Ventral nor-adrenergic tract, role in
    control of CRF secretion, 129

Yoga
  effect on adrenocortical function,
    273–277
  in control of body functions, 273–
    277
  effect on psychological parameters,
    274–5